Common Symptoms in the Ambulatory Setting

Editor

DOUGLAS S. PAAUW

MEDICAL CLINICS
OF NORTH AMERICA

www.medical.theclinics.com

Consulting Editors
DOUGLAS S. PAAUW
EDWARD R. BOLLARD

May 2014 • Volume 98 • Number 3

ELSEVIER

1600 John F. Kennedy Boulevard • Suite 1800 • Philadelphia, Pennsylvania, 19103-2899

http://www.theclinics.com

MEDICAL CLINICS OF NORTH AMERICA Volume 98, Number 3
May 2014 ISSN 0025-7125, ISBN-13: 978-0-323-29715-8

Editor: Jessica McCool
Developmental Editor: Yonah Korngold

Medical Clinics of North America (ISSN 0025-7125) is published bimonthly by Elsevier Inc., 360 Park Avenue South, New York, NY 10010-1710. Months of publication are January, March, May, July, September, and November. Business and editorial offices: 1600 John F. Kennedy Boulevard, Suite 1800, Philadelphia, PA 19103-2899. Periodicals postage paid at New York, NY, and additional mailing offices. Subscription prices are USD $255.00 per year (US individuals), $471.00 per year (US institutions), $125.00 per year (US Students), $320.00 per year (Canadian individuals), $612.00 per year (Canadian institutions), $200.00 per year (Canadian and foreign students), $390.00 per year (foreign individuals), and $612.00 per year (foreign institutions). To receive student/resident rate, orders must be accompanied by name of affiliated institution, date of term, and the signature of program/residency coordinator on institution letterhead. Orders will be billed at individual rate until proof of status is received. Foreign air speed delivery is included in all Clinics' subscription prices. All prices are subject to change without notice. **POSTMASTER:** Send address changes to *Medical Clinics of North America*, Elsevier Health Sciences Division, Subscription Customer Service, 3251 Riverport Lane, Maryland Heights, MO 63043. **Customer Service: Telephone: 1-800-654-2452** (U.S. and Canada); **1-314-447-8871** (outside U.S. and Canada). **Fax: 314-447-8029. E-mail: journalscustomerserviceusa@elsevier.com** (for print support); **journalsonlinesupport-usa@elsevier.com** (for online support).

Reprints. For copies of 100 or more of articles in this publication, please contact the Commercial Reprints Department, Elsevier Inc., 360 Park Avenue South, New York, NY 10010-1710. Tel.: 212-633-3874; Fax: 212-633-3820; E-mail: reprints@elsevier.com.

Medical Clinics of North America is also published in Spanish by McGraw-Hill Interamericana Editores S. A., P.O. Box 5-237, 06500 Mexico, D.F., Mexico.

Medical Clinics of North America is covered in *MEDLINE/PubMed (Index Medicus), Current Contents, ASCA, Excerpta Medica, Science Citation Index, and ISI/BIOMED.*

Printed in the United States of America.

PROGRAM OBJECTIVE
The goal of the *Medical Clinics of North America* is to keep practicing physicians up to date with current clinical practice by providing timely articles reviewing the state of the art in patient care.

TARGET AUDIENCE
All practicing physicians and other healthcare professionals.

LEARNING OBJECTIVES
Upon completion of this activity, participants will be able to:
1. Discuss treatment of shoulder, neck, back and leg pain.
2. Review diagnosis and treatment of headache in the ambulatory care setting.
3. Explain treatment of common dermatologic conditions.

ACCREDITATION
The Elsevier Office of Continuing Medical Education (EOCME) is accredited by the Accreditation Council for Continuing Medical Education (ACCME) to provide continuing medical education for physicians.

The EOCME designates this enduring material for a maximum of 15 *AMA PRA Category 1 Credit*(s)™. Physicians should claim only the credit commensurate with the extent of their participation in the activity.

All other health care professionals requesting continuing education credit for this enduring material will be issued a certificate of participation.

DISCLOSURE OF CONFLICTS OF INTEREST
The EOCME assesses conflict of interest with its instructors, faculty, planners, and other individuals who are in a position to control the content of CME activities. All relevant conflicts of interest that are identified are thoroughly vetted by EOCME for fair balance, scientific objectivity, and patient care recommendations. EOCME is committed to providing its learners with CME activities that promote improvements or quality in healthcare and not a specific proprietary business or a commercial interest.

The planning committee, staff, authors and editors listed below have identified no financial relationships or relationships to products or devices they or their spouse/life partner have with commercial interest related to the content of this CME activity:
Douglas B. Berger, MD Mlitt; Edward R. Bollard, MD, DDS, FACP; Ginger Evans, MD; Anna L. Golob, MD; Deborah L. Greenberg, MD; Natalie Hale, MPH, MDc; Brynne Hunter; Margaret L. Isaac, MD; Jared Wilson Klein, MD, MPH; Sandy Lavery; Jessica McCool; Jill McNair; Alexandra Molnar, MD; Kim M. O'Connor, MD; Maryann Katherine Overland, MD; Douglas S. Paauw, MD; Lindsay Parnell; Mark E. Pasanen, MD, FACP; Santha Priya; Eliza L. Sutton, MD; Genji Terasaki, MD; Jay C. Vary, MD, PhD; Christopher J. Wong, MD; Jennifer Wright, MD.

The planning committee, staff, authors and editors listed below have identified financial relationships or relationships to products or devices they or their spouse/life partner have with commercial interest related to the content of this CME activity:
Steven McGee, MD has royalties/patents with Elsevier.
Joyce E. Wipf, MD, FACP has royalties/patents with UpToDate.

UNAPPROVED/OFF-LABEL USE DISCLOSURE
The EOCME requires CME faculty to disclose to the participants:
1. When products or procedures being discussed are off-label, unlabelled, experimental, and/or investigational (not US Food and Drug Administration (FDA) approved); and
2. Any limitations on the information presented, such as data that are preliminary or that represent ongoing research, interim analyses, and/or unsupported opinions. Faculty may discuss information about pharmaceutical agents that is outside of FDA-approved labelling. This information is intended solely for CME and is not intended to promote off-label use of these medications. If you have any questions, contact the medical affairs department of the manufacturer for the most recent prescribing information.

TO ENROLL
To enroll in the *Medical Clinics of North America* Continuing Medical Education program, call customer service at 1-800-654-2452 or sign up online at http://www.theclinics.com/home/cme. The CME program is available to subscribers for an additional annual fee of USD $267.

METHOD OF PARTICIPATION
In order to claim credit, participants must complete the following:
1. Complete enrolment as indicated above.
2. Read the activity.
3. Complete the CME Test and Evaluation. Participants must achieve a score of 70% on the test. All CME Tests and Evaluations must be completed online.

CME INQUIRIES/SPECIAL NEEDS
For all CME inquiries or special needs, please contact elsevierCME@elsevier.com.

MEDICAL CLINICS OF NORTH AMERICA

RELATED INTEREST

Primary Care: Clinics in Office Practice, March 2014, (Vol 41, No. 1)
Primary Care ENT
Gretchen Dickson and Rick Kellerman, *Editors*
http://www.primarycare.theclinics.com/

NOW AVAILABLE FOR YOUR iPhone and iPad

Contributors

CONSULTING EDITORS

DOUGLAS S. PAAUW, MD, MACP
Professor, Division of General Internal Medicine, Department of Medicine; Rathmann Family Foundation Endowed Chair for Patient-Centered Clinical Education; Medicine Student Programs, University of Washington School of Medicine, Seattle, Washington

EDWARD R. BOLLARD, MD, DDS, FACP
Professor of Medicine, Associate Dean for Graduate Medical Education, Designated Institutional Official (DIO), Penn State University College of Medicine, Hershey, Pennsylvania

EDITOR

DOUGLAS S. PAAUW, MD, MACP
Professor, Division of General Internal Medicine, Department of Medicine; Rathmann Family Foundation Endowed Chair for Patient-Centered Clinical Education; Medicine Student Programs, University of Washington School of Medicine, Seattle, Washington

AUTHORS

DOUGLAS BERGER, MD, MLitt
Staff Physician; General Medicine Service, VA Puget Sound; Acting Instructor, Department of Medicine, University of Washington, Seattle, Washington

GINGER EVANS, MD
Acting Instructor, Department of Medicine, VA Puget Sound Health Care System, University of Washington, Seattle, Washington

ANNA L. GOLOB, MD
Acting Instructor, Department of Medicine, University of Washington; VA Puget Sound Healthcare System, Seattle, Washington

DEBORAH L. GREENBERG, MD
Associate Professor of Medicine; University of Washington School of Medicine, Seattle, Washington

NATALIE HALE, MPH, MDc
Department of Medicine, University of Washington School of Medicine, Seattle, Washington

MARGARET L. ISAAC, MD
Attending Physician, Harborview Medical Center; Assistant Professor, Department of Medicine, University of Washington School of Medicine, Seattle, Washington

JARED WILSON KLEIN, MD, MPH
Clinical Instructor, Division of General Internal Medicine, Department of Medicine, Harborview Medical Center, University of Washington, Seattle, Washington

STEVEN MCGEE, MD
Professor, Department of Medicine, Veterans Affairs Puget Sound Healthcare System–Seattle Division, University of Washington, Seattle, Washington

ALEXANDRA MOLNAR, MD
Clinical Assistant Professor, Department of Medicine, Harborview Medical Center, University of Washington, Seattle, Washington

KIM M. O'CONNOR, MD
Associate Professor, Division of General Internal Medicine, Department of Internal Medicine, General Internal Medicine Centre, General Internal Medicine Clinic, University of Washington, Seattle, Washington

MARYANN KATHERINE OVERLAND, MD
Acting Instructor, Division of General Internal Medicine, Primary Care Clinic, VA Puget Sound Health Care System, University of Washington, Seattle, Washington

DOUGLAS S. PAAUW, MD, MACP
Professor, Division of General Internal Medicine, Department of Medicine; Rathmann Family Foundation Endowed Chair for Patient-Centered Clinical Education; Medicine Student Programs, University of Washington School of Medicine, Seattle, Washington

MARK E. PASANEN, MD, FACP
Associate Professor of Medicine, Department of Medicine, University of Vermont College of Medicine, South Burlington, Vermont

ELIZA L. SUTTON, MD, FACP
Associate Professor, Department of Medicine, University of Washington, Seattle, Washington

GENJI TERASAKI, MD
Assistant Professor, Division of General Internal Medicine, Harborview Medical Center, University of Washington, Seattle, Washington

JAY C. VARY, MD, PhD
Division of Dermatology, Department of Internal Medicine; Assistant Professor, Dermatology Center, The University of Washington, Seattle, Washington

JOYCE E. WIPF, MD, FACP
Professor, Department of Medicine, University of Washington; VA Puget Sound Healthcare System, Seattle, Washington

CHRISTOPHER J. WONG, MD
Assistant Professor, Division of General Internal Medicine, Department of Medicine, University of Washington, Seattle, Washington

JENNIFER WRIGHT, MD
Assistant Professor, Division of General Internal Medicine, Department of Internal Medicine, General Internal Medicine Centre, University of Washington, Seattle, Washington

Contents

> Chronic cough is a common and frustrating problem for patients and health care providers that can result in a range of physical and psychological complications including exhaustion, urinary incontinence, vomiting, depression, and social isolation. A step-wise empiric approach to treatment will increase the likelihood of a successful resolution of the cough. Even with current treatment protocols, a subset of patients will continue to have chronic cough without a diagnosis. As understanding of the pathophysiology of chronic cough evolves particularly around the concept of cough reflex hypersensitivity, future research should lead to new diagnostic and therapeutic modalities for this challenging problem.

> Low back pain is one of the most frequent complaints for which patients are seen in primary care. Low back pain has a substantial economic impact, estimated at $100 billion per year including direct and indirect costs. The evaluation of low back pain involves a thorough history and physical examination. Imaging is only indicated when a more serious underlying cause or neurologic abnormality is suspected. Abnormalities detected on imaging do not strongly correlate with symptoms. Generally, a specific underlying cause for low back pain is not identified. Treatment consists of a multidisciplinary approach with goal to maintain function and minimize disability.

> Although discussions of leg pain usually begin with the hip, knee, and ankle, patients often present with leg symptoms unrelated to articular or periarticular structures. Pain, paresthesias, cramping, heaviness, or numbness may arise from a variety of vascular, neurologic, and musculoskeletal causes beyond the joints. This article describes the presentation, diagnosis, and treatment of common causes of such symptoms, including peripheral arterial disease, chronic venous insufficiency, deep vein thrombosis, lumbosacral radiculopathy, lumbar spinal stenosis, peripheral neuropathy, statin myalgia, cramps, and restless legs syndrome.

> This review discusses common dermatologic presentations as they would appear in a primary care office, exploring the differential diagnoses for

each. Tips are provided on choosing an appropriate topical drug and vehicle and advising patients on its use. Etiology, differential diagnosis, and treatment options are discussed for the following: alopecias including androgenetic alopecia, female pattern hair loss, alopecia areata, and telogen effluvium; facial rashes including acne vulgaris, acne rosacea, periorificial dermatitis, seborrheic dermatitis, erysipelas/cellulitis, and systemic lupus erythematosus; intertriginous rashes including infections, intertrigo, and inverse psoriasis; and the inflamed leg including cellulitis and erysipelas, stasis dermatitis, and contact dermatitis.

Deborah L. Greenberg

In the absence of trauma, most patients with shoulder pain will be found to have subacromial impingement syndrome. Control of discomfort and exercises to improve shoulder mechanics is the treatment of choice for most patients. Systematic history taking and physical examination will detect the uncommon, more urgent causes of shoulder pain.

Natalie Hale and Douglas S. Paauw

Headaches are the most common constellation of neurologic disorders observed in clinical practice. This article discusses the clinical features of the most common headache subtypes and helps elucidate the more nuanced features of newly recognized and frequently misdiagnosed headache disorders. The physical examination, recommendations regarding imaging, treatment, and the differentiation of primary from secondary headache disorders is discussed. Headache is one of the most commonly encountered clinical problems and this article aims to clarify diagnostic dilemmas and provide the most up-to-date recommendations with respect to treatment and long-term management.

Mark E. Pasanen

Symptoms related to colonic function are common and frequently related to functional issues. Possible presentations include constipation and either acute or chronic diarrhea. Because acute diarrhea is most commonly infectious, issues typically center on the role of stool testing and antibiotic treatment. For chronic diarrhea, the differential is much longer and the diagnostic options are many, making an efficient and focused evaluation a priority, whereas treatment is usually dictated by diagnosis. Constipation can be challenging and, like chronic diarrhea, an efficient and practical approach to diagnosis is critical. The role of newer laxative agents continues to be defined.

Maryann Katherine Overland

Dyspepsia is a common and complex condition consisting of chronic upper gastrointestinal symptoms. A rational approach to diagnosis and treatment of dyspepsia includes identifying those patients with alarm symptoms and referring them for prompt endoscopy. Those without alarm symptoms can be differentiated into patients who do and do not have symptoms consistent with gastroesophageal reflux disease. In the absence of predominant heartburn and regurgitation, patients should be tested and treated for *Helicobacter pylori*. Functional (nonulcer) dyspepsia is a multifactorial disorder with several possible pathophysiologic mechanisms, but no clear guidelines for therapy. There is some evidence of efficacy of proton pump inhibitors, antisecretory agents, antidepressants, and psychotherapy for functional dyspepsia.

Preface

Common Symptoms in the Ambulatory Setting

Evaluating Common Symptoms Correctly: The Core of Internal Medicine

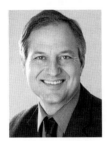

Douglas S. Paauw, MD, MACP
Editor

This issue is devoted to the evaluation and management of common symptoms seen in the ambulatory care setting. The art of medicine is recognizing when a symptom is a clue to an underlying disease and when a symptom is just a symptom. Recognizing when to aggressively work up a symptom, and when to patiently watch, is a crucial skill. The Choosing Wisely campaign was started by the American Board of Internal Medicine and has now been adopted by over 50 specialty societies. *Consumer Reports* has also become involved to share the campaign directly with patients. The goal of this campaign is to reduce unnecessary risk and costs in medical care. Initial evaluation of the most common symptoms patients present with is a key area of emphasis.

In a recent Mayo Clinic study, half of the 10 most common reasons for visiting a physician were for symptom-based visits (headache, back pain, joint/neck pain, skin problems, and upper respiratory symptoms).[1] Skin problems were present in 42% of patients, joint symptoms in 33%, back problems in 22%, respiratory symptoms in 21%, and headache in 13%. All these symptoms are covered in this issue. Active symptoms motivate patients to seek advice and treatment more than management of chronic, symptomless conditions.

Appropriate use of the history and physical examination is crucial in evaluating patients' symptoms. Most symptoms covered in this issue can be appropriately evaluated with appropriate history-taking and physical examination. Dizziness is an

Med Clin N Am 98 (2014) xi–xii
http://dx.doi.org/10.1016/j.mcna.2014.02.001
0025-7125/14/$ – see front matter
medical.theclinics.com

excellent example of a symptom where the use of history and physical examination is far superior to any form of imaging in making a diagnosis. The article in this issue on dizziness emphasizes the nuances in history-taking and physical examination that leads to accurate diagnosis. Accurate and confident diagnosis can reduce diagnostic testing.

No symptom has evolved in the approach to diagnosis and treatment more than back pain. In the 1960s and 1970s, back imaging with radiography was done on everyone with back pain. If patients had sciatica and evidence of disk herniation on examination, then back surgery was done. If surgery was not done, in the 1970s, then chymopapain injections into the disk space were given. By the 1970s, anyone presenting with significant back pain was advised to do a week of solid bed rest. As the 1980s came, CT scanning became widely available, and with it, even more surgery and chymopapain injections, as so many patients had herniated disks on CT scanning. In the 1990s, realization of the prevalence of disk herniations present in the asymptomatic population came to light, and much needed outcome studies of surgical interventions of back pain were published. Bed rest recommendations shrunk to 3 days, and eventually to no mandatory bed rest. In the last decade, well-established guidelines have been published that outline an evidence-based approach to imaging and therapy. Studies have shown early mobilization and activity are the best approach.

Evaluating and treating common symptoms is our bread and butter. For many of the symptoms covered in this issue, there have been significant advances in our understanding of the pathophysiology of the symptoms, and the diseases that commonly cause the symptoms. There has also been increased knowledge of what works and what doesn't work in treating these symptoms and the diseases that cause the symptoms. There is still a great deal to learn about why patients get certain symptoms, and what these symptoms mean. There is even an article on medically unexplained symptoms and how to appropriately care for the patients who suffer from multiple unexplained symptoms. To recognize rare symptoms is exciting in medicine, but to handle the common symptoms appropriately and skillfully is what defines our skillset.

Douglas S. Paauw, MD, MACP
Division of General Internal Medicine
Department of Medicine
University of Washington School of Medicine
Seattle, WA 98195, USA

E-mail address:
DPaauw@medicine.washington.edu

REFERENCE

1. St Sauver JL, Warner DO, Yawn BP, et al. Why patients visit their doctors: assessing the most prevalent conditions in a defined American population. Mayo Clin Proc 2013;88(1):56–67.

Evaluation and Treatment of Chronic Cough

Genji Terasaki, MD[a],*, Douglas S. Paauw, MD, MACP[b]

KEYWORDS

- Cough • Chronic cough • Primary care • Cough-variant asthma • Post nasal drip
- Upper airway cough syndrome • Gastroesophageal reflux

KEY POINTS

- Chronic cough is a common problem among adults that can result in a wide range of physical and psychological complications including urinary incontinence, insomnia, depression, and anxiety.
- The history should focus on the comorbid risk factors such as history of human immuno-deficiency virus and cancer, as well as red-flag symptoms (eg, weight loss, hemoptysis) suggesting a serious, life-threatening cause.
- Owing to its prevalence and relatively straightforward intervention, clinicians should ask about cigarettes and angiotensin-converting enzyme inhibitors (ACE-I).
- A 2-view chest radiograph is an essential part of the evaluation.
- A chronic cough in an otherwise healthy patient with a normal chest radiograph who is not taking ACE-I is mostly likely due to upper airway cough syndrome, asthma, or gastro-esophageal reflux disease, in that order.

INTRODUCTION

Cough is one of the most common symptoms for which patients seek medical care in the United States. In 2010, there were an estimated 30 million visits and $600 million spent on over-the-counter and prescription medications for cough.[1,2] As part of the body's defense mechanism against inhaled irritants and respiratory infections, cough is a natural and universal occurrence, and fortunately in most people it resolves soon after the inciting factor is gone, usually within 3 weeks (termed acute cough). However, at some point, many nonsmoking adults will experience a subacute cough lasting 4 to

Disclosures: The authors have no disclosures about conflicts of interest and funding.
[a] Division of General Internal Medicine, Harborview Medical Center, University of Washington, Box 359780, 325 Ninth Avenue, Seattle, WA 98104, USA; [b] Division of General Internal Medicine, University of Washington, Box 356420, BB527 Health Sciences Building, Seattle, WA 98195, USA
* Corresponding author.
E-mail address: terasaki@u.washington.edu

7 weeks and up to one-fourth of people will experience a chronic cough, defined as lasting more than 8 weeks.[3] Identifying a cause and managing a person with a chronic cough is challenging for clinicians, and in response in 1998 the American College of Chest Physicians (ACCP) developed evidence-based clinical practice guidelines to provide a systematic approach to diagnosing and managing chronic cough, which was subsequently updated and revised in 2006.

A FEW WORDS ON ACUTE COUGH

The most common, and most important, cause of acute cough is acute bronchitis, which is most often viral. *Mycoplasma* and *Chlamydia* pneumonia are the cause in 1% to 5% of young adults.[4,5] Many patients seek treatment for acute cough and believe they need antibiotics. Misperception of a "normal" duration of cough resulting from an upper respiratory infection (URI) may be part of the reason patients seek evaluation and ask for antibiotic treatment. In a study looking at patients' perception of how long a URI-associated cough lasts, cough was thought by subjects to last a mean of 7 to 9 days compared with the actual mean length of cough of 17.8 days in the published literature.[6] There are limited data showing any benefit of symptomatic relief for acute cough with suppressants such as dextromethorphan and codeine.[7] There is no evidence that β-agonists are helpful for cough related to acute bronchitis in the absence of asthma.[8] Most importantly, there is no evidence that antibiotics are beneficial in the treatment of acute bronchitis.[9]

> *Case Presentation. A 52-year-old woman presents to her primary care physician with a 3-month history of a dry cough. The cough has been worsening over the past month and is increasingly affecting her sleep. She reports feeling embarrassed by her coughing at work and social gatherings. Two days ago, she vomited following a severe bout of coughing, prompting a visit to the doctor.*

IMPACT OF CHRONIC COUGH

A wide range of complications can occur from coughing, including urinary incontinence, insomnia, exhaustion, headaches, vomiting, gastroesophageal reflux, loss of appetite, subconjunctival hemorrhage, rib pain, and throat pain. Rarely, vigorous coughing can result in serious problems such as syncope, rib fracture, inguinal or abdominal wall herniation, and diaphragmatic rupture.[10] Furthermore, the emotional and psychological impact can be profound. In a study of older adults with chronic cough, almost all reported feeling anxious that "something's wrong," and one-third expressed a specific fear of cancer. Almost half were self-conscious about their coughing.[11] Several studies of quality of life (QoL) have demonstrated that patients tended to have depression, anxiety, and social isolation associated with their chronic cough.[10,12,13] In particular, women experiencing stress urinary incontinence reported worse QoL scores and were more inclined to seek medical attention for their chronic cough.[14]

> *Case Presentation, Continued. Her primary care physician inquires further. She is a schoolteacher and has never smoked. She has no significant health conditions and is not currently on any medications. Specifically, the patient has no prior history of human immunodeficiency virus (HIV), cancer, recent foreign travel, or environmental exposures. In addition, she has had no associated hemoptysis, fevers, weight loss, or dyspnea. Her physical examination is normal, including no abnormalities of the mouth, nose, pharynx, neck, heart, and lungs. A 2-view chest radiograph is also normal.*

DIFFERENTIAL DIAGNOSIS AND INITIAL EVALUATION

A chronic cough can be the primary symptom of a variety of underlying conditions, including life-threatening diseases such as chronic obstructive lung disease (COPD), atypical pulmonary infections, malignancy, heart failure, and idiopathic pulmonary fibrosis (**Box 1**, **Fig. 1**). Clinicians should be aware of possible red flags and risk factors that would prompt further testing. For example, an expedited workup for tuberculosis is indicated in a patient from an endemic country who presents with

---

Box 1
List of potential causes of a chronic cough (duration of 8 weeks or more) in an adult

Common conditions

- ACE-I cough
- Chronic bronchitis caused by cigarette smoking
- Upper airway cough syndrome (formerly postnasal drip)
- Asthma
- Gastroesophageal reflux disease
- Nonasthmatic eosinophilic bronchitis

Less common conditions

- Postinfectious (pertussis, mycoplasma)
- Interstitial lung disease
- Bronchiectasis
- Obstructive sleep apnea
- Primary lung cancer
- Heart failure
- Tuberculosis
- Environmental exposures

Uncommon conditions

- Sarcoidosis
- Environmental exposures (eg, pneumoconiosis from asbestosis)
- Recurrent aspiration
- Chronic tonsillar enlargement
- Chronic irritation to auditory canal (cerumen or foreign body)
- Idiopathic pulmonary fibrosis
- Aspirated foreign body
- Endemic fungi
- Paragonimiasis
- Peritoneal dialysis
- Cystic fibrosis
- Tracheomalacia
- Aberrant innominate artery
- Habit or tic cough

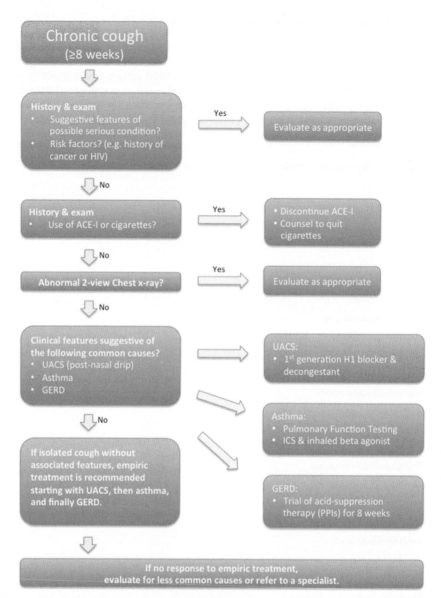

Fig. 1. Algorithm of the evaluation and management of chronic cough in adults. ACE-I, angiotensin-converting enzyme inhibitor; H1 blocker, H1-receptor blocker (antihistamine); HIV, human immunodeficiency virus; ICS, inhaled corticosteroid; PPI, proton-pump inhibitor; UACS, upper airway cough syndrome.

hemoptysis and unintentional weight loss. Similarly, an older patient with a history of tobacco use is at increased risk for primary lung cancer. Pulmonary metastases may be a consideration in a patient with a history of cancer. Moreover, immunosuppression and immune deficiency conditions, such as HIV infection, make patients susceptible to a wider spectrum of pulmonary infections including environmental fungi and bacteria. **Table 1** lists dangerous conditions and their possible associations that clinicians should be vigilant for.

Table 1
Potentially serious causes of a chronic cough (duration of 8 weeks or more) in an adult and suggestive features on history and physical examination

Condition	Suggestive Clinical Features
Asthma	Wheezing, triggers such as exercise, cold air
Tuberculosis	Fever, weight loss, night sweats, hemoptysis, from an endemic area
Primary lung cancer	Weight loss, hemoptysis, smoking history, older age
Metastases to lungs	History of cancer
Heart failure	History of cardiac disease, dyspnea, orthopnea, dependent edema
Chronic obstructive pulmonary disease	Smoking history, chronic sputum production
Interstitial lung disease	Dyspnea, possible environmental exposure, inspiratory crackles present on lung examination

Other elements of the history and physical examination may be helpful in suggesting a cause of a chronic cough. For instance, the finding of wheezing on a chest examination would warrant pulmonary function tests (PFTs) or, alternatively, empiric treatment directed at asthma. Moreover, significant sputum production is more likely to be associated with a primary lung disease.[15,16] The perception of the site from where the cough originates (eg, tickle in the throat vs the thorax) can be misleading and has little correlation with the actual pathologic location.[15] One study goes further, suggesting that the character, timing, or complications of a chronic cough is diagnostically unhelpful. However, it should be noted that participants in this study were recruited from a university-based specialty clinic and may not reflect the typical patient presenting to primary care.[17,18]

There are 2 high-yield elements of the history that clinicians need to be attentive to: the use of an angiotensin-converting enzyme inhibitor (ACE-I) and cigarette smoking. Approximately 10% of patients taking an ACE-I will be affected, but according to reports from China this figure can be as high as 44%.[19,20] Women and nonsmokers also seem to have a higher incidence.[21] The frequency or intensity of the cough does not seem to be dose related. Determining whether an ACE-I is the culprit can be challenging, but a temporal association can be helpful if it was initiated during the preceding year and before the onset of the cough. In predisposed persons, the cough frequently appears soon after the first dose, but has been reported to occur after weeks to months of regular use. Complicating the picture, however, is the possibility that the cough was originally triggered by an unrelated cause that has since resolved (eg, a respiratory infection or environmental irritant) but is potentiated and prolonged by the ACE-I, which may have been started later. For this reason, the ACCP guidelines recommend that an ACE-I be stopped regardless of the temporal relationship.[21] Angiotensin-receptor blockers (ARBs) infrequently cause a cough, making it a good alternative. One can expect the cough to resolve within 1 to 4 weeks of cessation of the ACE-I, although it can occasionally linger for several months afterward.[21]

Of equal importance is to inquire about current cigarette smoking or exposure to second-hand smoke, because it is highly prevalent and is a common cause of a chronic cough. Exposure to smoke can cause airway inflammation and excessive secretions in addition to varying degrees of airway obstruction. Clinically, chronic bronchitis is defined as a cough with sputum production present on most days for at least 3 months for 2 consecutive years. Although there is a dose-response relationship and cutting back on smoking can help, clinicians should counsel their patients to completely quit in light of the other well-known associated health risks. Adjunctive use of nicotine replacement therapy can be helpful.[22] In most patients who successfully quit, the chronic cough is expected to resolve. With advanced stages of COPD, however, the likelihood of full recovery to a baseline state diminishes.[23]

A 2-view chest radiograph is an essential part of the initial evaluation of a chronic cough. Statistically, most results will be normal, but a radiograph can potentially reveal a specific cause such as an atypical infection or the finding feared by patients, a lung mass. Pulmonary function testing can also be considered during the initial evaluation and may point toward a diagnosis of COPD, asthma, or a restrictive lung disease.[15]

With a normal chest radiograph in an otherwise healthy adult who does not use an ACE-I or cigarettes, chronic cough is most commonly caused by 3 conditions: upper airway cough syndrome (UACS), asthma, or gastroesophageal reflux disease (GERD). In fact, the current literature suggests that these 3 causes constitute more than 90% of cases of chronic cough.[17,24] Nonasthmatic eosinophilic bronchitis, postinfectious cough attributable to *Bordetella pertussis*, obstructive sleep apnea, and bronchiectasis from a variety of causes are reported less commonly.[24–26] Unfortunately, little research has been conducted in primary care settings where the prevalence of these diseases probably differs from the published reports, which are largely based on the experiences of secondary and tertiary care settings.[15,27] There also seem to be regional differences. Whereas studies from the United States and Europe report a high prevalence of GERD as the primary cause of the cough, this appears to be practically nonexistent in China and Japan, perhaps reflecting differences in diet, body habitus, or both.[28]

Case Presentation, Continued. The patient is greatly relieved to hear that her chest radiograph is normal. Contemplating the next step, her physician comments that the evaluation up to now has not revealed any obvious causes. Rather than pursuing further testing, however, he recommends empiric treatment directed at the 3 most common causes, starting with UACS. He gives her a prescription for diphenhydramine 25 mg and phenylephrine 20 mg, both to be taken every 8 hours.

He receives a phone call from the patient 3 weeks later stating that her cough is unchanged despite using the antihistamine and decongestant daily. He considers the possibility that she has cough-variant asthma and orders PFTs with pre- and postbronchodilator spirometry.

One week later, the patient returns to the office. He informs her that the PFT results were normal with no demonstration of reversible airflow obstruction. Despite this, he recommends to begin treatment directed at asthma. He gives her a prescription to use an albuterol inhaler, 2 puffs every 6 hours as well as beclomethasone, 2 puffs every 12 hours.

OVERVIEW OF TREATMENT

Treatment should be directed at the most likely condition based on the history, physical examination, and chest radiograph. However, when no cause of a chronic cough is apparent the guidelines from the ACCP recommend sequential targeting of the 3 most common conditions, UACS, asthma, and GERD, in order of prevalence, before embarking on a search for less common diagnoses. Of importance is that UACS, asthma, and GERD can each potentially present "silently" with cough as its only symptom. Given that more than 1 of the aforementioned causes may be present, the ACCP recommends that each subsequent empiric therapy be added onto the step prior. In clinical practice, however, the authors have found that patients often baulk at the increasing number of medications and accompanying concern for polypharmacy.

UPPER AIRWAY COUGH SYNDROME

UACS was previously referred to as postnasal drip syndrome, which typically presents with a sensation of secretions dripping down the posterior nasal passage and pharyngeal wall. Accompanying this may be nasal congestion, rhinorrhea, frequent throat clearing, or globus pharyngeus. The oropharyngeal examination may reveal mucopurulent secretions draining from the nasopharnyx or hypertrophy of lymphoid tissue (cobblestoning; **Fig. 2**).[29] That said, researchers have struggled with the fact that these signs and symptoms seem to correlate poorly with the complaint of cough. Given this uncertainty, experts advocate for the adoption of the newer term, UACS, in an attempt to separate the notion of postnasal drip from coughing attributable to an upper airway cause. Underlying inciting factors in the upper airway includes allergic rhinitis, vasomotor rhinitis, sinusitis, and rhinitis medicamentosa, which is a paradoxic rebound effect from the overuse of nasal decongestants. These inciting factors should be addressed as appropriate, but if none is evident during the initial evaluation, empiric therapy for UACS is recommended. The diagnosis of UACS is established in retrospect, by the resolution of the cough in response to empiric therapy.[30]

The initial treatment of UACS is a combination of a first-generation antihistamine (eg, diphenhydramine or chlorpheniramine) and decongestant (eg, pseudoephedrine or phenylephrine).[3] Second-generation antihistamines, though having a more favorable side-effect profile, seem to be less effective, perhaps because of their limited anticholinergic action that helps to reduce secretions.[30] For patients with rhinitis or nasal congestion, the addition of nasal corticosteroids, nasal anticholinergic agents, or nasal antihistamines may also be effective.[30]

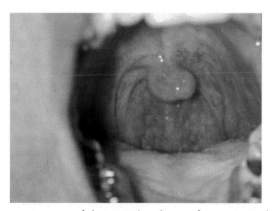

Fig. 2. Cobblestone appearance of the posterior pharynx from postnasal drip.

COUGH-VARIANT ASTHMA

The typical symptoms of asthma are intermittent episodes of wheezing, chest tightness, breathlessness, and cough. However, a subset of asthmatics will have cough-variant asthma, which manifests as a chronic cough as the only symptom with an otherwise normal physical examination. In studies of patients with chronic cough and a normal chest radiograph, asthma accounted for approximately one-third of all causes.[11,16,28] Cough-variant asthma is more common in studies done in China, where it is the most common cause of chronic cough.[28] In patients suspected of having cough-variant asthma, PFT is the initial test and should include forced expiratory volume in 1 second (FEV_1), forced vital capacity (FVC), and FEV_1-to-FVC ratio. The presence of an airway obstruction that improves after the administration of a bronchodilator agent is highly suggestive of asthma. The authors also recommend simultaneously assessing lung volume and diffuse capacity, in case the airway obstruction is irreversible, which would point toward a diagnosis of COPD. Obtaining accurate PFT measurements requires a high level of effort from the patient, and uncontrolled coughing during test makes it almost impossible. Failure to demonstrate a reversible airway obstruction does not exclude the diagnosis of asthma, and bronchoprovocation testing, such as the methacholine inhalation challenge, can be considered to confirm the diagnosis.[3] For safety reasons, a baseline FEV_1 of at least 70% predicted should be documented before bronchoprovocation testing.[31] The negative predictive value of a methacholine challenge test is reported to be close to 100, so a negative result essentially rules out asthma.[18] According to the ACCP, if methacholine challenge is not available or cannot be performed, empiric antiasthma treatment is indicated.

In terms of treatment, patients should be educated about potential triggers including cold air, occupational allergens, smoke, animal dander, pollen, physical exercise, and certain foods. Inhaled corticosteroids (ICSs) such as beclomethasone or fluticasone and a β-agonist such as albuterol are the recommended initial treatment. The evidence for empiric treatment of chronic cough, however, is less clear according to a recent Cochrane review. The investigators caution against empiric treatment and advocate a thorough investigation to confirm the diagnosis before starting inhaled corticosteroids.[32] In their clinical practice, the authors obtain full PFTs, but even if these are negative will prescribe a trial of ICS and a bronchodilator. The risk of side effects is low and patients generally experience improvement within 1 to 2 weeks of initiation if they indeed have cough-variant asthma.[18,33,34] In addition, the authors are careful to review the proper technique of using a metered dose inhaler and routinely offer an aerochamber to help maximize drug delivery to the lungs. Occasionally the addition of a leukotriene receptor inhibitor such as montelukast can help. For severe and refractory cough, a short course (1 week) of oral corticosteroids can be considered.[3,33] Failure to respond to these empiric therapies should prompt the clinician to consider another cause; in contrast to the ACCP recommendations, the authors rarely order bronchoprovocation challenge testing because it adds little diagnostically.

Case Presentation, Continued. The patient returns 4 weeks later. Unfortunately, neither inhaler offered any improvement in her cough. She has been living with the cough for almost 5 months and is very discouraged by the lack of improvement. Her physician again inquires about any symptoms related to the cough. She denies any associated dyspnea, pain, fevers, weight loss, heartburn, or dyspepsia. He explains that after addressing UACS and asthma, GERD remains a strong possibility as a cause of chronic cough even without any gastrointestinal symptoms. At his suggestion, she agrees to a trial of daily proton-pump inhibitor (PPI) medication. In addition, he offers her a referral to a consulting pulmonologist.

GASTROESOPHAGEAL REFLUX DISEASE

GERD is thought to trigger a cough when gastric contents flow back through a relaxed lower esophageal sphincter (LES) into the esophagus, larynx, and respiratory tract.

Physiologic reflux and microaspiration has been demonstrated in asymptomatic persons, and it is therefore unclear why certain individuals seem to have heightened cough sensitivity in response to this trigger. Intuitively, it is easy to imagine how the gastric acidity would irritate and trigger cough receptors located in the esophagus and respiratory tract. Several experiments have shown that infusing acid solution into the distal esophagus of normal subjects can produce a cough.[35] However, there is mounting evidence, including a 2011 Cochrane review, that acid-suppression therapy, though helpful for heartburn and dyspepsia, improves the symptom of cough in only a minority of patients.[36–40] With so many unanswered questions about the pathogenesis of GERD-related cough, use of the more general term reflux disease is favored over acid reflux disease.[41]

The frequency of GERD as the causative factor in chronic cough is unclear. Published reports vary widely, ranging between 0% and 73%, which may possibly reflect regional differences in prevalence and heterogeneity in the methods of diagnosis.[35] Establishing a causal connection is complicated by the fact the GERD can coexist with chronic cough as well as be the result of coughing.[35] Studies have demonstrated that reflux events following coughing are common, perhaps related to increased intra-abdominal pressures and relaxation of the LES, which may in turn perpetuate a cough-reflux cycle.[35,36]

The current guidelines for the management GERD-associated cough are largely driven by expert opinion. The ACCP recommends targeting GERD after UACS and asthma, even in patients with no heartburn, regurgitation, or sour taste. In lieu of testing, empiric treatment is recommended, beginning with lifestyle changes (eg, weight loss, smoking cessation, and limiting intake of fatty and acidic foods, alcohol, chocolates, coffee, and teas) and PPI therapy for at least 8 weeks. Prokinetic agents may also be added if there little response to initial therapy. The authors concur with the ACCP's empiric approach primarily because the available tests such as 24-hour pH monitoring would not necessarily alter the decision to recommend a course of antireflux therapy, of which there are relatively few options. Given the low likelihood of a significant response to PPIs, the authors do not wait 8 weeks for a response but rather concurrently pursue investigation into other causes. At this point, there is also a low threshold to refer the patient to a specialist. The authors' institution rarely offers antireflux surgery such as fundoplication for patients with the sole symptom of chronic cough, and certainly only after a sufficiently long trial on medical therapy and a thorough investigation including 24-hour pH monitoring, barium esophagography, and endoscopy.

LESS COMMON CAUSES OF CHRONIC COUGH

Chronic cough in adults who do not use cigarettes or ACE-I and have a normal chest radiograph is mostly like the result of UACS, asthma, or GERD. However, in those for whom the diagnosis remains undetermined, there are several important less common causes to be considered. A full discussion is beyond the scope of this review, but 2 important but underrecognized conditions are addressed here.

Nonasthmatic eosinophilic bronchitis (NAEB) is a common cause of chronic cough that in some series may be more common than GERD-related cough, especially in certain regions such as China and Japan.[24,28,42] Similar to asthma, it is characterized by eosinophilic inflammation of the airways but, importantly, reversible airway hyperresponsiveness is not present. Consequently, the primary treatment is ICSs but not β-agonist agents. In addition to a normal chest radiograph and PFTs, the presence of eosinophils on an induced sputum cell analysis is diagnostic according to the expert guidelines. Unfortunately, primary care offices and even many pulmonary clinics are not equipped to properly obtain an induced sputum sample.[18,40,43,44] The authors' approach is to address NAEB together with asthma, because the 2 conditions overlap in diagnosis and therapeutics. Patients are offered a trial of ICSs for at least 4 weeks, even if the PFTs are normal, and asthma and NAEB as a cause is considered unlikely if there is no improvement in the cough. Similarly to UACS and asthma, patients are asked about any possible environmental or occupational aggravating factors, especially those that can be easily avoided.

Whooping cough is increasingly recognized as a cause of a prolonged postinfectious cough. The etiologic agent is the bacterium *Bordetella pertussis*, which is highly contagious. Whereas it can cause serious disease and possibly death in unvaccinated infants and young children, adults rarely exhibit the classic symptoms including the characteristic inspiratory whooping sound between coughs and posttussive emesis. Instead, infected adults may manifest no symptoms or a range of milder symptoms, including nonspecific URI symptoms and prolonged cough.[26] Given how difficult it is to clinically assess adults' likelihood of having pertussis as the cause of a chronic cough, it is tempting to order laboratory testing, empirically treat with antibiotics, or both. Nasopharyngeal swabs for culture and the polymerase chain reaction both are diagnostic, but the window of usefulness is only during the first 4 weeks of illness. By contrast, serologic testing can be done in the later stages (4–12 weeks) and can confirm the diagnosis if there is a 4-fold increase in immunoglobulin G antibody levels; this would, however, require the forethought of obtaining an early serum sample during the acute phase.[45] Antibiotics are effective in eradicating the *B pertussis* and reducing transmission during the first several weeks of the illness. However, according to a Cochrane systematic review, treatment did not significantly alter the course of the illness, including cough.[46]

COUGH HYPERSENSITIVITY SYNDROME

There is growing evidence that the body can naturally modulate the sensitivity of the cough reflex sensors. This occurrence is commonly noticed after an acute URI when a person can experience a paroxysm of coughing in response to relatively minor triggers such cold air, inhaled aerosols, laughing, and taking a deep breath. This heightened cough sensitivity normally usually returns to baseline after 2 to 3 weeks.[43] For some people, however, this state of hypersensitivity persists long after the original stimulus is gone. Researchers are unclear as to which factors lead to cough reflex hypersensitivity, and some have hypothesized that it may be an underlying feature of all cases of chronic cough regardless of the aggravating conditions, whether GERD, asthma, or ACE-I use. Furthermore, it is uncertain whether these conditions cause cough hypersensitivity or serve as a trigger for an already sensitized person.[40]

While the concept of cough hypersensitivity syndrome continues to evolve we are increasingly recognizing the clinical implications, particularly for patients who, after an extensive evaluation and strict adherence to empiric therapies, are stuck with the label of "unexplained chronic cough." New treatment approaches, which attempt to reset the sensitivity of the cough reflex (peripheral and central), are under investigation.[42] For example, gabapentin, a central neuromodulator used in a variety of conditions including as an analgesic for neuropathic pain, is currently being studied and eventually may have a role in the management of a chronic cough.[47] Certain peripherally located transient receptor potential channels are also the potential targets for new antitussive agents.[43]

SUMMARY

Chronic cough is a frustrating and common problem, resulting in significant psychological and physical sequelae as well as enormous financial costs in terms of health care expense and time lost from work. Decreased QoL and depression are common. However, using a systematic approach, including assessing whether the patient uses ACE-I and cigarettes, excluding the presence of red flags and risk factors for life-threatening diseases, and obtaining and normal chest radiograph, more than 90% of cases of chronic cough are diagnosed as being caused by UACS, asthma, or GERD. It is recommended to address these conditions sequentially, starting with UACS. Nonasthmatic eosinophilic bronchitis and pertussis infections are unrecognized by primary care providers and should be considered after UACS, asthma, and GERD have been addressed. Finally, cough hypersensitivity syndrome is a new area of research and has been hypothesized to be the underlying factor in many cases of chronic cough, regardless of the inciting factor. More clinical research is needed to further elucidate the cough reflex pathway and the factors involved in modulating its sensitivity, which may eventually lead to new antitussive therapeutics.

REFERENCES

1. Sawin G, Pendleton M. Cough (subacute and chronic). In: D Slawson ME, Lin K, editors. Essential Evidence. John Wiley & Son, Inc; 2013. Available at: http://www.essentialevidenceplus.com. Accessed August 1, 2013.
2. National Hospital Ambulatory Medical Care Survey: 2010 Outpatient Department Summary Tables. Bureau USC. 2010.
3. Irwin RS, Baumann MH, Bolser DC, et al. Diagnosis and management of cough executive summary: ACCP evidence-based clinical practice guidelines. Chest 2006;129:1S–23S.
4. Wadowsky RM, Castilla EA, Laus S, et al. Evaluation of *Chlamydia pneumoniae* and *Mycoplasma pneumoniae* as etiologic agents of persistent cough in adolescents and adults. J Clin Microbiol 2002;40:637–40.
5. Grayston JT, Kuo CC, Wang SP, et al. A new *Chlamydia psittaci* strain, TWAR, isolated in acute respiratory tract infections. N Engl J Med 1986; 315:161–8.
6. Ebell MH, Lundgren J, Youngpairoj S. How long does a cough last? Comparing patients' expectations with data from a systematic review of the literature. Ann Fam Med 2013;11:5–13.
7. Bolser DC. Cough suppressant and pharmacologic protussive therapy: ACCP evidence-based clinical practice guidelines. Chest 2006;129:238S–49S.
8. Becker LA, Hom J, Villasis-Keever M, et al. Beta2-agonists for acute bronchitis. Cochrane Database Syst Rev 2011;(7):CD001726.
9. Smucny J, Fahey T, Becker L, et al. Antibiotics for acute bronchitis. Cochrane Database Syst Rev 2004;(4):CD000245.
10. Irwin RS. Complications of cough: ACCP evidence-based clinical practice guidelines. Chest 2006;129:54S–8S.
11. Smyrnios NA, Irwin RS, Curley FJ, et al. From a prospective study of chronic cough: diagnostic and therapeutic aspects in older adults. Arch Intern Med 1998;158:1222–8.
12. Polley L, Yaman N, Heaney L, et al. Impact of cough across different chronic respiratory diseases: comparison of two cough-specific health-related quality of life questionnaires. Chest 2008;134:295–302.

13. Birring SS, Prudon B, Carr AJ, et al. Development of a symptom specific health status measure for patients with chronic cough: Leicester Cough Questionnaire (LCQ). Thorax 2003;58:339–43.
14. French CT, Fletcher KE, Irwin RS. Gender differences in health-related quality of life in patients complaining of chronic cough. Chest 2004;125:482–8.
15. Morice AH, McGarvey L, Pavord I. Recommendations for the management of cough in adults. Thorax 2006;61(Suppl 1):i1–24.
16. Kastelik JA, Aziz I, Ojoo JC, et al. Investigation and management of chronic cough using a probability-based algorithm. Eur Respir J 2005;25:235–43.
17. Mello CJ, Irwin RS, Curley FJ. Predictive values of the character, timing, and complications of chronic cough in diagnosing its cause. Arch Intern Med 1996;156: 997–1003.
18. Pratter MR, Brightling CE, Boulet LP, et al. An empiric integrative approach to the management of cough: ACCP evidence-based clinical practice guidelines. Chest 2006;129:222S–31S.
19. Bangalore S, Kumar S, Messerli FH. Angiotensin-converting enzyme inhibitor associated cough: deceptive information from the Physicians' Desk Reference. Am J Med 2010;123:1016–30.
20. Woo KS, Nicholls MG. High prevalence of persistent cough with angiotensin converting enzyme inhibitors in Chinese. Br J Clin Pharmacol 1995;40:141–4.
21. Dicpinigaitis PV. Angiotensin-converting enzyme inhibitor-induced cough: ACCP evidence-based clinical practice guidelines. Chest 2006;129:169S–73S.
22. Stead LF, Perera R, Bullen C, et al. Nicotine replacement therapy for smoking cessation. Cochrane Database Syst Rev 2012;(11):CD000146.
23. Braman SS. Chronic cough due to chronic bronchitis: ACCP evidence-based clinical practice guidelines. Chest 2006;129:104S–15S.
24. Pratter MR. Overview of common causes of chronic cough: ACCP evidence-based clinical practice guidelines. Chest 2006;129:59S–62S.
25. Sundar KM, Daly SE, Willis AM. A longitudinal study of CPAP therapy for patients with chronic cough and obstructive sleep apnoea. Cough 2013;9:19.
26. Cornia PB, Hersh AL, Lipsky BA, et al. Does this coughing adolescent or adult patient have pertussis? JAMA 2010;304:890–6.
27. Hong Q, Bai C, Wang X. Characteristics of Chinese patients with cough in primary care centre. J Transl Med 2011;9:149.
28. Lai K, Chen R, Lin J, et al. A prospective, multicenter survey on causes of chronic cough in China. Chest 2013;143:613–20.
29. Ryan MW. The patient with "postnasal drip". Med Clin North Am 2010;94:913–21.
30. Pratter MR. Chronic upper airway cough syndrome secondary to rhinosinus diseases (previously referred to as postnasal drip syndrome): ACCP evidence-based clinical practice guidelines. Chest 2006;129:63S–71S.
31. Mottram CD. Bronchoprovocation testing. In: Ruppel's manual of pulmonary function testing. 10th edition. Maryland Heights (MO): Mosby, An imprint of Elsevier; 2013. p. 296–320.
32. Johnstone KJ, Chang AB, Fong KM, et al. Inhaled corticosteroids for subacute and chronic cough in adults. Cochrane Database Syst Rev 2013;(3): CD009305.
33. Dicpinigaitis PV. Chronic cough due to asthma: ACCP evidence-based clinical practice guidelines. Chest 2006;129:75S–9S.
34. Ribeiro M, Pereira CA, Nery LE, et al. High-dose inhaled beclomethasone treatment in patients with chronic cough: a randomized placebo-controlled study. Ann Allergy Asthma Immunol 2007;99:61–8.

35. Chung KF, Pavord ID. Prevalence, pathogenesis, and causes of chronic cough. Lancet 2008;371:1364–74.
36. Kahrilas PJ, Howden CW, Hughes N, et al. Response of chronic cough to acid-suppressive therapy in patients with gastroesophageal reflux disease. Chest 2013;143:605–12.
37. Chang AB, Lasserson TJ, Gaffney J, et al. Gastro-oesophageal reflux treatment for prolonged non-specific cough in children and adults. Cochrane Database Syst Rev 2011;(1):CD004823.
38. Shaheen NJ, Crockett SD, Bright SD, et al. Randomised clinical trial: high-dose acid suppression for chronic cough—a double-blind, placebo-controlled study. Aliment Pharmacol Ther 2011;33:225–34.
39. Faruqi S, Molyneux ID, Fathi H, et al. Chronic cough and esomeprazole: a double-blind placebo-controlled parallel study. Respirology 2011;16:1150–6.
40. Birring SS. Controversies in the evaluation and management of chronic cough. Am J Respir Crit Care Med 2011;183:708–15.
41. Irwin RS. Chronic cough due to gastroesophageal reflux disease: ACCP evidence-based clinical practice guidelines. Chest 2006;129:80S–94S.
42. Chung KF. Chronic 'cough hypersensitivity syndrome': a more precise label for chronic cough. Pulm Pharmacol Ther 2011;24:267–71.
43. McGarvey LP, Elder J. Future directions in treating cough. Otolaryngol Clin North Am 2010;43:199–211, xii.
44. Brightling CE. Chronic cough due to nonasthmatic eosinophilic bronchitis: ACCP evidence-based clinical practice guidelines. Chest 2006;129:116S–21S.
45. Pertussis (whooping cough): diagnosis confirmation. 2012. Available at: http://www.cdc.gov/pertussis/clinical/diagnostic-testing/diagnosis-confirmation.html. Accessed August 28, 2013.
46. Altunaiji S, Kukuruzovic R, Curtis N, et al. Antibiotics for whooping cough (pertussis). Cochrane Database Syst Rev 2007;(3):CD004404.
47. Ryan NM, Birring SS, Gibson PG. Gabapentin for refractory chronic cough: a randomised, double-blind, placebo-controlled trial. Lancet 2012;380:1583–9.

Low Back Pain

Anna L. Golob, MD[a,b,*], Joyce E. Wipf, MD[a,b]

KEYWORDS

- Acute low back pain • Chronic low back pain • Risk factors • Cause • Diagnosis
- Imaging • Treatment • Sciatica

KEY POINTS

- Low back pain is a common, frequently recurring condition that often has a nonspecific cause.
- History and physical examination should focus on evaluation for evidence of systemic or pathologic causes.
- Imaging is only indicated when there is evidence of neurologic deficits or red flags to suggest fracture, malignancy, infection, or other systemic disease, or when symptoms do not improve after 4 to 6 weeks.
- Most nonspecific low back pain will improve within several weeks with or without treatment.
- Back pain that radiates to the lower extremities, occurs episodically with walking or standing erect, and is relieved by sitting or forward spine flexion is typical of neuroclaudication and suggests central spinal stenosis.
- All patients with acute or chronic low back pain should be advised to remain active.
- The treatment of chronic nonspecific low back pain involves a multidisciplinary approach targeted at preserving function and preventing disability.
- Urgent surgical referral is indicated in the presence of severe or progressive neurologic deficits or signs and symptoms of cauda equina syndrome.

INTRODUCTION

Low back pain affects a significant proportion of the population.[1–5] The precise incidence and prevalence of low back pain are difficult to characterize due to significant heterogeneity in the epidemiologic studies. In a survey of Saskatchewan adults, 84% of participants reported experiencing at least one episode of back pain in their lifetime.[6] A 2002 US National Health Interview Study found that 26.4% of the 30,000 participants had experienced at least one full day of back pain in the past 3 months.[7] A 2010 review article reported 1-year incidences of first time, any time, and recurrent

Financial Disclosures: None (A.L. Golob); UpToDate chapter royalties (J.E. Wipf).
[a] Department of Medicine, University of Washington, Box 356420, 1959 NE Pacific Street, Seattle, WA 98195-6420, USA; [b] VA Puget Sound Healthcare System, General Medicine Service, S-123-PCC, 1660 South Columbian Way, Seattle, WA 98108, USA
* Corresponding author. VA Puget Sound Healthcare System, General Medicine Service, S-123-PCC, 1660 South Columbian Way, Seattle, WA 98108.
E-mail address: zilanna@uw.edu

low back pain episodes as ranging from 1.5% to 80%, and the 1-year prevalence of low back pain ranging from 0.8% to 82.5%.[8] These findings are summarized in **Table 1**.

The incidence of low back pain peaks in the third decade of life. The prevalence increases until age 60 to 65 and then gradually declines.

Commonly reported risk factors for low back pain include physical, psychological, social, and occupational factors and are summarized in **Table 2**.[2,6]

Low back pain has an enormous social and economic impact. It is a leading cause of work absenteeism globally and the second most common cause of missed work days in the United States.[9,10] Direct medical costs attributed to the evaluation and treatment of low back pain are estimated to exceed $33 billion annually in the United States. When the indirect costs of missed work and decreased productivity are added, the total costs exceed $100 billion each year.[2]

Primary care providers play a key role in the evaluation and treatment of low back pain. Indeed, low back pain is the chief complaint in about 2.3% of all ambulatory physician visits, representing about 15 million office visits per year, and is second only to upper respiratory symptoms as a symptom prompting office evaluation.[7]

PATHOPHYSIOLOGY
Anatomy

There are 5 lumbar vertebrae, each of which is composed of a vertebral body, 2 pedicles, 2 lamina, 4 articular facets, and a spinous process. Between each pair of vertebrae are the foramina, openings through which pass the spinal nerves, radicular blood vessels, and sinuvertebral nerves. The spinal canal is formed anteriorly by the posterior surface of the vertebral bodies, intervertebral discs, and posterior longitudinal ligament, laterally by the pedicles, and posteriorly by the ligamentum flavum and lamina (**Fig. 1**).

In the normal spine, the anterior structures including the vertebral bodies and intervertebral discs perform weight-bearing and shock-absorbing functions. The posterolateral structures, including the vertebral arches, lamina, transverse, and spinous processes, provide protection for the spinal cord and nerve roots. Balance, flexibility, and stability are provided by the facet joints and paraspinous muscles and ligaments.

Physiology

Low back pain is often characterized in terms of radiologic findings (spondylosis, spondylolisthesis, spondylolysis) and clinical and neurologic findings (lordosis, kyphosis, radiculopathy, sciatica). These terms are defined in **Table 3**.

Table 1 Incidence and prevalence of low back pain episodes	
Low Back Pain (LBP) Episode	**Incidence or Prevalence**
1-y incidence of first ever LBP episode	6.3%–15.4%
1-y incidence of any LBP episode	1.5%–36%
1-y incidence of recurrent LBP episode	24%–80%
Point prevalence of LBP episodes	1.0%–58.1% (mean 18.1%, median 15.0%)
1-y prevalence of LBP episodes	0.8%–82.5% (mean 38.1%, median 37.4%)

Data from Hoy D, Brookes P, Blyth F, et al. The epidemiology of low back pain. Best Pract Res Clin Rheumatol 2010;24(6):769–81.

	Psychological		
Physical Factors	Factors	Social Factors	Occupational Factors
Older age	Depression	Low educational achievement	Physically or psychologically strenuous work
Female gender Obesity Smoking	Anxiety Somatization disorder	Increased life stress	Sedentary work Whole body vibration Low social support in the workplace Job dissatisfaction Workers compensation insurance

Table 2
Risk factors for development of low back pain

Experimental studies indicate that mechanical low back pain can originate in one or more of the many structures of the spine, including ligaments, facet joints, intervertebral discs, paravertebral musculature and fascia, and spinal nerve roots.

Acute Low Back Pain

Acute low back pain occurring after physical activity most likely results from increased paraspinous muscle tension with resultant avulsion of tendinous attachments between the muscles and bone, or tearing of muscle fibers/sheaths. Persistent muscle overuse, particularly of untrained or poorly conditioned muscles, can cause tonic contraction (spasms).[11] Ligament sprains are another common cause of acute low back pain and occur when the ligament is stretched beyond its physiologic range.

Chronic Low Back Pain

In chronic low back pain, the most common source of pain is thought to be degenerative changes of the bony structures and ligaments. That said, arthritis of the spine, termed "spondylosis," seems to be a naturally occurring process. By age 49 years, 60% of women and 80% of men have osteophytes and other changes that indicate early spondylosis; by age 79, nearly all individuals have evidence of spondylosis on plain radiographs.[12,13] In addition, there is poor correlation between the presence of spondylosis, including disc herniation, on imaging studies, and clinical pain syndromes (**Fig. 2**).[12,13]

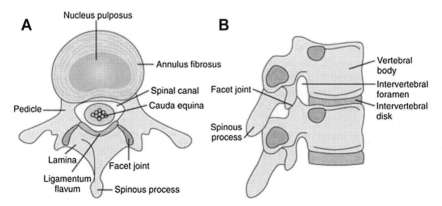

Fig. 1. Anatomy of the lumbar spine. (*A*) Cross-sectional view through a lumbar vertebra. (*B*) Lateral view of the lumbar spine. (*From* Firestein GS, Budd RC, Gabriel SE, et al. Kelley's textbook of rheumatology. Philadelphia: Saunders; 2013. p. 666; with permission.)

Table 3
Commonly used terms in low back pain

Term	Definition
Spondylosis	Osteoarthritis of the spine; evidenced by disc space narrowing and/or arthritic changes of the facet joints on radiographs
Spondylolisthesis	Anterior displacement of a vertebra in relation to the one beneath it. Displacement is graded 1–IV as follows: Grade I: 1%–25% slip; generally nonsurgical Grade II: 26%–50% slip; generally nonsurgical Grade III: 51%–75% slip; may be surgical Grade IV: 76%–100% slip; may be surgical
Spondylolysis	Fracture in the pars interarticularis of the vertebral arch (the joining of the vertebral body to the posterior structures), usually at L5. This is a congenital variant in 3%–6% of people
Spinal stenosis	Local, segmental, or generalized narrowing of the central spinal canal by bone or soft tissue elements, usually bony hypertrophy of the facet joints or thickening of the ligamentum flavum
Radiculopathy	Pain, sensory, and/or motor deficits resulting from compression of a spinal nerve root
Sciatica	Pain, numbness, or tingling in the sciatic nerve distribution, radiating down the posterior or lateral aspect of the leg often to the foot, due to compression of the sciatic nerve or its component nerve roots
Cauda equina syndrome	Loss of bowel or bladder control, numbness in the groin or saddle region of the perineum, and lower extremity weakness caused by compression of the inferior-most part of the spinal cord or spinal nerve roots due to canal stenosis or a large herniated disc
Kyphosis	Outward (convex) curve of the spine; there is a normal small thoracic kyphosis (at the level of the ribs)
Lordosis	Inward (concave) curve of the spine; there is a normal small lumbar lordosis
Scoliosis	Sideways (lateral) curve of the spine, always abnormal

The facet joints are true synovial joints and therefore are subject to develop degenerative or inflammatory changes. The resultant bony enlargement of these joints is thought to cause facet-mediated arthritic pain and can contribute to canal stenosis along with thickening of the ligamentum flavum.[14]

There is some debate about the role of internal disc degeneration or disruption, referring to degenerative changes of the annulus fibrosis (elastic collagen ring) and nucleus pulposus (gelatinous inner contents of the disc, surrounded by the annular fibrosis). Internal disc degeneration has been proposed to cause primary discogenic back pain. However, the nucleus pulposus has no nerve supply, and the nerve endings that enter the annulus fibrosis do not contain substance P and are not considered nociceptors,[15] leaving uncertainty regarding the pathophysiology of disc-related pain. Some have observed that new nerves and blood vessels can grow into the damaged annulosis fibrosis and propose that this neogrowth may be the source of discogenic pain.[16] Provocative discography, a procedure in which pain level is assessed while contrast material is injected into a disc, has been used to diagnose primary discogenic pain. However, this procedure can cause pain in people with normal discs and does not induce pain in all people with degenerated discs, leaving further questions regarding the clinical significance of internal disc degeneration and source of discogenic pain.[17]

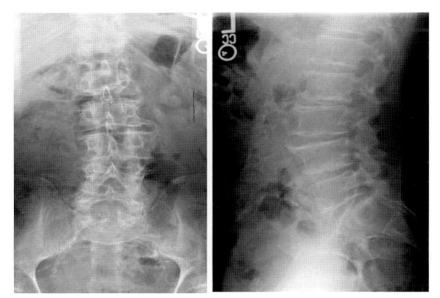

Fig. 2. Spondylosis and scoliosis of the lumbar spine. Anteroposterior and lateral radiographs of the lumbar spine showing mild levoconvex scoliosis with apex L2/3, multilevel disc space narrowing, endplate spurring, and lumbar facet arthropathy.

Radicular low back pain is pain that radiates into the lower extremity and is caused by compression and/or inflammation of a spinal nerve root. Sciatica refers to compression of the sciatic nerve, but is also commonly used to describe radicular back pain radiating into the lower extremities distal to the knee. Spinal nerve compression occurs most commonly from disc herniation or spondylosis, causing foraminal narrowing, and less commonly from benign or malignant tumors or epidural abscesses. The lumbar discs are at higher risk of herniation than cervical and thoracic discs partly because of the increased static and kinetic stress at this level, but also because the posterior longitudinal ligament, which forms the anterior wall of the spinal canal, is only half as wide along the lumbar vertebra as it is more superiorly, thus providing inadequate reinforcement of the lumbar discs. L5 and S1 radiculopathies are most common, comprising more than 90% of lumbosacral radiculopathies (**Figs. 3** and **4**).

Spinal stenosis refers to narrowing of the central spinal canal, most commonly caused by spondylosis, which is often asymptomatic. If symptomatic, the clinical manifestations of spinal stenosis vary by the degree of stenosis and its location. It is most commonly caused by degenerative spondylosis and as a result is usually seen in people over the age of 60. Symptomatic stenosis affecting the lateral aspect of the canal usually presents as a radiculopathy, whereas symptomatic stenosis affecting the central region of the canal presents as neurogenic claudication, also called "pseudoclaudication." This condition is characterized by aching pain or paresthesia in one or both lower extremities that comes on with standing upright or walking and is improved with rest or forward flexion (eg, relieved while pushing a shopping cart). It can be mistaken for vascular claudication, which also improves with rest. The two can be distinguished in that vascular claudication does not improve with forward flexion alone and should not include paresthesias, motor weakness, reflex changes, or intact distal pulses (**Fig. 5**).

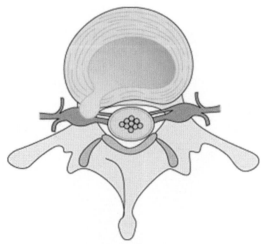

Fig. 3. Schematic drawing showing posterolateral disc herniation resulting in nerve root impingement. (*From* Firestein GS, Budd RC, Gabriel SE, et al. Kelley's textbook of rheumatology. Philadelphia: Saunders; 2013. p. 670; with permission.)

Spondylolisthesis is a condition in which a vertebra slips forward with respect to the vertebra beneath it. It is graded I–IV based on severity, as described in **Table 3**. Spondylolisthesis is caused by fractures or deformities of the pars interarticularis (congenital, traumatic, or pathologic), and degenerative changes. The lower lumbar vertebrae

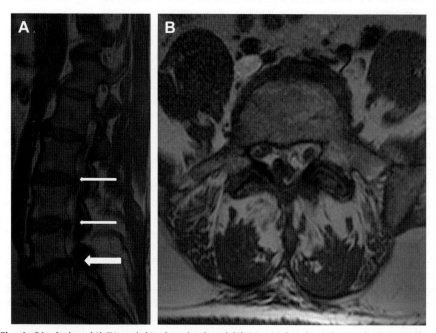

Fig. 4. Disc bulge. (*A*) T1-weighted sagittal and (*B*) T2-weighted axial MRI showing diffuse disc bulges at levels L3-4 and L4-5 (*thin arrows*) and posterior central disc extrusion at L5-S1 (*thick arrow*) resulting in narrowing of the left lateral recess that contacts the traversing left S1 nerve root.

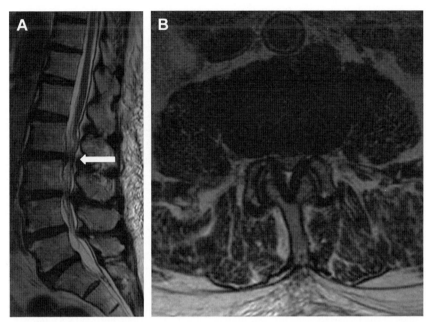

Fig. 5. Degenerative spinal stenosis. (*A*) T1-weighted sagittal and (*B*) T2-weighted axial MRI showing severe dural compression at L2-3 (*arrow*) secondary to severe facet and ligamentum flavum hypertrophy and circumferential disc bulge with caudal extension of the central disc extrusion. Severe dural compression at L3-4 and moderate dural compression at L4-5.

including L4-5 and L5-S1 are the most frequent sites of spondylolisthesis. If there are no neurologic signs or symptoms, and the grade of slippage is I or II, spondylolisthesis is treated conservatively, much like other causes of chronic mechanical low back pain. If there is neurologic compromise or grades III or IV slippage, the patient should be referred for surgical evaluation.

Spondylolysis refers to a defect in the pars interarticularis without vertebral slippage. It is common, is found in more than 5% of people older than age 7, and typically is asymptomatic. It is thought to result from a congenital defect in the pars with or without a stress fracture related to childhood activity (**Figs. 6** and **7**).[18]

Differential Diagnosis

One approach to organizing the differential diagnosis of low back pain is to consider it in terms of nonspecific "mechanical" low back pain versus back pain with lower extremity symptoms versus systemic and visceral diseases, as shown in **Table 4**.

By far the most common causes of low back pain are mechanical, representing about 97% of patients. In clinical practice, it is often difficult to determine the precise source of a patient's mechanical back pain. In fact, Deyo and Weinstein[17] have reported that a definitive diagnosis cannot be made in up to 85% of patients due to the weak association between symptoms, pathologic changes, and findings on imaging. The inability to make precise diagnoses results in the frequent use of nonspecific diagnostic terms, such as sprain, strain, spasm, and degenerative changes.

There are also nonmechanical causes of low back pain, including neoplasms, infections, and inflammatory conditions, as listed in **Table 4**. Nonmechanical causes of back pain are usually accompanied by systemic signs and symptoms or a severe,

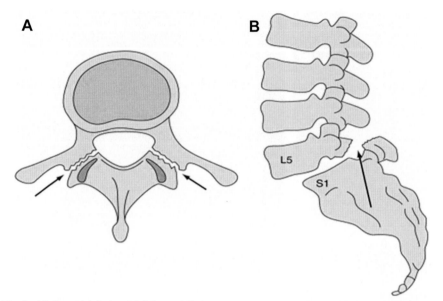

Fig. 6. (*A*) Spondylolysis with bilateral defects in the pars interarticularis (*arrows*). (*B*) Spondylolysis of the L5 vertebra (*arrow*) resulting in isthmic spondylolisthesis at L5-S1. (*From* Firestein GS, Budd RC, Gabriel SE, et al. Kelley's textbook of rheumatology. Philadelphia: Saunders; 2013. p. 672; with permission.)

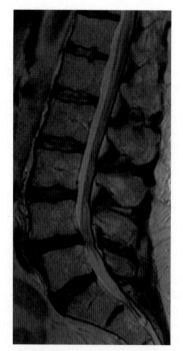

Fig. 7. Spondylolisthesis. T1-weighted sagittal MRI showing grade 1 anterolisthesis of L4 on L5, likely degenerative.

Table 4
Differential diagnosis of low back pain and estimated prevalence of each condition in primary care practice

Nonspecific "Mechanical" Low Back Pain (97%)	Back Pain with Lower Extremity Symptoms	Systemic and Visceral Diseases
Idiopathic musculoligamentous strain/ sprain (70%)	Disc herniation (4%)	Neoplasia (0.7%) • Multiple myeloma • Metastatic carcinoma • Lymphoma/leukemia • Spinal cord tumors • Retroperitoneal tumors
Disc/facet degeneration (10%)	Spinal stenosis (3%)	Infection (0.01%) • Osteomyelitis • Septic discitis • Paraspinous abscess • Epidural abscess • Shingles
Osteoporotic compression fracture (4%)	—	Inflammatory disease (0.03%) • Anklyosing spondylitis • Psoriatic spondylitis • Reactive arthritis • Inflammatory bowel disease
Spondylolisthesis (2%)	—	Visceral disease (0.05%)
Severe scoliosis, kyphosis, asymmetric transitional vertebrae (<1%)	—	• Prostatitis • Endometriosis • Chronic pelvic inflammatory disease • Nephrolithiasis • Pyelonephritis • Perinephric abscess • Aortic aneurysm • Pancreatitis • Cholecystitis • Penetrating ulcer
Traumatic fracture (<1%)	—	Other • Osteochondrosis • Paget's disease

Adapted from Wipf JE, Deyo RA. Low back pain. In: Branch WT, editor. The office practice of medicine. 3rd edition. Philadelphia: Saunders; 1994. p. 646.

rapidly progressing course. Visceral organ pain, including bowel, kidney, and pelvic organ pain, can also be referred to the spine. Overall, nonmechanical spine conditions and referred visceral organ pain are much less common causes of low back pain than mechanical causes. In fact, fewer than 5% of all primary care patients with low back pain will have a serious systemic pathologic condition.

DIAGNOSTIC EVALUATION

Given that a precise anatomic cause for low back pain usually cannot be found, the primary objectives in the diagnostic evaluation of the patient with low back pain are to evaluate for evidence of systemic disease or neurologic compromise that may require further workup or surgical evaluation, and to probe for factors that may predispose the patient to a prolonged course or chronic pain syndrome. These objectives can usually be met by taking a thorough history and physical examination.

Patient History

When assessing a patient with low back pain, providers should ask about time course, precipitating factors (trauma), location, character, severity, radiation, and exacerbating and alleviating factors. Most patients presenting with acute low back pain have a prior history of low back pain to which the current episode can be compared. Many, but not all, patients will recall an inciting activity that may have exacerbated the current flare. Most mechanical back pain is relieved by lying down and is not bothersome at night. Pain that is not relieved by lying down is more likely to be caused by malignancy or infection, but this is not a specific finding for these conditions. The likelihood of spinal infection is increased in patients with a history of injected drug use, skin or soft tissue infections, urinary tract infections, or fever.

Mechanical pain typically localizes to the paraspinal regions, occasionally spreading to the flanks or buttocks, but does not radiate into the legs. Radicular or sciatic pain radiates into the lower extremities and may be associated with paresthesias, sensory loss, motor weakness, or decreased reflexes. The distribution of pain and associated symptoms can help identify the nerve root involved. **Table 5** lists the signs and symptoms of the lumbar radiculopathies by nerve root. Radiculopathy syndromes caused by disc herniation often worsen with cough, sneeze, or Valsalva maneuvers.

Back pain that radiates to the lower extremities, occurs episodically with walking or standing erect, and is relieved by sitting or forward spine flexion is typical of neuroclaudication and suggests central spinal stenosis (must also consider vascular claudication).

The presence of radicular symptoms or neurogenic claudication suggests neurologic involvement, from either disc herniation or spinal stenosis, but can often be managed conservatively. However, the presence of bowel or bladder dysfunction may signal severe compression of the cauda equina, as do saddle anesthesia, bilateral leg numbness, and back pain. The cauda equina syndrome is usually caused by massive midline disc herniation, but can also be caused by tumor or abscess

Table 5
Signs and symptoms of lumbar radiculopathies by nerve root

Root	Pain Distribution	Dermatomal Sensory Distribution	Motor Weakness	Affected Reflex
L1	Inguinal region	Inguinal region	Hip flexion	Cremasteric
L2	Inguinal region Anterior thigh	Anterior thigh	Hip flexion Hip adduction	Cremasteric Thigh adductor
L3	Anterior thigh Knee	Distal anteromedial thigh including knee	Knee extension Hip flexion Hip adduction	Patellar Thigh adductor
L4	Anterior thigh Medial aspect leg	Medial leg	Knee extension Hip flexion Hip adduction	Patellar
L5	Posterolateral thigh Lateral leg Medial foot	Lateral leg Dorsal foot Great toe	Foot/toe dorsiflexion Knee flexion Hip adduction	—
S1	Posterior thigh Posterior leg Lateral foot	Posterolateral leg Lateral aspect of foot	Foot/toe plantar flexion Knee flexion Hip extension	Achilles

Data from Levin KH, Covington EC, Devereaux MW, et al. Neck and back pain. Continuum: Lifelong Learning Neurol 2001;7:16.

compressing the cauda equina. Of note, progressive neurologic deficits or suspected cauda equina syndrome or cord compression requires emergent surgical evaluation.

Historical red flags that may signal systemic disease include a personal history of cancer, advanced age, unexplained fever or weight loss, duration of pain greater than 4 weeks, pain occurring at night, or pain that has not responded to previous therapies. A list of these red flags is summarized in **Table 6**.

Even in the absence of neurologic compromise or systemic disease, some patients are more likely than others to have a prolonged pain and disability course, including patients with comorbid depression or anxiety, somatization disorder, substance abuse, job dissatisfaction, pursuit of disability compensation, and involvement in litigation.[19,20] When evaluating a patient with back pain, it is important to assess for the above psychosocial factors and emotional distress level as these factors are stronger predictors of outcomes than pain characteristics and physical examination findings.[21] Some authors now advocate using a prognostic tool to help determine which patients would benefit from earlier, structured treatments to decrease the development of prolonged pain and disability (see Treatment of Acute Back Pain section).[22]

Physical Examination

A general physical examination should be performed in all patients presenting with back pain, including careful examination of the abdomen given the possibility of visceral organ pain radiating to the spine, and special attention to potential malignant sources (breast, prostate, lymph nodes) or infectious sources (flank or suprapubic pain, skin or soft tissue infection, track marks, heart murmur) if the patient history raises concern for systemic disease.

The examination of the back should include inspection of the spine and patient posture, range of motion, and palpation of the spine and paraspinous structures. Spinal inspection may reveal scoliosis, kyphosis, or lordosis. Lumbar spine mobility is often reduced in patients presenting with low back pain. It is not useful as a tool to differentiate causes of low back pain because it varies widely between individuals, but may be useful to establish a baseline for the individual from which to compare response to therapies. Spinal pain that is reproduced by palpation or percussion may indicate spinal infection, but this is a sensitive, not specific, test, and interexaminer reproducibility is poor.[23]

For patients with lower extremity symptoms, a straight leg raising test and full neurologic assessment, as well as palpation of the pedal pulses to help distinguish neurologic from vascular claudication, should be performed.

Table 6
Red flags for serious or systemic cause of low back pain

Patient Factors	Pain Characteristics	Associated Signs/Symptoms
History of trauma	Nighttime pain	Unexplained weight loss
History of cancer	Duration greater than 4–6 wk	Unexplained fevers
Age >50 y	Unresponsive to conservative therapies	Comorbid infection such as urinary tract infection
History of osteoporosis or prolonged corticosteroid use		Focal neurologic deficits with progressive or disabling symptoms
Injection drug use Immunosuppression Diabetes		Cauda equina syndrome

The straight leg raising test helps to confirm radiculopathy. It is performed with the patient in a supine position. The examiner slowly raises the affected leg off the table with the foot dorsiflexed. The test is positive when radicular pain is reproduced between 30° and 70° of hip flexion (**Fig. 8**). The crossed straight leg raising test is performed by elevating the unaffected leg and is deemed positive when lifting the unaffected leg reproduces symptoms in the affected leg. The straight leg test is sensitive (73%–98% sensitivity), but not specific (11%–61% specificity), for herniated discs. The crossed straight leg test is less sensitive for herniated discs, but 90% specific.[24,25]

Other neuromechanical tests that may be performed in patients with pain radiating into the lower extremities are summarized in **Table 7**.

Neurologic testing for patients with lower extremity symptoms should focus on the L5 and S1 nerve roots, because more than 95% of disc herniations occur at these levels. Testing should include evaluation of muscle strength, sensation, and reflexes at each level (**Fig. 9** summarizes the signs and symptoms associated with compression of each lumbar nerve root).

The L5 nerve root motor function can be tested by evaluating the strength of foot and great toe dorsiflexion. The L5 nerve root sensory function can be tested by evaluating sensation of the medial foot and the space between the first and second toe. There is no reflex associated with the L5 nerve root.

The S1 nerve root function is tested by evaluating sensation at the posterior calf and lateral foot and by eliciting the Achilles reflex. Of note, loss of Achilles (ankle) reflexes often occurs with advancing age even in the absence of nerve root compression. In one study, bilateral ankle reflexes were found to be absent in 30% of individuals between the ages of 61 and 70, and in more than 50% of those aged 81 to 90.[26] Therefore, absent ankle reflex is more likely to be clinically meaningful if it is unilateral and affects the symptomatic leg. The S1 nerve root motor function is tested by evaluating strength of foot plantar flexion; however, weakness of plantar flexion is a late finding.

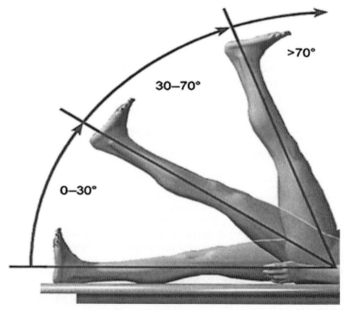

Fig. 8. Straight leg raising test. (*From* Levin KH, Covington EC, Devereaux MW, et al. Neck and back pain. Continuum: Lifelong Learning Neurol 2001;7:20; with permission.)

Table 7
Neuromechanical tests useful in evaluating the patient with back pain radiating into the lower extremities

Test	Description
Straight leg raising test	With the patient in the supine position, the examiner raises the symptomatic extremity slowly off the examining table. The test is positive when the radicular symptoms are reproduced when the extremity is elevated between 30° and 70°.
Lasegue test	With the patient in the supine position, the symptomatic lower extremity is flexed to 90° at the hip and knee. The knee is then extended slowly, which produces radiating pain as a result of L5 and S1 nerve root compression.
Bragard sign	A follow-up to a positive straight leg test. If pain is generated by straight leg raising, the symptomatic extremity is lowered until the pain recedes. At that point the foot is dorsiflexed. If this maneuver reproduces radicular pain, the test is positive.
Contralateral (crossed) straight leg raising test	With the patient in supine position, the examiner raises the unaffected extremity. The test is positive if this maneuver causes pain in the affected extremity.
Prone straight leg raising test	With the patient in prone position, the symptomatic extremity is slowly extended at the hip by the examiner. If this exacerbates pain in the anterior thigh, a high lumbar radiculopathy (L2-3) is suggested.
Valsalva test	The Valsalva maneuver increases intrathecal pressure, which accentuates radicular pain in the presence of spinal nerve compression and inflammation.
Brudzinski test	With the patient supine, the examiner flexes the patient's head. In the presence of spinal compression, this flexion exacerbates radicular pain.
Patrick (Faber) test	The lateral malleolus of the symptomatic extremity is placed on the patella of the opposite extremity, and the symptomatic extremity is slowly rotated externally. Accentuation of pain suggests that pain is caused by a hip or sacroiliac joint lesion rather than by radiculopathy.
Gaenslen test	With the patient supine and the symptomatic extremity and buttocks extending slightly over the edge of the examination table, the asymptomatic lower extremity is flexed at the hip and knee and brought to the chest. The symptomatic lower extremity is extended at the hip to the floor. Increased nonradiating low back and buttocks pain indicates sacroiliac joint disease.
Waddell test	Excessive sensitivity to light pinching of the skin in the region of low back pain suggests a functional component.

Adapted from Devereaux M. Low back pain. Med Clin North Am 2009;93(2):488–489; with permission.

Imaging and Additional Testing

A judicious approach to imaging in patients with low back pain is recommended for many reasons. First, most patients with nonspecific mechanical low back pain or radiculopathy will recover spontaneously within 4 to 6 weeks. Second, abnormalities on imaging have been shown to correlate poorly with clinical symptoms. In fact, imaging abnormalities have been found in about 20% of people in the absence of low back

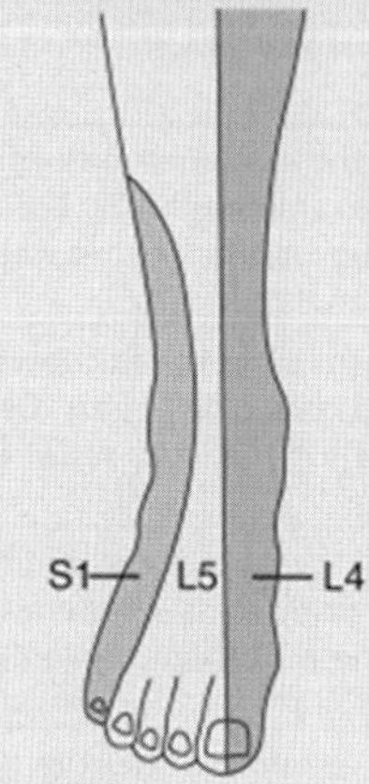

Lower extremity dermatome	Disc	Nerve root	Motor loss	Sensory loss	Reflex loss
	L3-4	L4	Dorsiflexion of foot	Medial foot	Knee
	L4-5	L5	Dorsiflexion of great toe	Dorsal foot	None
S1 L5 L4	L5-S1	S1	Plantarflexion of foot	Lateral foot	Ankle

Fig. 9. Neurologic features of lumbosacral radiculopathy. (*From* Firestein GS, Budd RC, Gabriel SE, et al. Kelley's textbook of rheumatology. Philadelphia: Saunders; 2013. p. 668; with permission.)

pain.[13] Given these findings, abnormalities detected on imaging may or may not be clinically relevant to the patient's current symptoms. Furthermore, they typically do not alter treatment strategy, may cause patient distress, and may lead to further unnecessary tests and procedures. In addition, obtaining unnecessary radiographs and computed tomography (CT) scans exposes patients to potentially harmful radiation and contributes to the economical burden of low back pain.

As a result, joint guidelines from the American College of Physicians (ACP) and the American Pain Society explicitly state: "Clinicians should not routinely obtain imaging or other diagnostic tests in patients with nonspecific low back pain."[27] The guidelines advise that diagnostic imaging is only indicated for patients with signs or symptoms of severe neurologic deficit or serious underlying disease (summarized in **Table 8**). Other patients may be imaged if they do not have improvement in their back pain after 4 to 6 weeks or if they develop any red flags.[27,28]

Table 8
Indications for diagnostic imaging in patients with low back pain and recommended initial imaging modality

Characteristic	Initial Imaging Modality
Progressive neurologic findings	Magnetic resonance imaging
Constitutional symptoms (fever, chills, weight loss)	Plain radiographs
History of traumatic onset	Plain radiographs
History of malignancy with new onset pain	Magnetic resonance imaging
Age >50 y	Plain radiographs
Infectious risk, such as injection drug use, immunosuppression, indwelling urinary catheter, prolonged steroid use, skin or urinary tract infection	Magnetic resonance imaging
Osteoporosis	Plain radiographs
Radiculopathy or pseudoclaudication persisting for more than 4–6 wk	Magnetic resonance imaging

If there is a concern for serious underlying pathologic condition or pain has not improved after 4 to 6 weeks, plain anteroposterior and lateral radiographs of the lumbosacral spine may be useful in evaluating for tumor, infection, spinal instability, spondylosis, and spondylolisthesis.

CT and magnetic resonance imaging (MRI) are more sensitive than plain radiographs in the early detection of malignancy and infection. Both modalities can also show herniated discs and stenosis; however, MRI is more sensitive for infections, metastatic cancer, and rare neural tumors and is preferred when available because of better visualization of soft tissues and avoidance of radiation. CT or MRI should be obtained when a patient has progressive neurologic deficits, findings highly concerning for malignancy or infection, or unexplained pain persisting for 12 weeks or longer. For patients with a typical radiculopathy syndrome persisting beyond 6 weeks, MRI should only be obtained if the patient is a candidate for a procedure such as corticosteroid injection or surgery.

For patients in whom an underlying serious or systemic cause for low back pain is suspected, it is also advisable to obtain specific blood and urine tests to aid in the diagnosis, which may include a complete blood count, erythrocyte sedimentation rate, antinuclear antibody with reflexive testing, prostate-specific antigen, a metabolic panel, blood cultures, urinalysis, and/or urine cultures.

For patients in whom there is a need to distinguish spinal stenosis or radiculopathy from a peripheral neuropathy syndrome, it may be helpful to obtain electromyography and nerve conduction testing. Ankle-brachial indices and arterial duplex studies may help differentiate vascular from neurogenic claudication.

Fig. 10 shows a diagnostic algorithm regarding the evidence-based evaluation and initial treatment of low back pain.

TREATMENT FOR ACUTE LOW BACK PAIN

It is important for providers to reassure their patients with acute nonspecific low back pain with or without radiculopathy that most people have significant improvement of their symptoms within 4 to 6 weeks without any specific treatment.[29] In fact, up to 90% of patients seen within 3 days of onset will recover after 2 weeks.[30] For patients with radiculopathy, prognosis is also generally favorable, although speed of recovery is usually slower: about one-third of patients are improved at 2 weeks, and about 75% by 3 months.[31] Patients with spinal stenosis are more likely to have chronic symptoms: in one small study of 32 patients with spinal stenosis followed for a mean of 49 months without surgical intervention, 15% had symptom improvement, 15% symptom worsening, and 70% unchanged symptoms.[32]

Although most patients have favorable outcomes without intervention, some are at higher risk for prolonged disability, including those with comorbid depression or anxiety, poor coping skills, job dissatisfaction, and higher initial disability levels. Recent studies have shown evidence for improvement in patient outcomes and resource utilization when initial treatment recommendations are stratified according to patient prognosis based on the above risk factors.[22] Therefore, it may be advisable for clinicians to use a prognostic tool to help identify patients who would benefit from earlier targeted interventions in addition to self-care advice. One validated prognostic tool is the Keele STarT Back Screening Tool,[33] shown in **Figs. 11** and **12**.

Hill and colleagues[22] found that patients randomized to targeted interventions based on the Keele prognostic score (low-risk patients received self-care advice, medium-risk patients were referred to physical therapy, and high-risk patients were referred to cognitive behavioral therapy-enhanced physical therapy) had statistically significant

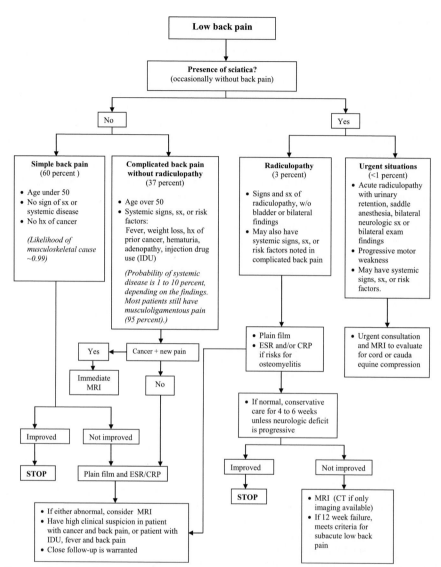

Fig. 10. Algorithm for the evaluation of low back pain. CRP, C-reactive protein; ESR, Erythrocyte sedimentation rate. (*Adapted from* Wipf JE, Deyo RA. Low back pain. Common medical problems in ambulatory care. Med Clin North Am 1995;79:239; with permission.)

improvements on a 1-year disability assessment compared with patients in the usual care group. In addition, care for the targeted intervention group was more cost-effective.

Activity Recommendations and Self-Care

All patients with acute nonspecific low back pain, including those with lower extremity symptoms, should be given general self-care advice including return to usual activity and the avoidance of prolonged bed rest. Studies indicate that bed rest does not increase the speed of recovery and in fact may delay it.[34] Self-care advice may also include heat application and self-education with evidence-based materials.

Keele STarT Back Screening Tool	No	Yes
Has your back pain spread down your leg(s) at some time in the last 2 weeks	○	○
Have you had pain in the shoulder or neck at some time in the last 2 weeks	○	○
Have you only walked short distances because of your back pain	○	○
In the last 2 weeks, have you dressed more slowly than usual because of back pain	○	○
Do you think it's not really safe for a person with a condition like yours to be physically active	○	○
Have worrying thoughts been going through your mind a lot of the time	○	○
Do you feel that your back pain is terrible and it's never going to get any better	○	○
In general have you stopped enjoying all the things you usually enjoy?	○	○

Overall, how bothersome has your back pain been in the last 2 weeks?

Not at all	Slightly	Moderately	Very much	Extremely
○	○	○	○	○

Fig. 11. Keele STarT back screening tool. Keele STarT back tool. (*Courtesy of* Keel University, Keele, Staffordshire, UK; with permission. The copyright (©2007) of the STarT Back Tool and associated materials is owned by Keele University, the development of which was part funded by Arthritis Research UK: i) the tool is designed for use by health care practitioners, with appropriate treatment packages for each of the stratified groups;ii) the tool is not intended to recommend the use of any particular product. No license is required for non-commercial use. If you would like to incorporate the tool in any way into commercial product materials, please contact Keele University for further advice.)

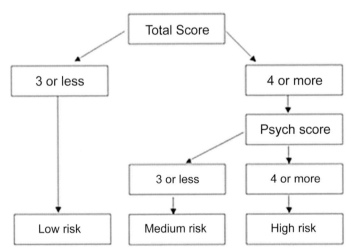

Fig. 12. Scoring the Keele STarT back screening tool. "Psych score" refers to score on questions 5 to 9. (*Courtesy of* Keel University, Keele, Staffordshire, UK; with permission. The copyright (2007) of the STarT Back Tool and associated materials is owned by Keele University, the development of which was part funded by Arthritis Research UK: i) the tool is designed for use by health care practitioners, with appropriate treatment packages for each of the stratified groups; ii) the tool is not intended to recommend the use of any particular product. No license is required for non-commercial use. If you would like to incorporate the tool in any way into commercial product materials, please contact Keele University for further advice.)

Analgesics

In addition to self-care advice, clinicians may recommend or prescribe analgesic medications to help alleviate pain in the short term. Several classes of medications have been shown to provide some pain relief when used for short time intervals for low back pain, including nonsteroidal anti-inflammatory drugs (NSAIDs), acetaminophen, skeletal muscle relaxants, tramadol, and opioids. When choosing a medication, clinicians should be mindful of effectiveness, tolerability, and side-effect profiles. The 2007 joint guidelines from the ACP and American Pain Society recommend either NSAIDs or acetaminophen as first-line analgesic agents for the treatment of low back pain.[27] **Table 9** lists the medication comparisons.

Of note, there is no good evidence supporting the use of systemic glucocorticoids,[37,38] lidocaine patches, anticonvulsants, or antidepressants in the treatment of acute low back pain, and therefore, their use is not recommended.

Nonpharmacologic Noninvasive Treatments

There is no high-quality evidence that nonpharmacologic therapies are superior to self-care advice in the treatment of acute low back pain, including spinal manipulation[39] and exercise therapy,[40] as well as massage, acupuncture, and yoga. However, these modalities may be of benefit in patients found to be at higher risk for prolonged pain and disability as discussed above.

For patients with acute low back pain who do not improve with self-care and short-term analgesics after 4 to 6 weeks, clinicians should first re-evaluate for an underlying serious condition (cancer or fracture) or systemic disease as per the algorithm in **Fig. 10**. If no serious cause is found, providers may begin to implement the treatments outlined in later discussion for subacute and chronic low back pain.

TREATMENT OF CHRONIC LOW BACK PAIN

If low back pain persists for more than 12 weeks and serious conditions have been ruled out, the focus of care should shift from pain-resolution to pain-management strategies that control pain while maximizing function and quality of life and preventing disability.

Treatment of chronic low back pain is often multidisciplinary, involving a combination of self-care, analgesics, spinal manipulation, physical therapy with or without cognitive behavioral therapy, massage, acupuncture, yoga, and in some cases, invasive interventions such as glucocorticoid injections and surgical procedures.

Analgesics

Regarding analgesics, most of the evidence for their benefit comes from short-term trials; therefore, the efficacy and safety for long-term use is unproven. Short-term courses of acetaminophen or NSAIDs are typically recommended for acute exacerbations of chronic low back pain if the side-effect profiles are acceptable for the patient. The long-term use of NSAIDs is limited by their potential gastric, renal, and cardiac toxicity.

Opioids have been increasingly used for chronic low back pain; however, evidence to support their use is minimal. A 2013 *Cochrane Review* found low- to moderate-quality evidence for short-term efficacy for pain and function when opioids were compared with placebo, but none of the trials persisted beyond 12 weeks.[41,42] In addition, the meta-analysis found that there is no high-quality evidence that long-term use of opiates is superior to other medications (NSAIDs, antidepressants) for pain relief and function. Furthermore, patients who use chronic opiates, especially in high doses,

Table 9
Pharmacotherapy for treatment of acute low back pain

Drug Class	Drug Names/Dose Regimens	Benefits/Evidence	Adverse Effects/Contraindications
NSAIDs	• Ibuprofen 400–600 mg po q6-8 h • Naproxen 250–500 mg po q12 h • Meloxicam 7.5–15 mg po daily • Diclofenac 50–75 mg po q12 h • Etodoloc 200–400 mg po q6-8 h • Ketorolac 30–60 mg im × 1	• 2008 *Cochrane Review* showed greater symptom improvement compared with placebo after 1 week: RR 1.19 (95% CI 1.07–1.35)[35] • Recommended as first-line therapy, along with acetaminophen, for acute LBP in the 2007 ACP/APS guidelines[27]	• Nephrotoxicity (avoid in patients with kidney disease or at high risk for renal injury) • Gastrointestinal toxicity (avoid in patients with a history of gastritis, upper GI bleed, or peptic ulcer disease; consider coadministration of a proton pump inhibitor in higher risk patients) • Increased risk of cardiovascular events (avoid in patients with known CAD and those at very high risk) • Higher risk in elderly patients • Use lowest dose for shortest duration
Acetaminophen	Acetaminophen 325–650 mg po q4-6 h (Not to exceed 4 g per 24 h or 2 g per 24 h in patients with underlying liver disease or heavy alcohol use)	• Similar to slightly less efficacy compared with NSAIDs • Less side effects than NSAIDs • Recommended as first-line therapy, along with NSAIDs, for acute LBP in the 2007 ACP/APS guidelines[27]	• Hepatotoxicity: risk varies by dose and patient; higher risk with concurrent alcohol use, underlying liver disease, or higher dose • May cause asymptomatic transaminase elevations at therapeutic doses
Centrally acting skeletal muscle relaxants	• Benzodiazepines • Cyclobenzaprine 5–10 mg po tid • Methocarbamol 1000 mg po qid • Carisoprodol 350 mg po tid and qhs • Baclofen 5–10 mg po tid • Tizanadine 4–8 mg po q6-8 h	• 2003 systematic review found that non-benzodiazepine muscle relaxants were more effective than placebo for short-term relief of LBP: RR 0.8, 95% CI 0.71–0.89[36]	• Sedation • Dizziness • Dependence/abuse potential (benzodiazepines and carisoprodol) • Hepatotoxicity and multiple drug interactions (tizanidine) • Use of muscle relaxants should generally be limited to 1-3 wk
Opioid agonists	• Tramadol (nonopiate that acts at opiate receptor) • Opioids (codeine, hydrocodone, oxycodone, hydromorphone, morphine, methadone, fentanyl)	• Data are limited for efficacy and safety in treatment of acute low back pain (most studies focus on chronic low back pain) • Avoid first line; if used, limit duration and consider scheduled rather than as needed administration	• Sedation • Confusion • Nausea • Constipation • Respiratory depression (at higher doses) • Dependence and abuse potential (higher risk with longer term use)

have a significant risk of adverse effects, including dependence, misuse, and overdose.[43] Therefore, the long-term use of opioids for chronic low back pain should be restricted to patients who demonstrate a functional improvement with opioid use, are at low risk for misuse, and can be monitored closely for adverse effects.

Antiepileptics and tricyclic antidepressants (TCAs) are frequently used to treat patients with radicular low back pain or spinal stenosis. However, a 2008 systematic review concluded there is not compelling evidence that antidepressants are superior to placebo in the treatment of nonspecific low back pain.[44] Similarly, a 2013 systematic

Table 10
Evidence-based nonsurgical treatments for chronic low back pain

Treatment	Benefit	Recommendation with Evidence Grade	Comments
NSAIDs	Moderate	Suggested as first-line therapy (2B)	Use limited by gastric and renal toxicity
Acetaminophen	Small	Suggested as first-line therapy (2B)	May cause asymptomatic liver enzyme elevation
Opioids	Small	Suggest not using as first-line therapy (2B)	Use limited by risk of side effects, dependency, misuse
Antidepressants	None to small	May be used to treat comorbid depression but not as sole back pain analgesic (2B)	—
Nonpharmacologic noninvasive therapies • Acupuncture[1] • Physical therapy • Massage therapy • Cognitive behavioral therapy • Spinal manipulation • Yoga[2] (viniyoga)	Moderate	Suggested (2B)	[1]Efficacy of sham acupuncture vs acupuncture inconsistent [2]Evidence insufficient to judge nonviniyoga
Nonsurgical invasive therapies • Epidural steroid injection	Moderate (short term only)	Suggested (2B)	Evidence for use in patients with disc herniations causing radiculopathy

Evidence Grade Explanation:

1A: Strong recommendation, high-quality evidence. Strong recommendation, can apply to most patients in most circumstances without reservation.

1B: Strong recommendation, moderate-quality evidence. Strong recommendation, likely to apply to most patients.

1C: Strong recommendation, low-quality evidence. Relatively strong recommendation; might change when higher-quality evidence becomes available.

2A: Weak recommendation, high-quality evidence. Weak recommendation, best action may differ depending on circumstances or patients or societal values.

2B: Weak recommendation, moderate-quality evidence. Weak recommendation, alternative approaches likely to be better for some patients under some circumstances.

2C: Weak recommendation, low-quality evidence. Very weak recommendation; other alternatives may be equally reasonable.

Data from Chou R, Qaseem A, Snow V, et al. Diagnosis and treatment of low back pain: a joint clinical practice guideline from the American College of Physicians and the American Pain Society. Ann Intern Med 2007;147:478.

review concluded there is only low-quality evidence for the use of antiepileptics given scarcity and poor methodology of existing trials.[45] Furthermore, the use of these medications is often limited by side effects, including somnolence, dizziness (antiepileptics and TCAs), and anticholinergic effects (TCAs).

Nonpharmacologic Noninvasive Treatments

Nonpharmacologic noninvasive evidence-based treatments for chronic low back pain include physical therapy, spinal manipulation, acupuncture, massage, yoga, and cognitive behavioral therapy. These treatments have B-grade evidence, meaning there is fair-quality evidence of moderate benefit, or small benefit but no significant harms, costs, or burdens.[27,46] All patients with chronic low back pain should be advised to remain active. Beyond that, use of the other nonpharmacologic treatments can be pursued based on provider and patient preferences and treatment availability.

Invasive Nonsurgical Treatments

Invasive nonsurgical treatments for chronic low back pain include epidural steroid injections, intradisc steroid injections, facet joint injections, medial branch blocks, and radiofrequency denervation. Of these, there is moderate-quality evidence only for epidural steroid injections in patients with sciatica or radiculopathy, and the benefit is short term (less than 6 weeks).[47] **Table 10** summarizes the evidence-based nonsurgical treatments for chronic low back pain.

Surgical Referrals

Urgent surgical evaluation is recommended for patients with severe or progressive motor weakness or evidence of cauda equina syndrome. In the absence of severe progressive neurologic deficits, surgery may be considered an elective treatment of patients with radiculopathy and spinal stenosis who have chronic disabling symptoms and have not responded to appropriate trials of nonsurgical treatments.[48] In general, surgical outcomes may be superior to nonsurgical management in the short term, but the difference does not persist after longer-term follow-up.

SUMMARY

Low back pain is a common, frequently recurring condition that often has a nonspecific cause. Most nonspecific acute low back pain will improve within several weeks with or without treatment. The diagnostic workup should focus on evaluation for evidence of systemic or pathologic causes. Psychosocial distress, poor coping skills, and high initial disability increase the risk for a prolonged disability course. All patients with acute or chronic low back pain should be advised to remain active. The treatment of chronic nonspecific low back pain involves a multidisciplinary approach targeted at preserving function and preventing disability. Surgical referral is indicated in the presence of severe or progressive neurologic deficits or signs and symptoms of cauda equina syndrome.

REFERENCES

1. Hart LG, Deyo RA, Cherkin DC. Physician office visits for low back pain. Frequency, clinical evaluation, and treatment patterns from a U.S. national survey. Spine (Phila Pa 1976) 1995;20:11.
2. Katz JN. Lumbar disc disorders and low-back pain: socioeconomic factors and consequences. J Bone Joint Surg Am 2006;88(Suppl 2):21.

3. Henschke N, Maher CG, Refshauge KM, et al. Prognosis in patients with recent onset low back pain in Australian primary care: inception cohort study. BMJ 2008; 337:a171.
4. Chou R, Shekelle P. Will this patient develop persistent disabling low back pain? JAMA 2010;303:1295.
5. Deyo RA, Tsui-Wu YJ. Descriptive epidemiology of low-back pain and its related medical care in the United States. Spine (Phila Pa 1976) 1987;12:264.
6. Cassidy JD, Carroll LJ, Côté P. The Saskatchewan health and back pain survey. The prevalence of low back pain and related disability in Saskatchewan adults. Spine (Phila Pa 1976) 1998;23:1860.
7. Deyo RA, Mirza SK, Martin BI. Back pain prevalence and visit rates: estimates from U.S. national surveys, 2002. Spine (Phila Pa 1976) 2006;31:2724.
8. Hoy D, Brookes P, Blyth F, et al. The epidemiology of low back pain. Best Pract Res Clin Rheumatol 2010;24(6):769–81.
9. Lidgren L. The bone and joint decade 2000-2010. Bull World Health Organ 2003; 81(9):629.
10. Levin KH, Covington EC, Devereaux MW, et al. Neck and low back pain. Continuum (NY) 2001;7:1–205.
11. Mense S, Simons D. Muscle pain: understanding its nature, diagnoses and treatment. Baltimore (MD): Lippincott Williams and Wilkins; 2001. p. 117–8.
12. Boden SD, Davis DO, Dina TS, et al. Abnormal magnetic resonance scans of the lumbar spine in asymptomatic subjects: a prospective investigation. J Bone Joint Surg Am 1990;72:403–8.
13. Jensen M, Brant-Zawadzki M, Obuchowski N, et al. Magnetic resonance imaging of the lumbar spine in people without back pain. N Engl J Med 1994;331: 69–73.
14. Meleger AL, Krivickas LS. Neck and back pain: musculoskeletal disorders. Neurol Clin 2007;25:419–38.
15. Korkala O, Grönblad M, Liesi P, et al. Immunohistochemical demonstration of nociceptors in the ligamentous structures of the lumbar spine. Spine 1985;10: 156–7.
16. Coppes M, Marani E, Thomeer R, et al. Innervation of "painful" lumbar discs. Spine 1997;22:2342–9.
17. Deyo RA, Weinstein JN. Low back pain. N Engl J Med 2001;344:363–70.
18. Fredrickson BE, Baker D, McHolick WJ, et al. The natural history of spondylolysis and spondylolisthesis. J Bone Joint Surg Am 1984;66:699–707.
19. Anderson GBJ. Epidemiologic features of chronic low back pain. Lancet 1999; 354:581–5.
20. Atlas SJ, Chang Y, Kammann E, et al. Long term disability and return to work among patients who have a herniated lumbar disc: the effects of disability compensation. J Bone Joint Surg Am 2000;82:4–15.
21. Pincus T, Burton AK, Vogel S, et al. A systematic review of psychological factors as predictors of chronicity/disability in prospective cohorts of low back pain. Spine 2002;27:E109–20.
22. Hill JC, Whitehurst DG, Lewis M, et al. Comparison of stratified primary care management for low back pain with current best practice (STarT Back): a randomized controlled trial. Lancet 2011;378:1560.
23. Chandrasekar PH. Low back pain and intravenous drug abusers. Arch Intern Med 1990;150:1125–8.
24. McGee S. Evidence-based physical diagnosis. Philadelphia: WB Saunders Company; 2001. Copyright 2001 Elsevier Science, Inc.

25. Van der Windt DA, Simons E, Riphagen II, et al. Physical examination for lumbar radiculopathy due to disc herniation in patients with low back pain. Cochrane Database Syst Rev 2010;(2):CD007431.

26. Bowditch MG, Sanderson P, Livesey JP. The significance of an absent ankle reflex. J Bone Joint Surg Br 1996;78:276.

27. Chou R, Qaseem A, Snow V, et al. Diagnosis and treatment of low back pain: a joint clinical practice guideline from the American College of Physicians and the American Pain Society. Ann Intern Med 2007;147:478.

28. Chou R, Qaseem A, Owens DK, et al. Diagnostic imaging for low back pain: advice for high value health care from the American College of Physicians. Ann Intern Med 2011;154:181.

29. Pengel LH, Herber RD, Maher CG, et al. Acute low back pain: systematic review of its prognosis. BMJ 2003;327:323.

30. Coste J, Delecoeuillerie G, Cohen de Lara A, et al. Clinical course and prognostic factors in acute low back pain: an inception cohort study in primary care practice. BMJ 1994;308:577.

31. Vroomen PC, de Krom MC, Knottnerus JA. Predicting the outcome of sciatica at short term follow-up. Br J Gen Pract 2002;52:119.

32. Johnsson KE, Rosén I, Udén A. The natural course of lumbar spinal stenosis. Clin Orthop Relat Res 1992;279:82.

33. Hill JC, Dunn KM, Lewis M, et al. A primary care back pain screening tool: identifying patient subgroups for initial treatment. Arthritis Rheum 2008;59(5):632–41.

34. Waddell G, Feder G, Lewis M. Systematic reviews of bed rest and advice to stay active for acute low back pain. Br J Gen Pract 1997;47:647–52.

35. Roelofs PD, Deyo RA, Koes BW, et al. Nonsteroidal anti-inflammatory drugs for low back pain. Cochrane Database Syst Rev 2008;(1):CD000396.

36. Van Tulder MW, Touray T, Furlan AD, et al. Muscle relaxants for non-specific low back pain. Cochrane Database Syst Rev 2003;(2):CD0044252.

37. Finckh A, Zufferey P, Schurch MA, et al. Short-term efficacy of intravenous pulse glucocorticoids in acute discogenic sciatica, a randomized controlled trial. Spine 2006;31:377–81.

38. Friedman BW, Holden L, Esses D, et al. Parenteral corticosteroids for Emergency Department patients with nonradicular low back pain. J Emerg Med 2006;31: 365–70.

39. Rubinstein SM, Terwee CB, Assendelft WJ, et al. Spinal manipulative therapy for acute low back pain. Cochrane Database Syst Rev 2012;(9):CD008880.

40. Hayden J, van Tulder MW, Malmivaara A, et al. Exercise therapy for treatment of nonspecific low back pain. Cochrane Database Syst Rev 2005;(3):CD000335.

41. Chaparro LE, Furlan AD, Deshpande A. Opioids compared to placebo or other treatments for chronic low back pain. Cochrane Database Syst Rev 2013;(8):CD004959.

42. Deshpande A, Furlan A, Mailis-Gagnon A, et al. Opioids for chronic low-back pain. Cochrane Database Syst Rev 2007;(3):CD004959.

43. Martell BA, O'Connor PG, Kerns RD, et al. Systematic review: opioid treatment for chronic back pain: prevalence, efficacy, and association with addiction. Ann Intern Med 2007;146:116.

44. Urquhart DM, Hoving JL, Assendelft WJ, et al. Antidepressants for non-specific low back pain. Cochrane Database Syst Rev 2008;(1):CD001703.

45. Ammendolia C, Stuber KJ, Rok E, et al. Nonoperative treatment for lumbar spinal stenosis with neurogenic claudication. Cochrane Database Syst Rev 2013;(8):CD010712.

46. Standaert CJ. Comparative effectiveness of exercise, acupuncture, and spinal manipulation for low back pain. Spine 2011;36:120–30.
47. Chou R, Atlas SJ, Stanos SP, et al. Nonsurgical interventional therapies for low back pain: a review of the evidence for an American Pain Society clinical practice guideline. Spine (Phila Pa 1976) 2009;34:1078.
48. Chou R, Baisden J, Carragee EJ, et al. Surgery for low back pain: a review of the evidence for an American Pain Society Clinical Practice Guideline. Spine (Phila Pa 1976) 2009;34:1094.

Leg Discomfort: Beyond the Joints

Douglas Berger, MD, MLitt

KEYWORDS

- Leg pain • Paresthesia • Claudication • Neuropathy • Myalgia • Cramp

KEY POINTS

- Although simple characterization of discomfort as cramps, heaviness, shooting pains, and so forth can be misleading, history and examination are key to accurate diagnosis.
- Absence of both dorsalis pedis and posterior tibial pulses strongly suggests peripheral arterial disease (PAD), and the presence of either pulse makes PAD less likely.
- Hydroxymethylglutaryl coenzyme A reductase inhibitors (statins) are a common cause of lower extremity myalgias.
- Restless legs syndrome causes nocturnal discomfort but must be distinguished from confounding "mimics."
- Neurologic causes of leg symptoms include lumbar spinal stenosis, radiculopathy, distal symmetric polyneuropathy, and entrapment neuropathy.
- Many common causes of leg discomfort can be managed conservatively.

INTRODUCTION

Discussions of leg pain usually begin with the hip, knee, and ankle. For each joint there are well-established differential diagnoses and physical examination maneuvers. Nonetheless, patients often present with discomfort that after brief history taking and examination seems unrelated to the joints and periarticular structures. Such symptoms are challenging for primary care providers because the range of possible causes is large, ill defined, and runs from benign cramps to life-threatening deep vein thrombosis (DVT). Moreover, leg symptoms can be difficult for patients to describe, and terms such as cramps or heaviness can lead clinicians to an overly narrow set of diagnostic considerations.

Leg discomfort is common, occurring in two-thirds of elderly Iowans[1] and outpatient veterans.[2] However, symptoms do not correlate well with disease. Carefully designed studies assessing the prevalence of lower extremity arterial[3] and venous[4] disease found background rates of exertional symptoms and "tired/heavy legs" as high as 40% to 60% with relatively small differences between those with and without evidence of vascular disease. Use of a survey designed to distinguish between cramps, restless

General Medicine Service, Department of Medicine, VA Puget Sound, University of Washington, 1660 South Columbian Way, Seattle, WA 98108, USA
E-mail address: douglas.berger@va.gov

Med Clin N Am 98 (2014) 429–444
http://dx.doi.org/10.1016/j.mcna.2014.01.004
0025-7125/14/$ – see front matter Published by Elsevier Inc.

legs syndrome (RLS), and peripheral neuropathy resulted in 20% of patients classified as having all 3 diagnoses.[2] Thus, simple symptom checklists are unlikely to yield an accurate diagnosis of leg symptoms.

Causes of leg discomfort are too numerous to list. Rather, this article presents common causes of leg pain, paresthesias, cramping, heaviness, and numbness arising outside the joints. The discussion is organized into vascular, neurologic, and musculoskeletal sources of pain; it is often helpful to consider each of these 3 categories when evaluating patients with leg discomfort.

VASCULAR CAUSES OF LEG DISCOMFORT
Lower Extremity Peripheral Arterial Disease

Atherosclerosis of arteries supplying the legs occurs in 3% to 10% of adults and up to 15% to 20% of those older than 70 years.[5] Risk factors are similar to those for coronary artery disease.

The classic symptom of peripheral arterial disease (PAD) is intermittent claudication: muscle fatigue, aching, cramping, numbness, or heaviness that comes with exertion and is relieved by rest within 10 minutes.[5] Severe PAD can cause critical limb ischemia: ulceration, gangrene, or constant pain when at rest that is worse with elevation and improved with dependency. Although claudication most commonly affects the calves, other areas may be affected depending on the location of stenosis:

- Aortoiliac occlusion: buttock and hip claudication, erectile dysfunction in men
- Iliofemoral occlusion: thigh claudication
- Femoral or popliteal occlusion: calf claudication
- Tibial or peroneal occlusion: foot claudication[6]

Only 20% of patients with PAD endorse classic claudication symptoms. Some are asymptomatic; many have atypical exertional symptoms.[3,7] Although a history of claudication increases the likelihood of PAD (likelihood ratio [LR] 3.3), the absence of classic claudication does not rule out even moderate to severe PAD (LR 0.57).[8] Physical examination is more helpful. Absence of both dorsalis pedis and posterior tibial pulses strongly suggests PAD (LR 14.9), and the presence of either pulse makes PAD less likely (LR 0.3).[9] A significant subset of healthy adults will lack one pulse, but usually the other vessel compensates, leaving only 1% to 2% of healthy adults lacking both pulses.[9] The presence of an iliac, femoral, or popliteal bruit is also suggestive of PAD (LR 5.9 for symptomatic patients), and absence of all 3 bruits reduces the likelihood of PAD (LR 0.38).[8,9] Wounds, skin discoloration, and temperature asymmetry increase the probability of PAD in symptomatic patients, but absence of these features is not helpful.[8,9] Bruits and pulses may also help clinicians locate the level of stenosis.[9]

Guidelines recommend that all patients with exertional leg symptoms be evaluated with an ankle-brachial index (ABI).[5,10] This noninvasive test (**Table 1**) has become standard for diagnosis and correlates exceptionally well with angiography (95% sensitivity and nearly 100% specificity).[5,10,11] Symptomatic patients with a normal or noncompressible ABI should be further investigated, usually with ABI after exertion or a toe-brachial index, respectively. Other tests may be used to diagnose PAD and identify the level of occlusion, but arterial imaging is usually reserved for preprocedural planning or investigating nonatherosclerotic causes of PAD.[10]

Symptomatic PAD without critical limb ischemia has a favorable prognosis in the leg: only 10% to 20% have progressive symptoms and only 1% to 2% develop critical limb ischemia over 5 years.[10] However, cardiovascular morbidity is high, with a 4% to

Table 1 Ankle-brachial index (ABI)	

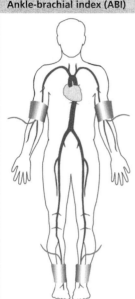	**Preparation:** Patient lies supine for 10 min in a warm room
	Measurement: Systolic pressures are measured at the brachial, dorsalis pedis (DP), and posterior tibial (PT) arteries bilaterally, usually using a handheld Doppler probe and appropriately sized sphygmomanometer cuffs
	Calculation:
	 Right ABI:
	  Higher of the right ankle pressures (DP or PT)
	  Higher of the brachial pressures (left or right)
	 Left ABI:
	  Higher of the left ankle pressures (DP or PT)
	  Higher of the brachial pressures (left or right)
	Interpretation: (revised 2011)[11]
	 • ≤0.9: Peripheral arterial disease
	 • 0.91–0.99: Borderline
	 • 1–1.4: Normal
	 • >1.4: Noncompressible arteries
	Variations:
	 • Exercise ABI: Repeat measurement after exercise (treadmill, stairs, pedal plantar flexion). Decrease in ABI of 15%–20% is considered diagnostic of PAD[5]
	 • Toe-brachial Index: Used in cases of noncompressible arteries (ABI>1.4); this procedure requires special equipment

Adapted from Norgren L, Hiatt WR, Dormandy JA, et al. Inter-Society Consensus for the Management of Peripheral Arterial Disease (TASC II). J Vasc Surg 2007;45(Suppl S):S5–67; with permission.

7% risk of nonfatal myocardial infarction or cardiovascular death annually.[5] Therefore, treatment is focused on reducing cardiovascular risk with aspirin or clopidogrel, statins, management of hypertension, and smoking cessation. For the leg, exercise, medications (eg, cilostazol), and revascularization reduce symptoms.[5,10] Data from an ongoing randomized trial suggest that for aortoiliac PAD, supervised exercise may yield larger gains in walking distance than endovascular intervention.[12] New evidence also suggests benefit from unsupervised home exercise.[13]

Chronic Venous Disease

Just as inadequate arterial supply to the legs can cause discomfort, so too can problems with venous return. Chronic venous insufficiency may be due to primary weakness of vein valves or walls. Secondary causes include prior DVT (postthrombotic syndrome) or other mechanical obstruction, such as occlusion of the left iliac vein by the right iliac artery (May-Thurner syndrome). Beyond a history of thrombosis or thrombophilia, risk factors include family history, female sex, age, obesity, greater height, prolonged standing, and multiple pregnancies.[14]

Venous disease is said to cause leg tingling, aching, burning, pain, cramps, throbbing, heaviness, pruritus, restlessness, and fatigue.[15] Empirically, aching, heaviness, and pruritus correlate best with ultrasonographic findings.[4,16,17] Symptoms are usually worse with dependency and improve with walking or elevation,[18] which facilitate venous return. Obstruction of deep veins rarely causes symptoms that worsen with activity, leading to the term "venous claudication".[5]

Most patients with discomfort attributable to venous disease will have visible vascular abnormalities or associated skin changes (**Fig. 1**).[18] Duplex ultrasonography is the preferred test to confirm the diagnosis as well as to identify and localize

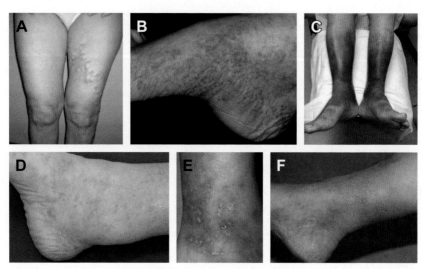

Fig. 1. Common skin changes associated with venous insufficiency. (*A*) Large varicose veins. (*B*) Venulectasias of the instep, sometimes called corona phlebectatica or ankle flare. (*C*) Hemosiderin deposition in the "gaiter area." (*D*) Edema localized to the ankle. Note also reticular veins in the instep and hemosiderin deposition above the ankle. (*E*) Atrophie blanche. (*F*) Lipodermatosclerosis. ([*A*] *From* Stoughton J. Venous ablation therapy: indications and outcomes. Prog Cardiovasc Dis 2011;54(1):63; with permission; [*B, E, F*] *From* Hafner A, Sprecher E. Ulcers. In: Bolognia JL, Jorizzo JL, Schaffer JV, et al, editors. Dermatology. 3rd edition. St. Louis, Mo: Saunders; 2012. p. 1729–46; [*C*] *From* Beckman JA, Creager MA. The history and physical examination. In: Vascular medicine: a companion to Braunwald's heart disease. 2nd edition. Philadelphia: W.B. Saunders; 2013. p. 139–47; with permission; and [*D*] *From* Hoffbrand AV, Pettit JE, Vyas P. Color atlas of clinical hematology. Philadelphia: Mosby/Elsevier; 2010. p. 474; with permission.)

underlying reflux or obstruction. Plethysmography and other tests may be used as adjuncts.[15]

Conservative treatments include compression (**Box 1**), weight loss, exercise, and elevation of the legs above the level of the heart.[18–21] Medical therapy is limited. Diuretics make little sense in the absence of systemic volume overload. Pentoxifylline provides limited benefit in venous ulceration but is not widely used.[18] Among several herbal preparations, horse chestnut seed extract (escin) has been shown to reduce symptoms and edema in short-term trials.[22] Surgical/interventional treatments include venous destruction with chemical sclerosants or thermocoagulation, ablation with radiofrequency or laser, stripping, or excision. In agreement with guidelines from surgical/interventional societies,[15,23] recent guidelines from the British National Institute for Health and Care Excellence[24] recommend ultrasonographic evaluation for patients with symptomatic varices, and interventional or surgical treatment rather than compression alone for symptomatic patients with truncal reflux.

Acute Deep Vein Thrombosis

Leg DVT is often asymptomatic but can cause pain, swelling, redness, and warmth. Risk factors can be as important diagnostically as symptoms or signs. Diagnosis usually relies on a combination of structured risk-stratification tools and noninvasive testing including serum D-dimer and ultrasonography. The most studied risk-stratification tool is the Wells score (**Table 2**).[25,26] In general, for patients with a low pretest probability

---

Box 1
Compression therapy for venous disease

Indications and Limitations for Use:

- Strong evidence for improved healing of venous ulcers[19] with limited evidence of symptomatic benefit in less severe disease.[20]

- Compression is contraindicated in patients with severe PAD for fear of decreasing arterial perfusion.[18]

- Risks include contact dermatitis and decreased venous return from bunching of poorly fit stockings.[20]

- Discomfort and difficulty donning stockings markedly limit adherence.[18]

Tips for Use of Compression Therapy in Chronic Venous Disease:

- Graduated compression (higher pressure distally) is preferred over fixed compression.[18] Multicomponent stockings with elastic may be more effective than single-component stockings.[19]

- Even in patients with proximal obstruction, compression is most important below the knee. Choice of height (knee, thigh, or waist) should be based on patient preference.[21]

- For edema caused by chronic venous disease, 20 to 30 mmHg pressure at the ankle typically suffices. Patients with venous dermatitis or ulcer may benefit from 30 to 40 mmHg if tolerable. Over-the-counter and antiembolic stockings used for DVT prophylaxis provide only 10 to 20 mmHg of pressure.

- Several varieties of stocking donners are available. Use of powder or liner hose may also help.

- Custom stockings are available if off-the-shelf stockings do not fit.

---

based on the Wells or similar validated score, a negative D-dimer is sufficient to rule out DVT without ultrasonography.[27] In higher-risk populations, depending on the details of the laboratory method, D-dimer may or may not be diagnostically helpful, and patients often need imaging.[27]

Table 2
Wells score for deep vein thrombosis

Clinical Feature	Score
Active cancer (treatment ongoing or within previous 6 mo or palliative)	1
Paralysis, paresis, or recent plaster immobilization of the lower extremities	1
Recently bedridden for 3 d or more, or major surgery within 4 wk	1
Localized tenderness along the distribution of the deep venous system	1
Entire leg swollen	1
Calf swelling by more than 3 cm when compared with the asymptomatic leg (measured 10 cm below tibial tuberosity)	1
Pitting edema (greater in the symptomatic leg)	1
Collateral superficial veins (nonvaricose)	1
Alternative diagnosis as likely or greater than that of deep vein thrombosis	−2
Risk scoring: low ≤0, moderate 1–2, high ≥3	

A revised Wells score[26] includes prior deep vein thrombosis as an additional risk factor, lengthened the postoperative risk period, and made several smaller textual changes. A revised score of <2 is considered low risk.

Adapted from Wells PS, Anderson DR, Bormanis J, et al. Value of assessment of pretest probability of deep-vein thrombosis in clinical management. Lancet 1997;350(9094):1795–8; with permission.

Although anticoagulation is the primary therapy for proximal DVT, in symptomatic patients compression therapy is an important adjunct. Initiating compression within 2 weeks and continuing for 2 years can reduce the incidence of postthrombotic syndrome by 50%.[27]

Other Vascular Causes of Leg Pain

Rare nonatherosclerotic causes of arterial obstruction include arterial dissection, aneurysm, embolism, arteritis, trauma, and external compression.[5] In the leg, arterial endofibrosis and popliteal artery entrapment may occur in athletes.[28]

NEUROLOGIC CAUSES OF LEG DISCOMFORT
Lumbosacral Radiculopathy and Lumbar Spinal Stenosis

Lumbosacral radiculopathy and lumbar spinal stenosis (LSS) often cause low back pain, but may present primarily or exclusively with leg symptoms.[29,30] Radiculopathy is most commonly caused by nerve-root compression from a herniated intervertebral disc. Bony disease, malignancy, epidural abscess, and even noncompressive etiologies such as herpes zoster also occur.[31] LSS is characterized by anatomic impingement of the spinal canal, recesses, or foramina owing to degenerative changes of the vertebrae or ligamentous hypertrophy.[30] Radiculopathy frequently presents in middle age.[32] LSS usually affects the elderly.[33]

Radiculopathy is defined by radiating pain, paresthesias, or other sensory changes in a dermatomal distribution, sometimes with weakness or reflex changes in the corresponding myotome (**Table 3**).[29] However, there are conceptual limits to dermatomal and myotomal mapping[34] and empirically, pain may not follow the classic dermatomes.[35,36] Other features, such as worsening with Valsalva, have not been validated. A host of examination maneuvers designed to stretch the nerve roots[34] are of limited value. The straight-leg raising (SLR, Lasègue) test, consisting of reproduction of radiating pain by passively elevating the affected leg of a supine patient, contributes little when positive (LR 1.5), but may argue against compressive radiculopathy when

Table 3				
Lumbosacral radiculopathies causing leg discomfort				
Root Level	**Dermatome**	**Myotome**	**Reflex Affected**	**Selected Mimics**[a]
L2	Anterolateral thigh	Hip flexion		Lateral femoral cutaneous neuropathy
L3	Medial thigh and knee	Hip flexion and adduction, knee extension	Knee jerk	
L4	Medial lower leg	Knee extension and hip adduction	Knee jerk	
L5	Lateral lower leg, dorsum of foot, great toe	Ankle dorsiflexion, foot inversion/eversion and toe flexion/extension		Peroneal neuropathy
S1	Lateral foot and toes, sole	Foot plantarflexion, knee flexion, hip extension	Ankle jerk	Sciatic neuropathy

Underlined findings have empirical support as useful in identifying the level of radiculopathy.
    [a] All can be mimicked by spinal stenosis or lumbosacral plexopathy.
    Data from Refs.[9,29,31]

absent (LR 0.4).[9] Pain on raising the unaffected leg (crossed SLR) suggests radiculopathy (LR 3.4), as do calf wasting and weak ankle dorsiflexion.[9,37]

Although LSS can also cause radiculopathy symptoms, it typically causes neurogenic claudication: a feeling of pain, weakness, or fatigue in the buttocks or legs provoked by walking and relieved by rest.[30] Patients may also describe numbness and tingling. Unlike radiculopathy, the symptoms are often bilateral.[38] Isolating leg exertion from spinal flexion can help distinguish arterial from neurogenic claudication (**Table 4**). Using expert opinion as the reference standard, bilateral buttock or leg pain, relief with sitting or bending, and rare urinary/anogenital symptoms increase the likelihood of spinal stenosis (LR>5). Absence of these key historical features decreases the likelihood of LSS (LR near 0.3):

- Age older than 65
- Neurogenic claudication
- Pain below the buttocks
- Pain in the thigh
- Aggravation by standing/walking and relief by sitting

On examination, wide-based gait and abnormal Romberg test are most helpful in identifying LSS (LR>4), with strength, sensory, and reflex abnormalities less helpful (LR 2–3).[39,40]

Magnetic resonance imaging is the diagnostic test of choice for LSS[30,40] and also when imaging is required for suspected radiculopathy.[41] Specificity is low; 20% to 30% of adults have imaging consistent with disc herniation,[32] and an equal proportion older than 55 years have radiographic evidence of LSS.[39] Electrodiagnostics can demonstrate and localize radiculopathy but may be normal in sensory-only radiculopathy.[29] The role for electrodiagnostics in diagnosis of LSS remains controversial.[30,42]

The prognosis of acute lumbosacral radiculopathy is good, with pain and weakness often resolving over days to weeks and more than two-thirds of patients recovering within a year.[41] Acute management is usually conservative and imaging unnecessary, unless there is abnormal perineal sensation, sexual, bladder, or bowel control suggestive of cauda equina syndrome; rapidly progressive neurologic deficits; or risk for epidural abscess or malignancy.[31,41] Similarly, the natural history of untreated spinal stenosis is favorable for many patients.[30] In a small study, over 4 years two-thirds of patients had no change in pain, with the remainder split between improvement and worsening.[43]

There is little evidence of benefit from conservative treatments for either condition including medications, physical therapy, traction, and transcutaneous electrical nerve stimulation (TENS).[30,41,44,45] Use of epidural steroid injections is controversial, with

Table 4	
Conceptual distinction between vascular and neurogenic claudication	
Vascular Claudication	**Neurogenic Claudication**
Triggered by increased demand across arterial stenosis. Relieved by rest	Triggered by lumbar extension worsening spinal stenosis. Relieved by lumbar flexion
Pain reliably comes after a fixed amount of exertion (eg, specific walking distance)	Pain may come with minimal exertion (eg, standing in line, going down stairs)
Pain comes with activity even if back is flexed (eg, riding a bicycle)	Pain does not occur with exertion in lumbar flexion (eg, leaning on a shopping cart)

statistically but perhaps not clinically significant benefit.[30,41,46] Surgery for radiculopathy and LSS likely yields at least short-term symptomatic benefit; analysis of randomized trials has been limited by crossover between surgical and nonsurgical arms.[47,48]

Entrapment Neuropathies

Most entrapment neuropathies of the leg are rare outside of surgical settings, or present primarily with weakness rather than pain or paresthesias.[49] Primary care providers will often encounter lateral femoral cutaneous neuropathy (LFCN, also called meralgia paresthetica from the Greek for "thigh pain"). LFCN is characterized by a sharply demarcated area of numbness and paresthesias on the anterolateral thigh. It is usually caused by compression of this sensory-only nerve as it travels under the inguinal ligament.[49] Obesity, diabetes, and older age are risk factors.[50] Mechanical causes include pregnancy, tight clothing, and heavy tool belts.[49] Diagnostic testing is rarely required, but imaging can be used to rule out rare intra-abdominal abnormality causing compression proximal to the inguinal ligament.[51,52] Reassurance, avoidance of tight clothing and belts, and weight loss are the mainstays of treatment. Neuropathic and other pain medications may be used. Local injections and surgery are rarely required.[53]

Peroneal neuropathy is the most common compression neuropathy of the leg.[49] It is characterized primarily by foot-drop and falls, although there may be pain changes over the lateral calf and dorsum of the foot. Peroneal neuropathy is typically caused by compression or entrapment at the fibular neck caused by leg crossing, squatting, or weight loss. Piriformis syndrome is a controversial diagnosis whereby the sciatic nerve is said to be compressed by the piriformis muscle at the sciatic notch.[52]

Distal Symmetric Polyneuropathy

Distal symmetric polyneuropathies (DSP) have a distribution that is length dependent rather than following a single nerve or dermatome.[54] Symptoms begin in the toes and progress proximally up the leg, eventually involving the hands (stocking-glove distribution) and anterior thorax.[55] Of the many metabolic, toxic, endocrine, inflammatory, genetic, and neoplastic causes, diabetes and alcohol misuse are the most commonly seen in primary care.[55,56] DSP affect 30% to 50% of diabetics, although only half are noticed by the patient.[57]

Patients may complain of neuropathic pain, numbness, or a tight, wooden leg, often worse at night or with standing.[58] Examination findings include decreased pain, touch, temperature, vibration, and proprioceptive sensation. In the leg, weakness usually begins in dorsiflexors before plantarflexors.[54] Atrophy may be visible directly or as muscular imbalance leading to hammertoes. Patients may lose the ability to walk on heels before tip-toe.[55] Ankle-jerk reflex may be diminished or absent, although this finding is common among elderly patients without DSP.[54] For diabetics, use of either a tuning fork to test vibratory sensation or a Semmes-Weinstein monofilament can accurately predict neuropathy on nerve conduction study; inability to walk on heels and abnormalities of deep tendon reflexes are less useful.[59]

Electrodiagnostics can confirm the presence of DSP and distinguish between axonal and demyelinating disase.[55,58] Basic laboratory tests include serum glucose/hemoglobin A_{1C}, vitamin B_{12}, serum protein electrophoresis, antinuclear antibody, erythrocyte sedimentation rate, and rapid plasma reagin, with tests for other infectious, autoimmune, toxic, and nutritional causes reserved for select patients or when the initial studies are unrevealing.[55,56] In diabetics with classic symptoms, testing may not be required.[58,60]

There is increasing recognition of DSP involving only the small fibers that transmit pain and touch, leaving other senses, strength, reflexes, and electrodiagnostics unaffected.[54] Such small-fiber neuropathy may be idiopathic in the elderly[58] but is also a cause of atypical diabetic neuropathy occurring in patients without microvascular complications, or even in patients with elevated glucose not meeting criteria for diabetes.[61]

Treatment of DSP is directed at the underlying cause. Multispecialty guidelines also support the use of pregabalin, gabapentin, sodium valproate, venlafaxine, duloxetine, amitriptyline, opioids, capsaicin, isosorbide spray, and percutaneous nerve stimulation.[62]

Other Neurogenic Causes of Leg Discomfort

Numerous neurologic conditions including amyotrophic lateral sclerosis, cervical myelopathy, and Guillain-Barré syndrome cause weakness, gait abnormalities, or sensory changes in the leg.[63] Plexopathies are less common in the leg than in the arm but can be caused by compression, trauma, radiation, and infection.[64] Lumbosacral radiculoplexopathy is a rare syndrome of disabling leg pain and weakness occurring primarily in patients with uncomplicated diabetes.[65]

MUSCULOSKELETAL CAUSES OF DISCOMFORT

Most musculoskeletal leg discomfort derives from the joints or periarticular structures (eg, arthritis, tendinopathy, bursitis) and is not discussed here. It is noteworthy that joint pain may radiate away from the joint; distal radiation of pain from hip arthritis is particularly common.

Stress Fracture

Diagnosis of fracture is clear in the setting of trauma and local tenderness, but pathologic and insufficiency fractures from malignancy and osteoporosis may occur with minimal trauma and cause more diffuse pain. Stress fractures occurring, for example, in the setting of increased athletic training also require a high index of suspicion. Not only can the onset of pain be insidious, but initial radiographs may be normal, necessitating repeat films or advanced imaging. For medial tibia stress fractures, rest, perhaps with immobilization or non–weight bearing, is the primary treatment, although fractures of the anterior cortex may require surgical management.[66]

Statin Myalgia

3-Hydroxy-3-methylglutaryl coenzyme A reductase inhibitors (statins) cause myalgia (muscle pain) with or without myopathy (muscle damage) in 5% to 10% of users.[67,68] Myalgia may occur in any part of the body but the legs are most commonly affected, usually the calves and thighs.[69,70] The pain is described as heaviness, stiffness, cramping, and sometimes weakness. It is often exertional, causing patients to limit physical activity. Symptoms start on average 1 month after statin initiation, but can be delayed for 6 to 12 months[69] and can last 2 months after cessation of the medication.[67] Risk of myalgias and myopathy are increased by drug interactions including fibrates and cytochrome P450 3A4 (CYP 3A4) inhibitors (eg, amiodarone, cyclosporine, protease inhibitors, macrolide antibiotics, and calcium-channel blockers). Pravastatin, fluvastatin, and rosuvastatin are less prone to the CYP 3A4 interactions.[67] Low levels of grapefruit consumption are unlikely to be problematic.[71]

Workup of statin myalgias usually includes measurement of serum creatinine kinase (CK) and thyroid stimulating hormone, as thyroid abnormalities can cause hyperlipidemia and myalgia.[68] Statin myalgias in the absence of CK elevations are not dangerous and need not prompt management changes if they are not of significant concern. Large elevations of CK (>5–10 times the upper limit of normal) may require modification or cessation of statin therapy independent of myalgias.[67] Strategies to address statin myalgia include:

- Cessation of the statin or interacting drugs
- Dose reduction
- Use of an alternative statin (eg, pravastatin, fluvastatin, or rosuvastatin)
- Alternate-day dosing
- Addition of coenzyme Q (limited evidence)[67,68]

Cramps

Cramps are sudden, involuntary, painful, electrically active contractions of skeletal muscle.[72] Leg cramps usually occur in the posterior calf but may involve the foot or the thigh. Cramps often occur at night and last seconds to minutes but may result in prolonged soreness. During the cramp, muscle contraction is usually visible or palpable.[63]

There are long lists of medical conditions said to cause cramps, including pregnancy, dialysis, hypothyroidism, hypovolemic hyponatremia, cirrhosis, radiculopathies, and peripheral neuropathies.[63,73] Many of the associations are based on surveys and must be interpreted cautiously, especially in light of a reported cramp prevalence of 30% to 95% in the general population.[63] One study looking at Canadian pharmacy data suggests a strong association with inhaled long-acting β2-agonists and potassium-sparing and thiazide diuretics, with a weaker association for statins and loop diuretics.[74] Alcohol and calcium-channel blockers are also frequently cited.[63,75–77]

Cramps are diagnosed by history taking, with physical examination and diagnostic testing used to exclude other conditions. Routine evaluation of thyroid function and electrolytes remains controversial, based in part on data suggesting that electrolyte abnormalities do not predict cramps among endurance athletes.[63,75,77] Stretching or massage of the affected muscle can bring acute relief. There is new evidence for prophylactic stretching,[78] which has long been advocated based on anecdotal evidence.[79] As nocturnal cramps have been attributed to shortening of the calf and plantar foot muscles by pressure from bedclothes,[63,76] one might also suggest a blanket lift or other strategy to reduce this pressure. A review by the American Academy of Neurology (AAN) found no evidence for hydration in the prevention of cramps.[72] Quinine, once the mainstay of the pharmacologic treatment of cramps, has modest benefit usually outweighed by the risk of thrombocytopenia, hypersensitivity, and QT prolongation. In 2006 the Food and Drug Administration added a black-box warning advising against off-label use of quinine for cramps, and the AAN review argues that quinine should be avoided for routine treatment and considered only for disabling cramps after specific discussion and informed consent.[72] There is no evidence regarding use of tonic water for cramping. Small studies have suggested that vitamin B6 (even in nondeficient patients), diltiazem, and natridrofuryl (a vasodilator not approved in the United States) may be helpful.[72] A Cochrane review concluded that magnesium is not helpful in nonpregnant adults.[80]

RESTLESS LEGS SYNDROME

RLS (also called Willis-Ekbom disease) is defined by discomfort and an urge to move the legs that occurs at rest, is relieved by movement, and occurs primarily in the evening or at night. It is often associated with periodic limb movements of sleep. Patients describe the discomfort as creepy-crawly, jittery, throbbing, tight, tearing, and electric current. RLS affects 1% to 3% of the population and is often familial. An association with age has been shown in some but not all studies. It is associated with iron deficiency, end-stage renal disease, and medications including antidopaminergic neuroleptics and antiemetics, antihistamines, and antidepressants (selective serotonin reuptake inhibitors and selective norepinephrine reuptake inhibitors, but not bupropion).[81]

Although RLS is defined by symptoms, patients with various "mimics" (including cramps, arthritis, and peripheral neuropathies) may meet the original diagnostic criteria.[82] RLS must be distinguished from positional discomfort (eg, crossed legs) and unintentional movements such as hypnic jerks or unconscious foot tapping. Patients with RLS have symptoms in various rest positions and consciously move the leg to relieve symptoms.[82]

Multiple groups have reviewed treatment of RLS,[83–86] including a federally funded analysis[87] free from industry-related conflict of interest. Nonpharmacologic treatments are often favored for mild to moderate disease, with some evidence to support exercise and cognitive-behavioral therapy.[84,87] Mental-alerting activities (eg, crosswords or video games) and avoidance of caffeine are suggested based on expert opinion.[85] It is reasonable to assess iron stores and replete patients with low iron stores. There is less consensus on iron supplementation in patients with low to normal iron levels.[83–86] Dopaminergic medications (eg, pramipexole, ropinirole, rotigotine) are effective but limited by augmentation, the iatrogenic development of more severe symptoms or spread to other limbs earlier in the day, as well as concerns about impulse-control problems. $\alpha2\delta$ ligands (gabapentin, gabapentin encarbil, and pregabalin) are increasingly considered as first-line agents. Opioids, benzodiazepines, and their respective agonists are used without high-quality supporting evidence.[83–87]

Other Musculoskeletal Causes of Leg Discomfort

Diffuse myalgia may be caused by medications other than statins and a host of infectious, endocrine, metabolic, and rheumatologic diseases.[63] Polymyalgia rheumatica perhaps deserves special mention as a cause of bilateral proximal leg pain and stiffness, sometimes in the absence of shoulder symptoms. Localized myalgias are commonly caused by muscle strain. Acute compartment syndrome, raised pressure in a closed fascial space, is a surgical emergency that usually occurs in the setting of trauma,[88] although a chronic form occurs in athletes.[28] Medial tibial stress syndrome (shin splints) is also associated with athletic training, and causes symptoms similar to those of stress fracture.[28] Other causes of bone pain include malignancy and osteomyelitis.[89] Questions have been raised about the association between vitamin D deficiency and chronic musculoskeletal pain including lower extremity pain, but vitamin D supplementation has not been associated with pain relief.[90,91]

SUMMARY

Leg pain is common, and patients may have more than one cause. Although simple questionnaires or descriptors (eg, cramps, aching) are inadequate to distinguish between etiologies, history plays a key role in diagnosis. Timing and triggers of symptoms as well as lateralization can narrow the differential. Nocturnal symptoms are likely to be cramps, RLS, or DSP. Exertional symptoms suggest PAD, whereas symptoms caused by standing may be LSS or venous insufficiency. DVT and radiculopathy are usually unilateral, whereas DSP, RLS, and statin myalgia tend to be bilateral.

Fortunately, few of the diagnoses discussed constitute medical emergencies. DVT, acute compartment syndrome, pyomyositis, and malignancy all require prompt diagnosis and treatment. However, PAD (without rest pain, ulceration, or gangrene) is unlikely to progress rapidly, and routine radiculopathy and spinal stenosis (with no cauda equina syndrome or rapidly progressive neurologic deficit) can safely be managed conservatively. That said, accurate diagnosis of leg discomfort can afford patients a prognosis and, in some cases, effective therapy.

REFERENCES

1. Herr KA, Mobily PR, Wallace RB, et al. Leg pain in the rural Iowa 65+ population. Prevalence, related factors, and association with functional status. Clin J Pain 1991;7(2):114–21.
2. Oboler SK, Prochazka AV, Meyer TJ. Leg symptoms in outpatient veterans. West J Med 1991;155(3):256–9.
3. Hirsch AT, Criqui MH, Treat-Jacobson D, et al. Peripheral arterial disease detection, awareness, and treatment in primary care. JAMA 2001;286(11): 1317–24.
4. Chiesa R, Marone EM, Limoni C, et al. Chronic venous disorders: correlation between visible signs, symptoms, and presence of functional disease. J Vasc Surg 2007;46(2):322–30.
5. Norgren L, Hiatt WR, Dormandy JA, et al. Inter-Society Consensus for the Management of Peripheral Arterial Disease (TASC II). J Vasc Surg 2007;45(Suppl S): S5–67.
6. Wilson JF. Peripheral arterial disease. Ann Intern Med 2007;146(5):ITC3-1.
7. Newman AB, Naydeck BL, Sutton-Tyrrell K, et al. The role of comorbidity in the assessment of intermittent claudication in older adults. J Clin Epidemiol 2001; 54(3):294–300.
8. Khan NA, Rahim SA, Anand SS, et al. Does the clinical examination predict lower extremity peripheral arterial disease? JAMA 2006;295(5):536–46.
9. McGee SR. Evidence-based physical diagnosis. Philadelphia: Elsevier/Saunders; 2012.
10. Hirsch AT, Haskal ZJ, Hertzer NR, et al. ACC/AHA 2005 guidelines for the management of patients with peripheral arterial disease. J Am Coll Cardiol 2006; 47(6):1239–312.
11. Rooke TW, Hirsch AT, Misra S, et al. 2011 ACCF/AHA focused update of the guideline for the management of patients with peripheral artery disease (updating the 2005 guideline): a report of the American College of Cardiology Foundation/American Heart Association Task Force on Practice Guidelines. J Am Coll Cardiol 2011;58(19):2020–45.
12. Murphy TP, Cutlip DE, Regensteiner JG, et al. Supervised exercise versus primary stenting for claudication resulting from aortoiliac peripheral artery disease: six-month outcomes from the claudication: exercise versus endoluminal revascularization (CLEVER) study. Circulation 2012;125(1):130–9.
13. McDermott MM, Liu K, Guralnik JM, et al. Home-based walking exercise intervention in peripheral artery disease: a randomized clinical trial. JAMA 2013; 310(1):57–65.
14. Bergan JJ, Schmid-Schönbein GW, Smith PD, et al. Chronic venous disease. N Engl J Med 2006;355(5):488–98.
15. Gloviczki P, Comerota AJ, Dalsing MC, et al. The care of patients with varicose veins and associated chronic venous diseases: clinical practice guidelines of

the Society for Vascular Surgery and the American Venous Forum. J Vasc Surg 2011;53(Suppl 5):2S–48S.

16. Langer RD, Ho E, Denenberg JO, et al. Relationships between symptoms and venous disease: the San Diego population study. Arch Intern Med 2005; 165(12):1420–4.

17. Bradbury A, Evans CJ, Allan P, et al. The relationship between lower limb symptoms and superficial and deep venous reflux on duplex ultrasonography: The Edinburgh Vein Study. J Vasc Surg 2000;32(5):921–31.

18. Raju S, Neglén P. Clinical practice. Chronic venous insufficiency and varicose veins. N Engl J Med 2009;360(22):2319–27.

19. O'Meara S, Cullum N, Nelson EA, et al. Compression for venous leg ulcers. Cochrane Database Syst Rev 2012;(11):CD000265.

20. Palfreyman SJ, Michaels JA. A systematic review of compression hosiery for uncomplicated varicose veins. Phlebology 2009;24(Suppl 1):13–33.

21. Prandoni P, Noventa F, Quintavalla R, et al. Thigh-length versus below-knee compression elastic stockings for prevention of the postthrombotic syndrome in patients with proximal-venous thrombosis: a randomized trial. Blood 2012; 119(6):1561–5.

22. Pittler MH, Ernst E. Horse chestnut seed extract for chronic venous insufficiency. Cochrane Database Syst Rev 2012;(11):CD003230.

23. Rochon P, Vu C, Ray C, et al. ACR appropriateness criteria: radiologic management of lower-extremity venous insufficiency. 2009. Available at: acr.org. Accessed August 15, 2013.

24. National Institute for Health and Care Excellence (NICE). Varicose veins in the legs: full guideline. Available at: nice.org.uk. Accessed September 6, 2013.

25. Wells PS, Anderson DR, Bormanis J, et al. Value of assessment of pretest probability of deep-vein thrombosis in clinical management. Lancet 1997;350(9094): 1795–8.

26. Wells PS, Anderson DR, Rodger M, et al. Evaluation of D-dimer in the diagnosis of suspected deep-vein thrombosis. N Engl J Med 2003;349(13):1227–35.

27. Kearon C, Akl EA, Comerota AJ, et al. Antithrombotic therapy for VTE disease: antithrombotic therapy and prevention of thrombosis, 9th ed: American College of Chest Physicians Evidence-Based Clinical Practice Guidelines. Chest 2012; 141(Suppl 2):e419S–94S.

28. Brewer RB, Gregory AJ. Chronic lower leg pain in athletes: a guide for the differential diagnosis, evaluation, and treatment. Sports Health 2012;4(2): 121–7.

29. Daroff RB, Fenichel GM, Jankovic J, et al. Lower back and lower limb pain. In: Bradley's Neurology in clinical practice. Philadelphia, London: Saunders; 2012. p. 349–60.

30. Kreiner DS, Shaffer WO, Baisden JL, et al. An evidence-based clinical guideline for the diagnosis and treatment of degenerative lumbar spinal stenosis (update). Spine J 2013;13(7):734–43.

31. Tarulli AW, Raynor EM. Lumbosacral radiculopathy. Neurol Clin 2007;25(2): 387–405.

32. Koes BW, van Tulder MW, Peul WC. Diagnosis and treatment of sciatica. BMJ 2007;334(7607):1313–7.

33. Katz JN, Harris MB. Clinical practice. Lumbar spinal stenosis. N Engl J Med 2008;358(8):818–25.

34. De Luigi AJ, Fitzpatrick KF. Physical examination in radiculopathy. Phys Med Rehabil Clin N Am 2011;22(1):7–40.

35. Taylor C, Coxon A, Watson P, et al. Do L5 and S1 nerve root compressions produce radicular pain in a dermatomal pattern? Spine 2013;38(12):995–8.
36. Beattie PF, Meyers SP, Stratford P, et al. Associations between patient report of symptoms and anatomic impairment visible on lumbar magnetic resonance imaging. Spine 2000;25(7):819–28.
37. Van der Windt DA, Simons E, Riphagen II, et al. Physical examination for lumbar radiculopathy due to disc herniation in patients with low-back pain. Cochrane Database Syst Rev 2010;(2):CD007431.
38. Chad DA. Lumbar spinal stenosis. Neurol Clin 2007;25(2):407–18.
39. Suri P, Rainville J, Kalichman L, et al. Does this older adult with lower extremity pain have the clinical syndrome of lumbar spinal stenosis? JAMA 2010;304(23):2628–36.
40. De Schepper EI, Overdevest GM, Suri P, et al. Diagnosis of lumbar spinal stenosis: an updated systematic review of the accuracy of diagnostic tests. Spine 2013;38(8):E469–81.
41. Van Tulder M, Peul W, Koes B. Sciatica: what the rheumatologist needs to know. Nat Rev Rheumatol 2010;6(3):139–45.
42. Haig AJ, Tomkins CC. Diagnosis and management of lumbar spinal stenosis. JAMA 2010;303(1):71–2.
43. Johnsson KE, Rosén I, Udén A. The natural course of lumbar spinal stenosis. Clin Orthop Relat Res 1992;279:82–6.
44. Dahm KT, Brurberg KG, Jamtvedt G, et al. Advice to rest in bed versus advice to stay active for acute low-back pain and sciatica. Cochrane Database Syst Rev 2010;(6):CD007612.
45. Clarke JA, van Tulder MW, Blomberg SE, et al. Traction for low-back pain with or without sciatica. Cochrane Database Syst Rev 2007;(2):CD003010.
46. Deyo RA. Commentary: clinical practice guidelines: trust them or trash them? Spine J 2013;13(7):744–6.
47. Bruggeman AJ, Decker RC. Surgical treatment and outcomes of lumbar radiculopathy. Phys Med Rehabil Clin N Am 2011;22(1):161–77.
48. Kovacs FM, Urrútia G, Alarcón JD. Surgery versus conservative treatment for symptomatic lumbar spinal stenosis: a systematic review of randomized controlled trials. Spine 2011;36(20):E1335–51.
49. Katirji B, Wilbourn A. Mononeuropathies of the lower limb. In: Dyck PJ, Thomas PK, editors. Peripheral neuropathy. 4th edition. Philadelphia: W.B. Saunders; 2005. p. 1487–510.
50. Parisi TJ, Mandrekar J, Dyck PJ, et al. Meralgia paresthetica: relation to obesity, advanced age, and diabetes mellitus. Neurology 2011;77(16):1538–42.
51. Harney D, Patijn J. Meralgia paresthetica: diagnosis and management strategies. Pain Med 2007;8(8):669–77.
52. Shapiro BE, Preston DC. Entrapment and compressive neuropathies. Med Clin North Am 2009;93(2):285–315, vii.
53. Haim A, Pritsch T, Ben-Galim P, et al. Meralgia paresthetica: a retrospective analysis of 79 patients evaluated and treated according to a standard algorithm. Acta Orthop 2006;77(3):482–6.
54. England JD, Gronseth GS, Franklin G, et al. Distal symmetric polyneuropathy: a definition for clinical research: report of the American Academy of Neurology, the American Association of Electrodiagnostic Medicine, and the American Academy of Physical Medicine and Rehabilitation. Neurology 2005;64(2):199–207.
55. England JD, Asbury AK. Peripheral neuropathy. Lancet 2004;363(9427):2151–61.

56. Hughes R. Peripheral nerve diseases: the bare essentials. Pract Neurol 2008; 8(6):396–405.
57. Lindsay TJ, Rodgers BC, Savath V, et al. Treating diabetic peripheral neuropathic pain. Am Fam Physician 2010;82(2):151–8.
58. Mendell JR, Sahenk Z. Clinical practice. Painful sensory neuropathy. N Engl J Med 2003;348(13):1243–55.
59. Kanji JN, Anglin RE, Hunt DL, et al. Does this patient with diabetes have large-fiber peripheral neuropathy? JAMA 2010;303(15):1526–32.
60. Rutkove SB. A 52-year-old woman with disabling peripheral neuropathy: review of diabetic polyneuropathy. JAMA 2009;302(13):1451–8.
61. Dyck PJ, Albers JW, Andersen H, et al. Diabetic polyneuropathies: update on research definition, diagnostic criteria and estimation of severity. Diabetes Metab Res Rev 2011;27:620–8.
62. Bril V, England J, Franklin GM, et al. Evidence-based guideline: treatment of painful diabetic neuropathy: report of the American Academy of Neurology, the American Association of Neuromuscular and Electrodiagnostic Medicine, and the American Academy of Physical Medicine and Rehabilitation. Neurology 2011;76(20):1758–65.
63. Miller TM, Layzer RB. Muscle cramps. Muscle Nerve 2005;32(4):431–42.
64. Donaghy M. Lumbosacral plexus lesions. In: Dyck PJ, Thomas PK, editors. Peripheral neuropathy. 4th edition. Philadelphia: W.B. Saunders; 2005. p. 1375–90.
65. Dyck PJ. Radiculoplexus neuropathies: diabetic and nondiabetic varieties. In: Dyck PJ, Thomas PK, editors. Peripheral neuropathy. 4th edition. Philadelphia: W.B. Saunders; 2005. p. 1993–2015.
66. Patel DS, Roth M, Kapil N. Stress fractures: diagnosis, treatment, and prevention. Am Fam Physician 2011;83(1):39–46.
67. Joy TR, Hegele RA. Narrative review: statin-related myopathy. Ann Intern Med 2009;150(12):858–68.
68. Jacobson TA. Toward "pain-free" statin prescribing: clinical algorithm for diagnosis and management of myalgia. Mayo Clin Proc 2008;83(6):687–700.
69. Bruckert E, Hayem G, Dejager S, et al. Mild to moderate muscular symptoms with high-dosage statin therapy in hyperlipidemic patients—the PRIMO study. Cardiovasc Drugs Ther 2005;19(6):403–14.
70. Parker BA, Capizzi JA, Grimaldi AS, et al. Effect of statins on skeletal muscle function. Circulation 2013;127(1):96–103.
71. Reddy P, Ellington D, Zhu Y, et al. Serum concentrations and clinical effects of atorvastatin in patients taking grapefruit juice daily. Br J Clin Pharmacol 2011; 72(3):434–41.
72. Katzberg HD, Khan AH, So YT. Assessment: symptomatic treatment for muscle cramps (an evidence-based review): report of the therapeutics and technology assessment subcommittee of the American academy of neurology. Neurology 2010;74(8):691–6.
73. Parisi L, Pierelli F, Amabile G, et al. Muscular cramps: proposals for a new classification. Acta Neurol Scand 2003;107(3):176–86.
74. Garrison SR, Dormuth CR, Morrow RL, et al. Nocturnal leg cramps and prescription use that precedes them: a sequence symmetry analysis. Arch Intern Med 2012;172(2):120–6.
75. Kanaan N, Sawaya R. Nocturnal leg cramps: clinically mysterious and painful—but manageable. Geriatrics 2001;56(6):34.
76. McGee SR. Muscle cramps. Arch Intern Med 1990;150(3):511–8.

77. Allen RE, Kirby KA. Nocturnal leg cramps. Am Fam Physician 2012;86(4): 350–5.
78. Hallegraeff JM, van der Schans CP, de Ruiter R, et al. Stretching before sleep reduces the frequency and severity of nocturnal leg cramps in older adults: a randomised trial. J Physiother 2012;58(1):17–22.
79. Blyton F, Chuter V, Walter KE, et al. Non-drug therapies for lower limb muscle cramps. Cochrane Database Syst Rev 2012;(1):CD008496.
80. Garrison SR, Allan GM, Sekhon RK, et al. Magnesium for skeletal muscle cramps. Cochrane Database Syst Rev 2012;(9):CD009402.
81. Allen RP, Picchietti D, Hening WA, et al. Restless legs syndrome: diagnostic criteria, special considerations, and epidemiology. A report from the restless legs syndrome diagnosis and epidemiology workshop at the National Institutes of Health. Sleep Med 2003;4(2):101–19.
82. Hening WA, Allen RP, Washburn M, et al. The four diagnostic criteria for restless legs syndrome are unable to exclude confounding conditions ("mimics"). Sleep Med 2009;10(9):976–81.
83. Garcia-Borreguero D, Ferini-Strambi L, Kohnen R, et al. European guidelines on management of restless legs syndrome: report of a joint task force by the European Federation of Neurological Societies, the European Neurological Society and the European Sleep Research Society. Eur J Neurol 2012;19(11):1385–96.
84. Garcia-Borreguero D, Kohnen R, Silber MH, et al. The long-term treatment of restless legs syndrome/Willis-Ekbom disease: evidence-based guidelines and clinical consensus best practice guidance: a report from the International Restless Legs Syndrome Study Group. Sleep Med 2013;14(7):675–84.
85. Silber MH, Becker PM, Earley C, et al. Willis-Ekbom Disease Foundation revised consensus statement on the management of restless legs syndrome. Mayo Clin Proc 2013;88(9):977–86.
86. Aurora RN, Kristo DA, Bista SR, et al. The treatment of restless legs syndrome and periodic limb movement disorder in adults-an update for 2012: practice parameters with an evidence-based systematic review and meta-analyses: an American Academy of Sleep Medicine Clinical Practice Guideline. Sleep 2012;35(8):1039–62.
87. Wilt TJ, MacDonald R, Ouellette J, et al. Treatment for restless legs syndrome. Rockville (MD): Agency for Healthcare Research and Quality (US); 2012.
88. Tiwari A, Haq AI, Myint F, et al. Acute compartment syndromes. Br J Surg 2002; 89(4):397–412.
89. Barr KP. Review of upper and lower extremity musculoskeletal pain problems. Phys Med Rehabil Clin N Am 2007;18(4):747–60, vi–vii.
90. Plotnikoff GA, Quigley JM. Prevalence of severe hypovitaminosis D in patients with persistent, nonspecific musculoskeletal pain. Mayo Clin Proc 2003; 78(12):1463–70.
91. Warner AE, Arnspiger SA. Diffuse musculoskeletal pain is not associated with low vitamin D levels or improved by treatment with vitamin D. J Clin Rheumatol 2008;14(1):12–6.

Common Dermatologic Conditions

Jay C. Vary, MD, PhD[a],*, Kim M. O'Connor, MD[b]

KEYWORDS

- Alopecia • Facial rashes • Intertriginous rashes • Leg rashes • Acne

KEY POINTS

- The most common causes of alopecia are non-scarring and non-inflammatory and can be distinguished by the pattern of hair loss and the presence of ongoing shedding.
- Age of onset, distribution of the rash, presence or absence of comedones or systemic symptoms can help distinguish between the causes of facial rash.
- The utilization of the KOH prep and Wood's lamp examination can aid in the diagnosis of intertriginous rashes.
- Stasis dermatitis and contact dermatitis on the legs are commonly mistaken for infection but history and examination findings can usually quickly exclude infection.

INTRODUCTION

The skin serves many functions other than simply wrapping and containing all the deeper structures.[1,2] It is composed of an uppermost self-renewing epidermis of primarily keratinocytes that becomes scaly and red in response to superficial inflammation from irritation or infection. Immediately subjacent is the dermis, which contains not only connective tissues and vasculature but also the skin appendages. These appendages are derived from buds of the epidermis that grow down into the dermis early in development and result in the eccrine and apocrine sweat glands, nails, and the pilosebaceous unit that is the target of inflammation in alopecia, acne vulgaris, and rosacea. Below the dermis, the subcutaneous tissue lies above muscular fascia in most areas of the body, and is composed of adipocytes as well as the larger trunks of vessels and nerves passing through.

Conflict of Interest Disclosures: The authors have no conflicts of interest to report including no financial conflicts of interest.
Role in Authorship: All authors had access to the data and had a role in writing the article.
[a] Division of Dermatology, Department of Internal Medicine, The University of Washington, Box 354697, 4225 Roosevelt Way Northeast, 4th Floor, Seattle, WA 98195, USA; [b] Division of General Internal Medicine, Department of Internal Medicine, Box 354760, 4245 Roosevelt Way Northeast, Seattle, WA 98195, USA
* Corresponding author.
E-mail address: jvary@u.washington.edu

Med Clin N Am 98 (2014) 445–485
http://dx.doi.org/10.1016/j.mcna.2014.01.005
0025-7125/14/$ – see front matter © 2014 Elsevier Inc. All rights reserved.

Dermatologic diseases can all be thought of as perturbations of the components of these 3 layers of cells and structures. Loss of the barrier function, exuberant inflammation or autoinflammation, aberrant neurologic signals, infection, or metabolic disruptions in normal function account for virtually all of the more than 3000 dermatologic diagnoses. Identifying the specific causes can be challenging, and the causes of many dermatologic diseases remain unknown. Many diseases can appear similar to each other, and it is common for skin diseases to present uncommonly. Traditional texts and atlases of dermatology often present only 1 or 2 images of any skin disease, whereas newer Internet-based sources can produce hundreds of images of a single diagnosis to allow a better appreciation of how a disease can vary in its presentation. However, trying to match a patient's skin to a picture or set of pictures can be time consuming and prone to error.

This review attempts to approach the subject as a clinician would: exploring the differential diagnosis for common complaints. The authors start with the hair and briefly describe how to approach the patient with hair loss to reach a diagnosis. Next, the 4 most common causes of hair loss, namely androgenetic alopecia, female pattern hair loss (FPHL), alopecia areata (AA), and telogen effluvium (TE), are discussed in depth. The discussion then turns to the patient with a facial rash. Differentiation of acne vulgaris from rosacea, periorificial dermatitis, and seborrheic dermatitis is covered, as is differentiation of erysipelas and cellulitis, and the malar rash of systemic lupus erythematosus (SLE). Axillary and inguinal rashes are presented in the section on intertriginous rash, and include candidal intertrigo, tinea, erythrasma, inverse psoriasis, and the common frictional and irritant contact dermatitis referred to as intertrigo. Finally, the authors provide quick and reliable signs and symptoms to differentiate infectious causes of an edematous red leg that may require immediate antibiotics or admission from subacute mimics such as contact and stasis dermatitis. A brief discussion of deep vein thrombosis (DVT) is also included.

ALOPECIA

One of the more common dermatologic complaints seen by dermatologists and primary care physicians alike is alopecia or hair loss. The term alopecia is usually used to refer to loss of hairs at the follicle, although often patients will complain of hair loss that is in fact due to breakage of the hair shaft resulting from congenital or acquired causes of hair-shaft fragility instead of true loss of the entire hair. These entities are usually easily differentiated by an initial examination of the scalp and a hair-pull test. The hair-pull test is done by grasping hairs within approximately 1 cm^2 of scalp and pulling firmly between the thumb and forefinger (violent pulling such as with the aid of a clamp is not recommended); more than 5 hairs per location is considered abnormal. Examination of the ends of the hair can further differentiate between broken hairs that will end abruptly or hairs that have come from the follicle and will have some remnant of a follicle. Normally only resting telogen or "club" hairs can be pulled, which have a small spherical follicular remnant at the end. Actively growing anagen hairs will keep part of the root sheath, which appears like a sheath on the end of the hair (**Fig. 1**). Anagen hairs should never normally be released with a firm pull unless there is an underlying disease process.

The potential causes of alopecia are many (**Table 1**), but the differential diagnoses can be focused by an examination of the scalp to determine if there is evidence of scarring or inflammation. Unlike some mammals that can regenerate the pilosebaceous unit, human hair follicles never regenerate if destroyed. Scarring can be subtle in early stages, but close examination shows a complete loss of the follicular os and

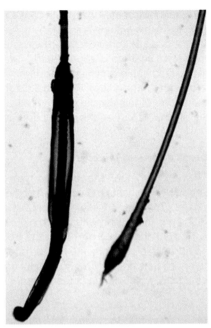

Fig. 1. Hair-shaft examination from hair-pull test. Note the anagen hair (*left*) has an attached rumpled inner root sheath still attached while the telogen hair (*right*) is often referred to as a club hair because of its shape and lack of attached root sheath. (*From* James WD, Berger TG, Elston DM. Andrews' diseases of the skin: clinical dermatology. Philadelphia: Elsevier/Saunders; 2011; with permission.)

Table 1
Classification of alopecia diagnoses based on clinical findings

	Scarring	Nonscarring
Inflammatory	Lupus erythematosus (discoid or subacute cutaneous) Lichen planopilaris Frontal fibrosing alopecia Chronic suppurative folliculitis Folliculitis decalvans Dissecting cellulitis of the scalp Sarcoidosis Favus Acne keloidalis nuchae	Alopecia areata (early lesions) Tinea capitis (can scar if very inflammatory, a "kerion") Syphilis Early lupus
Noninflammatory	Central centrifugal scarring alopecia (follicular degeneration syndrome) Pseudopelade Inactive "burnt-out" scarring alopecia Scleroderma	Androgenetic alopecia Female pattern hair loss Alopecia areata Telogen effluvium Trichotillomania Traction alopecia Metabolic causes (thyroid, dietary deficiencies or excesses, etc) Medications Alopecia neoplastica Congenital triangular alopecia

replacement with smooth epidermis, occasionally with "doll's hairs" clustering of multiple hairs through a single os. As this change is permanent, scarring alopecia must be treated quickly to stabilize the disease and prevent further loss. Referral to a dermatologist is strongly recommended if scarring is appreciated.

The presence of erythema and scale is clinically apparent in many causes of alopecia, and can be used to further narrow the differential diagnoses. A full discussion of alopecia is beyond the scope of this article; however, the 3 most common diagnoses are covered here, all of which are nonscarring and usually noninflammatory (**Table 2**).

Androgenetic Alopecia/Female Pattern Hair Loss

Male pattern baldness is very common, although the term androgenetic alopecia (AGA) is preferred, as it correctly suggests the causes as being androgen dependent and genetically predisposed. There is an estimated prevalence of nearly 50% in Caucasian men by age 50 years, increasing with age to plateau at about 80% prevalence in those older than 70, such that a lack of AGA in the elderly may be considered the abnormal state.[3] An androgenic cause for AGA was recognized early as it is not found in eunuchs lacking androgens, in those without functional androgen receptors, or in those lacking 5α-reductase, which converts testosterone to dihydrotestosterone

Table 2 Differential diagnoses for alopecias		
Condition	**History/Demographics/Risk Factors**	**Physical Examination Findings**
Androgenetic alopecia	Common in males (about 50% by age 50), usually with a family history May occur in women because of hyperandrogenism Asymptomatic and slowly progressive, usually no shedding Associated with metabolic syndrome and cardiovascular disease	Bitemporal or vertex thinning that may progress to total crown alopecia Miniaturization of hairs present
Female pattern hair loss	Occurs in women, usually with a family history Hormonal influence is unclear Asymptomatic and slowly progressive, usually no shedding Associated with metabolic syndrome and cardiovascular disease	Crown diffusely thins without preference to temples or vertex, but does not appear totally bald as in advanced AGA Miniaturization of hairs present
Alopecia areata	Occurs in children and adults Associated with other autoimmune diseases such as thyroid disease or vitiligo Usually self-resolving but can progress	Circular patches of complete alopecia Spares white hairs initially Exclamation-point hairs often present
Telogen effluvium	More common in women Usually asymptomatic shedding of hair with abrupt onset several months after a trigger Triggers include childbirth, significant physical or psychological stress, or dietary changes Usually resolves spontaneously within months but can be chronic	Diffuse shedding of scalp hairs that does not spare the parietal and occipital areas Hair-pull test positive for telogen club hairs

(DHT), the androgen most directly responsible for AGA. It is odd that DHT causes follicular miniaturization only in AGA-susceptible follicles on the crown, while the same hormone is responsible for development of secondary sexual hair in the axilla, groin, chest, back, and face. Transplantation of uninvolved follicles from the occiput to the crown results in hairs that do not undergo miniaturization, which is why hair transplants for AGA can be successful.

FPHL is also much more common than is generally believed, with a prevalence of 20% to 30% by age 50 years although, like AGA, it can start in the 20s.[3,4] Though still controversial, a hormonal basis for FPHL has been more difficult to establish, hence the separate diagnostic term for the similar process in women. Although increased androgen levels can induce FPHL, androgen levels are not abnormal in most women with FPHL, nor do most have other evidence of androgen excess such as hirsutism or irregular menses.[5,6] Antiandrogens are sometimes successful in treatment, however, suggesting a role in the etiopathogenesis of FPHL.

Genetics also play a strong role, but AGA and FPHL are likely polygenic and not well characterized. Not surprisingly, most candidate genes are involved in the production or binding of testosterone and DHT. Most commonly there is a family history of AGA, but phenotypic variation in families and variable penetrance owing to this likely polygenic inheritance often results in a patient feeling they are the "only one in the family" to be so affected, and should not be used as a reason to dismiss the diagnosis.[7]

Contrary to popular belief and the clinical appearance, individuals with AGA do not have true alopecia but rather miniaturization of the affected hairs. In affected pilosebaceous units of AGA and FPHL, the hair-follicle growth phase, anagen, shortens drastically, resulting in miniaturized hairs appearing on the scalp, with thinner shafts, much shorter length (sometimes too short to reach the follicular os), and often a lighter color, giving the appearance of no hair at all.[7] Patterns in AGA and FPHL are similar but distinctly different (**Fig. 2**). AGA results in initial bitemporal recession of the frontal hairline or vertex thinning, often developing into complete apparent loss of the hair on the crown, but completely spares the horseshoe distribution of the inferior parietal and occipital scalp.[3] By contrast, FPHL results in a more uniform apparent thinning of the entire crown owing to miniaturization of many, but not all of the hairs in the involved area. FPHL shares the same horseshoe distribution as in male AGA. Comparison of part width on the crown to the sides or occiput can be helpful in early cases of FPHL.[4,8]

More recently, associations of AGA and FPHL with other comorbid diseases have become apparent. Metabolic syndrome is highly correlated with both AGA and FPHL (odds ratio = 10.5 and 10.7, respectively) as well as the presence of atherosclerotic plaques and cardiovascular disease in males with AGA and possibly in women with FPHL, although this is less established.[9] The mechanisms by which these associations may occur are still unclear.

Though less common, conditions of androgen excess can also result in AGA or FPHL. In women, androgen excess should be suspected if alopecia is of a more male pattern and is accompanied by hirsutism, deepening of the voice, clitoral enlargement, hormonal acne, or irregular menses. Clinical or laboratory assessment for polycystic ovarian syndrome, congenital adrenal hyperplasia, or an androgen-secreting tumor should be considered in these cases. Sudden-onset AGA or FPHL in either sex should also prompt consideration of such tumors.[8]

Diagnosis is by recognition of the common pattern of involvement and the presence of miniaturized hairs on close inspection, often with the aid of magnification. Eliciting a history of effluvium (hair shedding) rather than simply slow apparent disappearance of hair is important, as other causes of alopecia will unmask AGA or FPHL, leading to a similar initial appearance. For example, a person with previously subclinical

A

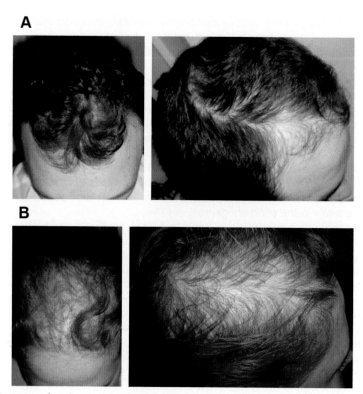

B

Fig. 2. Patterns of androgenetic alopecia (AGA) and female pattern hair loss (FPHL). Note the bitemporal and vertex predominance of alopecia in AGA (*A*), whereas FPHL is associated with generalized thinning in the entire crown (*B*). (*From* Restrepo R, Calonje E. Diseases of the hair. In: Calonje E, Bremm T, Lazar AJ, et al, editors. McKee's pathology of the skin. Philadelphia: Saunders; 2012. p. 967–1050; with permission.)

FPHL who has their patterned alopecia unmasked only when 10% of the entire scalp hair is lost for an unrelated reason may appear clinically to have FPHL until a hair-pull test shows effluvium from all areas of the scalp.

Any discussion of treatment should include acceptance, as AGA and FPHL are common. Techniques to disguise the appearance without actively altering the disease are also important, alone or in combination with medical therapy, including the "comb-over," aerosolized powders or fibers to coat remaining hairs making them appear thicker, volumizing shampoos, artificial hairpieces, or hair transplantation.

There are several medical treatments in common use for AGA and FPHL, but it must be stressed at the time of initiation that none are a cure but rather are treatments that must be continued, or reversion to the initial state will occur.

Minoxidil is an antihypertensive medication that results in generalized hypertrichosis by an unknown mechanism if taken orally, but is much more commonly used as a topical preparation to encourage growth of hairs with thicker diameter and length. It is relatively inexpensive, is available without a prescription in the United States, and has a favorable side-effect profile in both men and women. The most common side effect is local irritation caused by propylene glycol in the solution formulation, but this is absent in the foam.[10] As minoxidil lowers blood pressure when taken orally, topical application can be associated with compensatory symptoms (eg, tachycardia, presyncopal symptoms), but in blinded trials hypotension occurs at the same rate as in the vehicle.[10] Accidental application to other areas can result in localized hypertrichosis, but discontinuation usually normalizes this. When compared with twice-daily 5% solution, the 2% solution applied twice a day has a lower incidence of side effects, as does the once-daily application of 5% solution, though both at the expense of lesser efficacy.[11,12] A temporary effluvium 1 to 3 months after initiation is common, as many follicles in telogen are stimulated to enter anagen, resulting in an effluvium of the hair shafts already residing in those follicles when treatment is begun. Educating patients to expect this paradoxic sign of medication efficacy will help adherence and prevent panicked phone calls. It will then take another few months for the new hairs to grow long enough that the hair appears denser.

Antiandrogens such as finasteride, spironolactone, flutamide, and cyproterone are also often used for AGA and FPHL, although finasteride is the only medicine approved by the Food and Drug Administration (FDA) for this indication, and only in males. Finasteride is a type II 5α-reductase inhibitor, resulting in less conversion of testosterone to DHT. Finasteride is available in the United States as a 1-mg once-daily treatment of AGA in males, although often for cost-saving reasons it is prescribed as one-quarter tablet once daily of the 5-mg dose (resulting in a 1.25-mg final dose) produced to treat prostate disease. In a double-blind, placebo-controlled crossover study, hair count, patient self-assessment, and investigator assessment were significantly greater in the treatment cohorts. The most significant side effects are sexual, with decreased libido, erectile dysfunction, or decreased ejaculate volume.[13] A recent meta-analysis of 12 studies of finasteride in men showed that patient self-report of improvement with long-term use was significantly more favorable than with placebo (relative risk [RR] = 1.71, 95% confidence interval [CI] 1.15–2.53) with a number needed to treat of 3.4. Interestingly the relative risk of sexual side effects was actually higher than that for hair growth (RR = 2.22, 95% CI 1.03–4.78), although this complaint was uncommon even in placebo, so the number needed to harm was 82.1 and the number who discontinued the medication because of sexual side effects when compared with placebo was not significant.[14] Recent concern in the lay press arose after a publication describing persisting sexual side effects in 71 men after discontinuation of finasteride; however, this descriptive case series was not part of a larger cohort, so an incidence estimate cannot be made. In addition, men never on finasteride complain of sexual side effects, so without a placebo group, causation by finasteride has yet to be established.[15]

Initially there was concern that use of finasteride may delay early detection of prostate cancer, and early studies suggested an increased incidence of high-grade malignancies in those taking the 5-mg dose, prompting an FDA warning. However, subsequent analysis shows it is associated with a nearly 30% reduction in low-grade prostate cancer, with no effect on high-grade prostate cancer.[16] Dutasteride is a similar inhibitor of both type I and type II 5α-reductase and has also shown efficacy in AGA without significant adverse events when compared with placebo, although admittedly in a relatively small study.[17] Use in AGA or FPHL is currently off-label. Finasteride and dutasteride are not recommended in women of child-bearing potential given the high risk of hormone-related birth defects, and are FDA pregnancy category X. Use in postmenopausal women to treat FPHL has been mixed.[18]

Other antiandrogens are not typically used in males owing to the risk of feminization, although they are used in FPHL. Well-designed studies examining effectiveness of antiandrogens in FPHL have been lacking thus far to allow firm conclusions as to their effectiveness, but small case series sometimes support their use.[19] A recent Cochrane review of hormonal and nonhormonal treatments found minoxidil was the only medication for which evidence of treatment effect could be demonstrated in FPHL, possibly in part due to this lack of studies. Though used sometimes in FPHL, flutamide use is often limited because of concerns about hepatotoxicity, and cyproterone is not available in the United States. On the contrary, spironolactone is commonly used off-label to treat hormonal acne, hirsutism, and FPHL in doses from 50 to 200 mg daily.[8] Spironolactone both decreases testosterone production and competitively blocks the androgen receptor. Hypotension and hyperkalemia can occur, but with normal renal function these are uncommon. At higher doses, irregular menses and breast tenderness occur, although this can often be mitigated by concurrent use of oral contraceptive pills.[8,18] As expected by its effect on androgen activity, spironolactone is contraindicated in pregnancy. An FDA warning was issued because of an increased risk of malignancy based on animal studies, but it is unclear as to whether this is relevant in humans. A large retrospective matched cohort study of more than 1 million women aged 55 years and older showed no increased incidence of breast cancer in those who took spironolactone,[20] but no such studies have been done in premenopausal women who might be expected take the medication for years.

Alopecia Areata

AA is the most common inflammatory cause of alopecia, with an estimated prevalence of approximately 0.1%, while the lifetime risk approaches 2% based on those seeking medical attention. It is perhaps slightly more common in children than in adults.[21,22] Its course is unpredictable, but typically self-resolving, so patients are often told that treatment is not necessary, and it is often viewed as strictly a cosmetic problem. However, its sudden onset and apparently random patchy areas can be very distressing to patients.

AA is an autoimmune process that appears to be a result of, or is associated with, loss of the immunologically privileged site of the hair bulb where pigment is produced. There is a predominantly T-cell rich infiltrate at the hair bulb that results in cessation of hair-shaft production but, importantly, it does not scar or permanently damage the follicle itself.[22]

Most commonly, patients complain of 1 or a few patches of complete hair loss overlying otherwise normal skin while the rest of the scalp is unaffected (**Fig. 3**A). Early in its course, the involved skin can be subtly pink but not scaly. The beard is commonly affected in men, while involvement of the body hair without concomitant scalp involvement is either uncommon or uncommonly comes to medical attention.[23] It is usually otherwise asymptomatic, and many people are unaware of the condition until a hairdresser or relative points it out. Areas of involvement start as a circular patch of near complete alopecia that gradually increases in diameter, often growing back centrally as it continues to expand peripherally. Often at the periphery of these patches are exclamation-point hairs, which are short hairs (<1 cm) named for the characteristic tapering diameter as they approach the follicular ostia (see **Fig. 3**B).[23] New patches in other areas of the scalp may also occur and sometimes coalesce. Like another common autoimmune pigmentary disease, vitiligo, it mysteriously affects small areas of skin that enlarge rather than being generalized in most cases. Like vitiligo, it can often wax and wane in its course. There is often a history of white hairs growing back during recovery, even in patients without normal graying. Similarly, in those with graying hair the already white hairs are usually spared initially while the darker hairs fall out, leading to the myth of people's hair turning white overnight when diffuse involvement occurs. It is the only type of alopecia that preferentially spares white hairs, so this is a pathognomonic finding. More extensive (and less responsive) patterns are uncommon and include the ophiasis pattern (loss of all but the crown), the sisaipho pattern (loss of

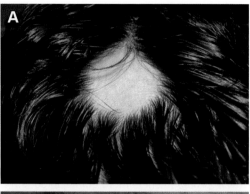

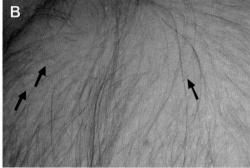

Fig. 3. Alopecia areata. Note the isolated area of smooth alopecia with trace pink to peach-colored erythema of acute alopecia areata in (*A*) and the exclamation-point hairs (*arrows*) in (*B*). ([*A*] *Data from* Restrepo R, Calonje E. Diseases of the hair. In: Calonje E, Bremm T, Lazar AJ, et al, editors. McKee's pathology of the skin. Philadelphia: Saunders; 2012. p. 967–1050; with permission; and [*B*] *Adapted from* Sperling LC, Sinclair RD, Shabrawi-Caelen LE. Alopecias. In: Bolognia JL, Jorizzo JL, Schaffer JV, editors. Dermatology. 3rd edition. Philadelphia: Elsevier/Saunders; 2012; with permission.)

the crown only), AA totalis (loss of all scalp hair sparing the face and body), or AA universalis (loss of all scalp, facial, and body hair).[23]

Diagnosis is by recognition of the common circular patterns without scaliness or scarring of the underlying skin, presence of exclamation-point hairs, and apparent sparing or regrowth of white hairs. The differential diagnosis includes secondary syphilis, SLE, tinea capitis, and trichotillomania when localized and nonscarring patches are seen. When diffuse, the differential includes trichotillomania, telogen effluvium (see later discussion), and metabolic or drug-induced causes, and can be more difficult to diagnose without biopsy. Hair-pull tests are often positive near involved skin and will show anagen hairs, which are otherwise not a normal finding.

AA affects only the hair, nails, and rarely the eyes, without any other systemic manifestations. Comorbid conditions include thyroid disease in 8% to 28% of patients as well as, less commonly, vitiligo, lupus, atopy, and other autoimmune conditions.[23,24] A review of systems should be done to evaluate for these, although testing is not typically cost-effective in the absence of symptoms as they are not thought to be causal or temporally associated.[25]

Treatment can consist of the "tincture of time," as approximately 80% of cases spontaneously resolve within a year, although resolution is less common in extensive disease.[25] Providing information as to what to expect by directing patients to resources such as the National Alopecia Areata Foundation (www.naaf.org) can be as valuable as any treatment offered. Localized involvement often responds fairly well to topical or intralesional corticosteroids. High-potency topical corticosteroids are effective in approximately 25% of patients but can take up to 6 months to see regrowth, while monthly intralesional injection (usually triamcinolone) throughout affected patches into the deep dermis (to the base of the follicles) allows for more rapid regrowth, although both treatments need to continue until the disease has run its course.[22,23] Aside from steroid atrophy and folliculitis, these are very safe options. When atrophy is seen and treatment is halted, it usually will resolve; if appropriately informed, many patients will tolerate mild atrophy if it occurs under a blanket of regrown hair. In more widespread disease, use of contact immunotherapy by application of a contact dermatitis sensitizer to involved skin will also allow regrowth, but referral to a dermatologist is recommended for this approach, as it is more complicated and can result in severe allergic or irritant contact dermatitis even in experienced hands. There is also a role for minoxidil as an adjunct topical therapy with any of the aforementioned treatments. Aside from systemic steroids, whose chronic use is not recommended for the months to years of expected disease, systemic agents have been disappointingly ineffective in most cases.[22,23,25]

Telogen Effluvium

TE is a very common, usually temporary, shedding (effluvium) of hairs of the telogen-phase hair follicles. It is much more common in women than in men, and is the most common cause of effluvium in adult women.[26,27] It usually starts abruptly, causing significant concern to the patient. Hair is easily pulled out at the root and patients will describe it collecting in their beds, on their brushes or combs, or in the shower drain. A decreased thickness of the ponytail is also a common complaint, as is a pile of shed hair offered to the provider as proof of a problem.[26,28] Hair is lost uniformly throughout the scalp rather than in discrete circles as in AA, or just from the crown as in FPHL or AGA. As preexisting FPHL and AGA are common in the population, however, TE may unmask clinically subtle cases, resulting in a generalized effluvium that leaves the crown, vertex, or temples apparently more affected, as discussed in the section on AGA/FPHL.[26]

The hair-follicle cycle is composed of a growth phase (anagen), an involution phase (catagen), and a resting phase (telogen), which occurs asynchronously among the 100,000 or so hair follicles on the scalp. After completing the telogen phase, the hair cycle restarts and produces a new anagen hair, releasing the old club telogen hair currently occupying that follicle. After a triggering event, an increased number of hairs leave anagen phase and enter catagen and then telogen phase in synchrony (anagen release), resulting in a sharp increase in shedding of club hairs approximately 3 months later as telogen ends.[26,27,29]

Common triggers include childbirth (postpartum effluvium or telogen gravidarum), or any significant physical or emotional trigger such as trauma, major surgery, strict diets, or emotional stress such as divorce or death of a loved one. However, approximately one-third of cases have no identifiable trigger, making TE sometimes a diagnosis of exclusion.[28]

Diagnosis is by recognition of a generalized effluvium that is sudden in onset, generally after a clear trigger. A hair-pull test will produce club hairs and will be positive in all areas of the scalp examined, rather than just the crown or in discrete patches. A skin biopsy can help distinguish TE from a diffuse form of AA, or from FPHL, AGA, and other less common causes of alopecia. An increased proportion of telogen-phase hairs is seen by histology with lack of inflammation or scar, confirming the diagnosis.[28]

Treatment is reassurance that the patient will not lose all of the hair as the hairs are being pushed out by new ones growing in. TE is self-limited, so doing nothing is appropriate. Highly concerned patients can be instructed to collect and count all of their fallen hairs daily from the sources mentioned earlier and elsewhere in their environment. Patients can track the number of hairs and thus be reassured when it returns to a normal amount (about 50–100 hairs per day is a normal average number of hairs to shed).[29]

A chronic form of TE also exists whereby the condition persists for more than 6 months.[28] This form may result from a chronic systemic medical or emotional disease, essentially an ongoing trigger. Exclusion of reversible causes is of course required to treat this condition, although it is commonly idiopathic. Again, patients can be reassured that their hair is regrowing constantly and will not all be lost, but it may not be possible to predict when it may normalize if a trigger is not identified, and may often persist for years.[26]

FACIAL RASHES

Facial rash is a fairly common complaint in the primary care setting. Learning how to approach the evaluation of facial rashes is a valuable skill. This section discusses the common presentations of facial rashes and how to distinguish between clinical conditions, and discusses treatments for primary care providers to appropriately manage rashes and recognize clues to more severe illness that may require hospitalization or subspecialty management. The conditions addressed are acne vulgaris, acne rosacea, periorificial dermatitis, seborrheic dermatitis, erysipelas, cellulitis, and SLE (**Table 3**). In general, when evaluating a facial rash the first question to ask is whether the patient appears ill or complains of systemic symptoms. If the response is affirmative then erysipelas, cellulitis, or SLE moves to the top of the list.[30] When considering the rashes of acne vulgaris, acne rosacea, periorificial dermatitis, or seborrheic dermatitis, age of onset of symptoms may help narrow the differential. The presence of symptoms during adolescence suggests acne vulgaris, whereas acneiform conditions developing sometime after the age of 30 years are more likely to be acne rosacea. Finally, the distribution of the rash as well as its characteristics (acneiform, eczematous, comedonal, and so forth) will further aid in proper diagnosis.

Acne Vulgaris

Acne vulgaris is the most common skin condition affecting young adults. Estimates of prevalence rates range from 35% to 90% in adolescents.[31] Although most cases of acne vulgaris start in adolescence and resolve by the mid 20s, there is evidence that up to 50% of patients will have persistent symptoms into later adulthood.[32] It is important for the primary care provider to recognize that this is a chronic, inflammatory condition that significantly affects quality of life and often results is anxiety, depression, and social withdrawal. Acute treatment followed by maintenance therapy can improve dermatologic and quality-of-life outcomes.

Understanding the pathogenesis of acne vulgaris helps to differentiate this from other acneiform facial rashes. It starts with androgen-induced increased sebum production in the pilosebaceous unit followed by abnormal keratinization, which occludes the follicle and leads to the development of a microcomedone. Bacterial colonization of the hair follicle with *Propionibacterium acnes* triggers a host immune response, leading to the development of inflammatory lesions.[32,33] Understanding that the microcomedone is the base lesion for all types of acne vulgaris aids in the differentiation of acne vulgaris from acne rosacea and periorificial dermatitis, and

Table 3
Differential diagnoses for facial rashes

Condition	History/Demographics/Risk Factors	Physical Examination Findings
Acne vulgaris	Starts in adolescence	Comedones (whiteheads or blackheads) should always be present Inflammatory papules
Acne rosacea	Tends to present between ages 30 and 60 y More common in light-skinned individuals or Celtic or Northern European descent	Flushing Nontransient erythema Telangiectasias Inflammatory papules No comedones Sebaceous gland hypertrophy
Periorificial dermatitis	More common in women ages 16–45 y History of topical or inhaled corticosteroid exposure	1–2 mm clustered erythematous papules, papulovesicles or papulopustules with or without mild scale Located around mouth and/or the eyes Spares the vermillion border
Seborrheic dermatitis	Peak incidence third to fourth decades Human immunodeficiency virus (HIV) associated with severe cases of seborrheic dermatitis	Greasy-looking, yellowish or erythematous scale affecting scalp, nasal ala, eyebrows, glabella, nasolabial fold
Erysipelas	Often complain of fevers and chills	Well-demarcated, shiny, erythematous, painful plaque with associated swelling and perifollicular edema
Systemic lupus erythematosus	Indolent and intermittent presentation of rash Most often affects young African American women	Flat or raised Painful or pruritic No comedones, papules, or pustules Triggered by sun exposure Butterfly pattern sparing the upper lip and nasolabial fold. The nose acts as a sun shade to these areas

also helps explain why keratinolytics are necessary in the treatment of all types of acne vulgaris (comedonal and inflammatory). When evaluating a patient with acneiform lesions of the face, the most important thing to look for is the presence of comedones (closed comedones are known as whiteheads, open comedones as blackheads) (**Fig. 4**). These lesions will be present in acne vulgaris but not in acne rosacea or periorificial dermatitis, as the microcomedone is not involved in the pathogenesis of the latter conditions. In addition to affecting the face, acne vulgaris can involve the back, chest, shoulders, and torso, which are the areas with the highest sebaceous gland activity.

Acne vulgaris can range in severity from mild comedonal, to inflammatory (**Fig. 5**), to severe nodulocystic (see **Fig. 5**; **Fig. 6**); however, addressing the issue of abnormal keratinization with a topical keratinolytic is mandatory for the management of this chronic condition regardless of the type of acne. Setting appropriate expectations for improvement is also important. Treatments for acne vulgaris do not address the lesions that are already present, but rather prevent the development of new lesions. It takes approximately 8 weeks for a microcomedone to mature, so patients should

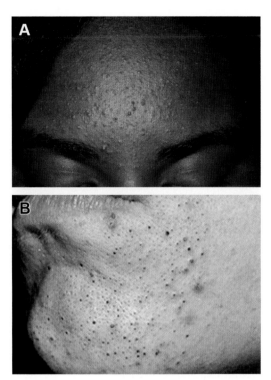

Fig. 4. Comedonal acne. Note the closed comedones in (*A*) and open comedones in (*B*), most of which are noninflammatory. ([*A*] *From* Brinster NK, Liu V, Diwan AH, et al. Dermatopathology: high-yield pathology. Philadelphia: Saunders; 2011; with permission; and [*B*] *From* Benner N, Sammons D. Overview of the treatment of acne vulgaris. Osteopathic Family Physician 2013;5(5):185–90; with permission.)

be advised that they may not see any improvement in their skin for several months. Topical keratinolytics are available over the counter or by prescription. Over-the-counter options include tea-tree oil, benzoyl peroxide, and salicylic acid. Prescription agents include topical retinoids and topical azeleic acid. Recent recommendations

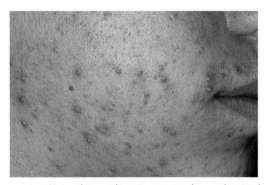

Fig. 5. Inflammatory acne. Note the erythematous papules and pustules. (*From* Habif TP, Campbell JL, Chapman MS. Skin disease: diagnosis and treatment. Philadelphia: Elsevier/ Saunders; 2011; with permission.)

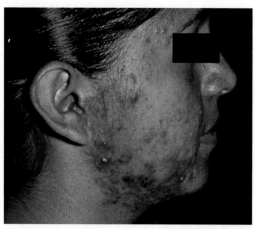

Fig. 6. Nodulocystic acne. Note the deeper papulonodules and cystic lesions along the jawline and scarring on the malar cheeks. (*From* Paller AS, Mancini AJ. Hurwitz clinical pediatric dermatology. Philadelphia: Elsevier/Saunders; 2011; with permission.)

from the Global Alliance Improve Outcomes in Acne Group recommend using topical retinoids as first-line agents when possible.[32] This recommendation is based on the fact that topical retinoids are more efficacious than the over-the-counter options or azeleic acid, and that topical retinoids also improve penetration of other topical agents such as antibiotics if they become necessary.

Topical retinoids should only be applied at night because they can be deactivated by light and increase the risk of photosensitivity. Side effects include redness, dry skin, peeling, and burning. Starting at a lower potency and working up to the highest potency tolerated will improve efficacy and decrease the risk of side effects. Warning patients that they may have a pustular flare on initiating treatment is also important, as adherence rates are likely to decrease if patients are unaware that their skin may worsen before it improves. Cost and side-effect profile will influence the choice of topical retinoid. The least expensive option is tretinoin (Retin-A, Atralin, and so forth), the most potent is tazarotene (Tazorac), and the least likely to irritate the skin is adapelene (Differin). If patients cannot afford or cannot tolerate a topical retinoid, one of the other over-the-counter or prescription options should be considered. Tea-tree oil, salicylic acid, and benzoyl peroxide are similarly efficacious for the treatment of comedonal acne. Benzoyl peroxide or tea-tree oil can also be used as a single agent for the treatment of inflammatory acne. Tea-tree oil is generally well tolerated but may cause an allergic contact dermatitis. Salicylic acid is useful in patients with sensitive skin. Benzoyl peroxide may bleach clothes, towels, and sheets, so patients should be warned to wash off the product entirely or make sure it is dry or fully rubbed into the skin so that clothes or bedding are not ruined. Linens and towels made with benzoyl peroxide–resistant dyes are also available. Azeleic acid (Azelex, Finacea) is a prescription agent that can be used as a single agent for comedonal or inflammatory acne. It is generally well tolerated in patients with sensitive skin, but is more costly. It has the potential of causing hypopigmentation of the skin, which may be beneficial in patients with postinflammatory hyperpigmentation.

If patients have primarily inflammatory acne, an antibiotic may need to be added to the keratinolytic. Recent evidence has demonstrated the development of *Propionibacterium acnes* antibiotic resistance; therefore, limiting the use of topical and oral antibiotics to patients who really need them and for the least amount of time possible is recommended.[32,34,35] Ideally antibiotics would be limited to 3 months of therapy. Evidence suggests that if antibiotics are needed for longer than 2 months, patients should also be started on topical benzoyl peroxide or azelaic acid to minimize the development of resistance at sites of application.[32,36] Benzoyl peroxide or azelaic acid can be applied continuously to prevent this resistance. In addition, oral and topical antibiotics should never be used as monotherapy for acne; they should always be combined with a keratinolytic.[35] Once a patient's inflammatory acne has improved, the antibiotics should be halted and the keratinolytic continued for maintenance therapy, with benzoyl peroxide or azelaic acid added for antimicrobial effect if needed.[32]

The latest studies suggest that anti-inflammatory action of antibiotics is the most likely mechanism in the treatment of acne vulgaris and acne rosacea.[36] With this information, the focus has shifted to using topical antibiotics or considering the use of sub–antimicrobial dose oral antibiotics. At this point, data demonstrate that sub–antimicrobial doses are effective in treating acne, but there is not enough known about whether these lower doses also decrease the risk of antibiotic resistance.[35] Topical antibiotic options include clindamycin, erythromycin, dapsone, or sulfur/sulfacetamide These products come alone or in some cases are combined with a retinoid or benzoyl peroxide, and studies have demonstrated that such combinations are more effective in the treatment of inflammatory acne than any of the agents used alone.[36] Clindamycin or dapsone topicals can be stored at room temperature. Erythromycin-containing products must be refrigerated. Topical dapsone 5% (Aczone) is a relatively new agent used in the treatment of acne. Despite its risk when used in the oral formulation, topical dapsone is safe in patients with glucose-6-phosphate dehydrogenase deficiency or sulfonamide allergies.[36,37] There have been no direct comparisons of topical dapsone with topical clindamycin or erythromycin. The cost of dapsone in comparison with these other agents likely outweighs any benefits of the product at present.

Oral antibiotics may be needed for moderate to severe inflammatory acne. Tetracyclines such as doxycycline or minocycline are mainstays of therapy. There is no difference in efficacy between these 2 antibiotics[36]; however, because of the side-effect profiles of both, doxycycline is generally recommended as the first-line agent. Side effects of doxycycline include gastrointestinal upset, pill esophagitis, and photosensitivity. Minocycline may cause vestibular symptoms, irreversible bluish-gray skin discoloration, and drug-induced lupus. Traditional dosing for both is 100 mg once or twice a day; however, there may be future recommendations for sub–antimicrobial dosing regimens such as 20 mg twice a day. There are variations in brand name, which are enteric coated (Doryx) or extended release (Oracea or Solodyn). For those who are allergic to tetracyclines, the macrolide azithromycin may be an option. Randomized controlled trials comparing azithromycin with doxycycline, minocycline, and tetracycline demonstrate that it is at least equally effective and in some cases even more effective.[36] In these studies azithromycin was dosed in some form of pulsed dosed therapy. However, a recommended dosing regimen has yet to be determined. (Usual dosing options: 500 mg 3 times per week for 1 month followed by 500 mg twice weekly for 1 month, followed by once weekly for 1 month; or 500 mg on the first day followed by 4 consecutive days of 250 mg, repeated on the 1st and 15th of every month.)[36] Azithromycin is a safe option during pregnancy and breastfeeding, whereas all the tetracyclines are contraindicated. Not enough data exist to determine whether cephalosporins or fluoroquinolones are effective in the treatment of acne.[36] Finally, patients with moderate acne who do not respond to other therapies or those with severe/nodulocystic acne should be referred to Dermatology to discuss treatment with oral isotretinoin (formerly known by the brand Accutane).

Acne Rosacea

Like acne vulgaris, acne rosacea is a chronic inflammatory disorder with periods of exacerbation and remission. Unlike acne vulgaris, it tends to present in the 30s to 60s rather than during adolescence.[38] It most commonly affects light-skinned individuals of Celtic and Northern European descent. Rosacea can affect the central face, nose, cheeks, eyelids, forehead, and chin. Symptoms include flushing, nontransient erythema, telangiectasias, papules, pustules, nodules, cysts, or sebaceous gland hypertrophy (eg, rhinophyma) (**Fig. 7**). A patient may have any one of these findings or a combination, and symptoms can range from mild to severe. Ocular involvement with blepharitis or conjunctivitis is present in more than 50% of patients, and may be found in the absence of other skin manifestations of rosacea.[38] To differentiate rosacea from acne vulgaris one should look for the presence of comedones; acne vulgaris will have comedones whereas rosacea will not. The pathogenesis of rosacea is not well understood but seems to be a combination of factors including abnormalities in innate immunity, inflammatory reactions to cutaneous microorganisms, ultraviolet damage, and vascular dysfunction. Advising patients to avoid excessive sun exposure is important, as is setting clear expectations for the benefits of therapy. Topical and oral therapies work well for papules and pustules, but less so or not at all for flushing, redness, or telangiectasias. It may take 2 to 3 months before one sees any benefit from therapy, and because this is a chronic condition maintenance therapy is recommended.

Randomized controlled trials demonstrate equal efficacy for topical metronidazole 0.75% to 1% and azeleic acid 15% to 20%, although topical metronidazole is better tolerated and less expensive.[39] Other options include topical sulfacetamide 10%/sulfur 5% or combination benzoyl peroxide/clindamycin; however, the data for efficacy are less robust. Data supporting the use of monotherapy with topical clindamycin or erythromycin are limited, and because of the potential risk of antibiotic resistance should be avoided.[36] Only one small study of 50 patients evaluated the topical retinoid adapalene in comparison with topical metronidazole. Adapalene was better at reducing inflammatory lesions, although the metronidazole-treated patients had less erythema. There was no difference in the scores for erythema or telangiectasia.[40]

Oral antibiotic therapies are similar to those used in the treatment of acne vulgaris, and include doxycycline, minocycline, and tetracycline. Oral antibiotics should be considered in patients with moderate to severe rosacea, ocular rosacea, and in those not responding to topical therapies. Whether traditional dosing versus sub-antimicrobial dosing should be used is not yet clear. The only systemic FDA-approved therapy for rosacea is once-daily sub–antimicrobial dose doxycycline (Oracea). Two double-blind, randomized, placebo-controlled trials demonstrated an average 61% reduction in inflammatory lesions, compared with 29% with placebo.[36] Again, duration of use of antibiotics should be limited to the shortest time course possible. A few studies demonstrate added benefit when combining oral antibiotics with topical metronidazole.[41,42] Maintenance therapy with a topical agent such as metronidazole or azeleic acid should be continued long term. The efficacy of oral isotretinoin in the treatment of rosacea has not been well established, but referral to Dermatology should be considered for patients with moderate to severe disease or the development of focal enlargement resulting from sebaceous gland hypertrophy (eg, rhinophyma) in an attempt to prevent poor cosmetic outcomes.

Unfortunately there are few pharmacologic options for the treatment of flushing. A variety of agents have been tried, including clonidine, β-blockers, antidepressants, gabapentin, topical oxymetazoline, and the newly approved topical brimonidine gel, but the data are limited and the side-effect risks are significant. Avoidance of triggers

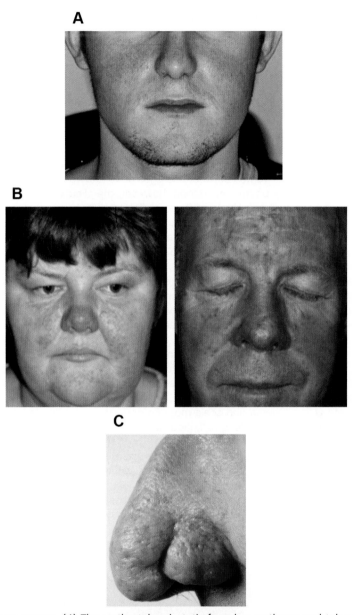

Fig. 7. Acne rosacea. (*A*) The erythrotelangiectatic form has erythema and telangiectasias predominantly on the malar cheeks and nose. (*B*) The papulopustular form has inflammatory lesions in this area as well as the forehead and chin. (*C*) The phymatous form results in glandular enlargement of tissue, most commonly on the nose (rhinophyma). ([*A*] *From* James WD, Berger TG, Elston DM. Andrews' diseases of the skin: clinical dermatology. Philadelphia: Elsevier/Saunders; 2011; with permission; [*B, left*] *From* Wollina, U. Rosacea and rhinophyma in the elderly. Clin Dermatol 2011;29(1):61–8; with permission; [*B, right*] *From* Habif TP. Clinical dermatology: a color guide to diagnosis and therapy. 5th edition. Philadelphia: Elsevier; 2010; with permission; and [*C*] *From* Powell F, Raghallaigh SN. Rosacea and related disorders. In: Bolognia JL, Jorizzo JL, Schaffer JV, editors. Dermatology. 3rd edition. Philadelphia: Elsevier/Saunders; 2012. p. 561–9; with permission.)

such as extremes of temperature, sunlight, spicy foods, and alcohol may be effective, but difficult to adhere to in most cases. Referral to Dermatology for pulsed-light therapy and laser therapy can be considered for the treatment of telangiectasias and nontransient erythema.[43]

Periorificial Dermatitis

Periorificial dermatitis, also called perioral dermatitis, typically presents with multiple small inflammatory papules around the mouth, nose, or eyes. Although the name suggests that the condition may have an eczematous appearance, it most closely resembles an acneiform or rosacea-like eruption with or without eczematous features. This condition can occur in individuals of all ethnic and racial backgrounds, with more than 90% of cases affecting women between the ages of 16 and 45 years.[44,45] Pathogenesis of this condition is poorly understood; however, the clinical and histologic features of the lesions resemble those of rosacea. Exposure to external elements likely triggers these lesions, the strongest association being with topical or inhaled corticosteroids. Other triggers may include fluorinated toothpastes, heavy face creams and moisturizers, especially those with a petrolatum or paraffin base, and certain cosmetics such as lipsticks.[44]

The classic patient history may describe a mild papular or slightly scaly facial rash that initially improves with topical corticosteroid use, but either recurs or worsens with continued use or attempts to discontinue corticosteroid therapy. Periorificial dermatitis manifests with 1- to 2-mm clustered erythematous papules, papulovesicles, or papulopustules with or without mild scale. It most often affects the perioral region, but can also involve the nasolabial fold and area around the eyes or eyelids. The absence of comedones will rule out acne vulgaris. The presence of vermillion border sparing (a clear zone of 3–5 mm near the edge of the lip) around the perioral region argues for periorificial dermatitis and against acne rosacea (**Fig. 8**). Seborrheic dermatitis presents with erythema and scale most commonly around the nasal ala, scalp, eyebrows, and nasolabial folds. Small papules are not a feature of seborrheic dermatitis, nor is a perioral distribution.

The most important intervention is to stop the use of the inciting agent. Periorificial dermatitis may resolve on its own without therapy within a few months if topical corticosteroids or other triggers can be eliminated. Most patients will request therapy, however, as the initial flare of their rash can be distressing once the steroids or other triggers are stopped. Tapering from a higher-potency steroid to a lower-potency

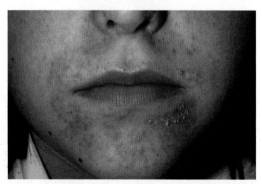

Fig. 8. Periorificial dermatitis. Note the papules surrounding an area of sparing around the vermillion border of the perioral area. (*From* Habif TP. Clinical dermatology: a color guide to diagnosis and therapy. 5th edition. Philadelphia: Elsevier; 2010; with permission.)

steroid such as hydrocortisone 1% over a few months, and then discontinuing entirely, may reduce the likelihood of a significant flare, but this approach has not been well studied.[45] For mild to moderate cases, topical calcineurin inhibitors (pimecrolimus or tacrolimus) should be considered. Most of the placebo-controlled randomized trial data support the use of pimecrolimus 1% cream twice a day, with most benefit shown in the first few weeks of therapy.[46,47] Therapy should continue for about 4 weeks, then be either discontinued if effective or changed to a different therapy if ineffective. The data supporting the use of topical antibiotics such as erythromycin or metronidazole are limited, but if cost is an issue with pimecrolimus it might be worth trying one of these agents for up to 8 weeks for mild to moderate cases.

The use of an oral tetracycline has also demonstrated efficacy in small, randomized controlled trials. One trial of 120 patients comparing placebo with oral tetracycline 500 mg twice daily × 10 days then 250 mg twice daily × 10 days or topical erythromycin 1% demonstrated similar increased rates of improvement in the oral tetracycline and topical erythromycin groups compared with placebo.[48] Another multicenter randomized trial of 108 patients compared oral tetracycline 250 mg twice daily with twice-daily application of metronidazole 1% cream for 8 weeks.[49] Both groups showed improvement in lesion counts, although the oral antibiotic group improved faster. There are no studies examining the efficacy of doxycycline or minocycline; however, these regimens are often tried for 8 weeks because of their advantage of fewer restrictions on timing of administration. Small, uncontrolled studies or case reports have shown some benefit with azeleic acid 20% cream, topical tetracycline, topical adapalene 0.1% gel, topical clindamycin with or without hydrocortisone 1%, and topical sulfacetamide-sulfur plus oral tetracycline.

Seborrheic Dermatitis

Erythema accompanied by greasy-looking, yellowish scale in the eyebrows, glabella, lateral nasal areas, and nasolabial folds is characteristic of seborrheic dermatitis (**Fig. 9**). The mustache and beard (if present), scalp, external ear canals, chest, axilla, and groin may also be affected. Seborrheic dermatitis may begin in infancy (cradle cap) but typically resolves, often recurring later in life with the peak incidence during the third and fourth decades of life. Most individuals are healthy; however, there is a relationship between human immunodeficiency virus (HIV) infection and seborrheic dermatitis, with 35% of early HIV patients and up to 85% of patients with AIDS affected. Severe seborrheic dermatitis is more common with advancing HIV disease. If a patient presents with severe seborrheic dermatitis and risk factors for HIV infection, screening for HIV is appropriate.[50,51] Other causes of immunosuppression such as lymphoma, or neurologic conditions such as Parkinson disease or unilateral involvement after a cerebrovascular accident, can occur as well. The cause of seborrheic dermatitis is unknown but is likely related to overgrowth of *Malassezia* species that thrive on the oils in sebum, possibly explaining why areas rich in sebaceous gland activity are predisposed to this condition. Seborrheic dermatitis can mimic rosacea, but rosacea is associated with telangiectasias and papulopustular lesions, has minimal or no scale, and more often affects the nose, malar, and perioral regions. However, seborrheic dermatitis and rosacea often occur concurrently.

Seborrheic dermatitis is a chronic, relapsing condition that flares with psychological stress, changes in weather, or lack of regular shampooing; therefore, acute treatment followed by maintenance therapy is required. For acute treatment, either topical low-potency corticosteroids or antifungals are effective. For facial symptoms, a low-potency steroid (group 6 or 7) or antifungal creams such as ketoconazole 2% or ciclopirox may be used once or twice a day until symptoms resolve. For maintenance

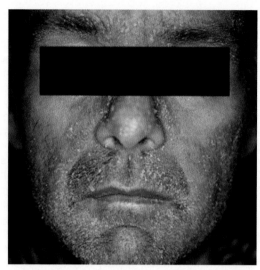

Fig. 9. Seborrheic dermatitis: Note the erythema and "greasy" scale on the midface with preference for skin creases. (*From* Dhanireddy S, Harrington R. Human immunodeficiency virus infection and the acquired immunodeficiency syndrome. In: Morse SA, Ballard RC, Holmes KK, et al, editors. Atlas of sexually transmitted diseases and AIDS. 4th edition. Philadelphia: Elsevier; 2010. p. 256–86; with permission.)

therapy for facial symptoms, intermittent use of topical antifungals (weekly ketoconazole 2% cream or shampoo wash to the face) or emollient therapies is effective. Long-term use of topical steroids should be avoided for maintenance therapy to prevent telangiectasias and atrophy. Randomized controlled trials have demonstrated equal efficacy between pimecrolimus cream, topical steroids, and topical antifungals; however, topical calcineurin inhibitors are costly, associated with short-term side effects, and not FDA approved for the treatment of seborrheic dermatitis. For scalp symptoms, antifungal shampoos such as selenium sulfide 2.5%, ketoconazole 2%, or ciclopirox 1% are effective. The shampoo should be left on for 5 to 10 minutes before rinsing off. Daily or thrice-weekly use until symptoms are improved should then be followed by weekly maintenance therapy. Tachyphylaxis is common with these shampoos, so rotating to a different type every few months can help maintain remission. A high-potency steroid (groups 1–3) shampoo, lotion, or foam may be added daily to control severe itching, although treatment should be limited to 4 weeks. Fluocinolone acetonide 0.01% shampoo is approved by the FDA for the treatment of seborrheic dermatitis.

Erysipelas and Cellulitis

Erysipelas (also known as St Anthony's fire) and cellulitis are skin infections most often caused by β-hemolytic streptococci (groups A, B, C, G, and F) followed by methicillin-sensitive *Staphylococcus aureus* (MSSA) or methicillin-resistant *S aureus* (MRSA) in high-risk populations. The lower extremities are most often involved, although facial infections can occur. Erysipelas affects the upper dermis and superficial lymphatics, and classically presents with a rapidly expanding, well-demarcated, shiny, erythematous, painful plaque associated with swelling and perifollicular edema (peau d' orange) often in a malar distribution (**Fig. 10**). Systemic symptoms such as fever, chills, and

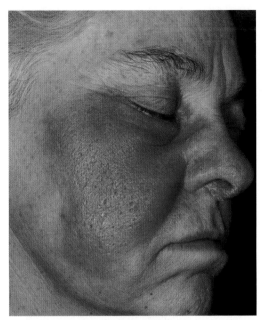

Fig. 10. Erysipelas on the malar cheek. (*From* Habif TP. Clinical dermatology: a color guide to diagnosis and therapy. 5th edition. Philadelphia: Elsevier; 2010; with permission.)

malaise are often present.[30] Cellulitis affects the deeper dermis and subcutaneous fat, and differs from erysipelas in that it is generally less well demarcated, will have little or no edema, and few if any systemic symptoms early in the course. Infection involving the ear or "Milian's ear sign" is a finding unique to erysipelas and does not occur in cellulitis because the ear does not contain deeper dermis tissue (**Fig. 11**). Antecedent breaks in the skin allowing portals of entry are common for these infections when they involve the lower extremities but not when they occur on the face. Treatment with antibiotics such as dicloxacillin or cephalexin that cover both β-hemolytic streptococci and MSSA are necessary. If the patient is penicillin allergic, a broad-spectrum quinolone can be used. If there is concern for MRSA (purulent discharge or abscess), the addition of trimethoprim-sulfamethoxazole or doxycycline may be added. Clindamycin alone may treat both *Streptococcus* species and community-acquired MRSA in some communities, although inducible resistance is common in MRSA. Linezolid alone should cover streptococci and MRSA, but this is a costly alternative. Parenteral antibiotics should be used if patients have systemic symptoms.

Systemic Lupus Erythematosus

The presence of a malar rash is a classic finding in SLE (**Fig. 12**). The rash can be raised or flat, and may be pruritic or painful. The absence of papules, pustules, and comedones helps to differentiate it from acne rosacea or acne vulgaris. The indolent and intermittent presentations of the SLE rash differentiate it from erysipelas and cellulitis. The malar rash of SLE is triggered by sun exposure and is described as a butterfly pattern. The butterfly appearance is due to the angle at which the sun's ultraviolet rays land on the skin with the nose acting as a sunshade, thus sparing the upper lip and nasolabial fold. Seborrheic dermatitis commonly affects the nasolabial fold, hence aiding in the differentiation between these 2 conditions.[30] Treatment of the SLE rash may

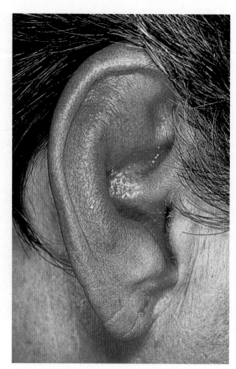

Fig. 11. Milian's ear sign of erysipelas. (*From* Habif TP, Campbell JL, Chapman MS. Skin disease: diagnosis and treatment. Philadelphia: Elsevier/Saunders; 2011; with permission.)

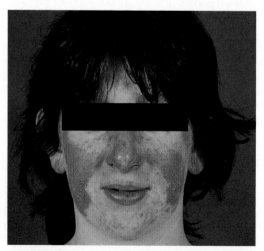

Fig. 12. Malar rash of SLE. Rash predominantly involves the malar cheeks and nose but spares the upper lip and nasolabial folds. (*From* Doherty M, Ralston SH. Musculoskeletal disease. In: Colledge NR, Walker BR, Ralston SH, editors. Davidson's principles and practice of medicine. 21st edition. Philadelphia: Elsevier; 2010. p. 1053–129; with permission.)

require systemic therapies targeting the underlying disorder along with topical steroids, although sun protection is a mandatory prophylactic measure.

INTERTRIGINOUS RASHES

In the primary care setting, patients often present with rashes in their intertriginous areas. The word intertrigo comes from the Latin *inter* (between) and *terer* (to rub), and refers to a condition involving friction and maceration caused by skin against skin. It often is used to refer to this irritant dermatitis without superinfection of any type, but the term may be also be used when infection is present.[52] The most commonly involved sites include axilla, groin, anogenital region, web spaces of toes and fingers, and skin folds of the breast or pannus. These moist areas provide an ideal breeding ground for yeast, fungal, or bacterial superinfections. Other noninfectious inflammatory conditions may also develop in these areas and are often misdiagnosed. Because treatments differ depending on the etiology, some clinical pearls are presented here to help determine the cause and allow tailoring of appropriate therapy (**Table 4**).

Table 4 Differential diagnoses for intertriginous rash		
Condition	**History/Demographics/Risk Factors**	**Physical Examination Findings**
Candidiasis	Usually complain of severe pruritus Higher risk in moist skin folds, such as in obesity Higher risk in immunosuppressed states such as HIV or diabetes mellitus	Erythematous, macerated, plaque or erosion Severe pruritus and satellite papulopustular lesions are most helpful in diagnosis Simultaneously involve thigh and scrotum in men KOH prep may demonstrate oval budding yeast with pseudohyphae
Tinea cruris	More common in men Often multiple sites infected simultaneously (tinea cruris, tinea pedis, tinea manus)	Slightly elevated, erythematous, sharply demarcated borders with partial central clearing No papulopustular satellite lesions Generally start on inner thigh and spread outward from center. First down the leg, then to the pubic region Generally spares the scrotum in men KOH prep may show filamentous and segmented hyphae
Erythrasma	Usually asymptomatic or only mild itching	Well-demarcated red or brown patch or plaque Fine-scale with cigarette-paper appearance May fluoresce coral-red after 5–10 s with Wood's lamp examination
Inverse psoriasis	One-third of patients will report family history of psoriasis	Uniformly and evenly erythematous, well-demarcated, shiny plaques lacking scale No pruritic papulopustular or satellite lesions May have associated nail findings: pitting, subungual keratosis, oil-drop sign, onycholysis KOH negative

In addition to a clear history of risk factors and symptoms and the appearance of the rash, the regular use of a potassium hydroxide (KOH) prep and a Wood's lamp can help in the diagnosis. A general approach to all types of intertrigo is to educate patients about keeping skin folds dry and avoiding friction. Drying the intertriginous areas thoroughly with a cool hairdryer if possible; wearing light, nonconstricting, absorbent clothing; and avoiding wool and synthetic fibers can be helpful. Absorptive powders or barrier creams may also help decrease moisture or limit friction.[53] Cornstarch rather than talcum powder should be used as a drying agent in women in the genital area, as there has been an association reported between use of talcum powder and an increased risk of ovarian cancer.[54]

KOH preps can easily be done in the primary care setting. Use a clean glass slide to collect scale that falls while scraping material from a lesion using the edge of another glass slide, or wet with an alcohol swab and then use a #15 blade to scrape. The highest-yield areas for hyphae are from the leading edge of the lesion, papule, pustule, or vesicle. Apply a coverslip to the slide to transport to the microscope area, then 1 to 2 drops of KOH to one edge of the coverslip: it will wick under the coverslip by capillary action. Gently heat the slide over an alcohol burner or with a lighter for a few seconds until just before it starts to boil. This technique breaks down cell-membrane components and makes it easier to see yeast or fungal elements. Repetitive gentle pressure to the top of the coverslip with a pen or probe will help flatten the specimen once it starts digesting, and will make examination easier. Examine the slide at 10× magnification and increase to 20× if needed to confirm the presence of the pseudohyphae or yeast forms of candida or the hyphae of dermatophytes. It is important to be aware that KOH preps can often yield false-negative results and that many structures (hair fibers, clothing fibers, KOH crystals, or the edges of folds of the sheets of cells) can mimic hyphae and cellular debris from digestion can mimic yeast forms (**Fig. 13**). Gram stains, if available, will highlight yeast forms.

Candidiasis

The warm moist environment of intertriginous areas provides an ideal location for the growth of candida. Obesity, hyperhidrosis, incontinence, and tight clothing lead to increased friction, and moisture in the area and immunosuppression secondary to either medical conditions or medications may promote fungal overgrowth. Refractory candidal intertrigo without a clear explanation may raise the possibility of an underlying condition such as malnutrition, endocrinopathy, malignancy, or HIV infection.

The classic description of candidal intertrigo is an erythematous, macerated plaque with erosions, delicate peripheral scale, and satellite papulopustules (**Fig. 14**). Patients generally describe severe pruritus or burning, and may develop painful skin breakdown. The diagnosis can be made clinically, but KOH prep or culture of skin scrapings can be helpful. Pruritus and satellite lesions are the most clinically helpful for diagnosis of candida. KOH prep may reveal oval budding yeasts with pseudohyphae (see **Fig. 13**B).

There are few data from controlled trials comparing the different topical antifungal agents for the treatment of candida. In general, twice-daily treatment until symptom resolution with any of the following agents is acceptable: nystatin, the azoles (clotrimazole, ketoconazole, miconazole, econazole, sertaconazole), or hydroxypridone (ciclopirox). Of note, all of these agents will also work for dermatophyte infections except for nystatin, which is only effective against candida. By contrast, the allylamines (teribinafine and naftifine) and benzylamines (butenafine) are the most effective topical agents against dermatophytes, but have less activity against yeasts.[55] Some patients may benefit from twice-weekly applications in preventing recurrence. In general cream

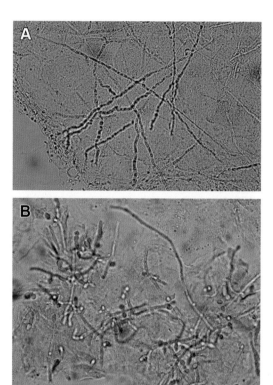

Fig. 13. (*A*) Hyphae of dermatophytes after KOH digestion. (*B*) Pseudohyphae and yeast forms of *Candida* after KOH digestion. ([*A*] *From* Habif TP, Campbell JL, Chapman MS. Skin disease: diagnosis and treatment. Philadelphia: Elsevier/Saunders; 2011; with permission; and [*B*] *From* Elewski BE, Hughey LC, Sobera JO, et al. Fungal diseases. In: Bolognia JL, Jorizzo JL, Schaffer JV, editors. Dermatology. 3rd edition. Philadelphia: Elsevier/Saunders; 2012. p. 1251–84; with permission.)

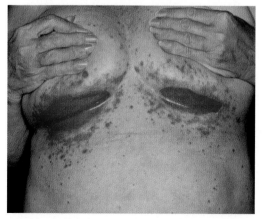

Fig. 14. Candidal intertrigo. Erythematous, well-demarcated plaques with satellite papules and pustules. (*From* Habif TP. Clinical dermatology: a color guide to diagnosis and therapy. 5th edition. Philadelphia: Elsevier; 2010.)

formulations are more potent, although antifungal powders may have the added benefit of providing a drying effect. Consider using creams for treatment of acute infections and powders for maintenance therapy. In most cases, treatment with an antifungal will lead to rapid resolution of symptoms, but the addition of a low-potency topical steroid may help with the pruritus, pain, and burning. Moderate-potency and high-potency topical steroids should be avoided in intertriginous areas because of their increased potency and side effects when used under occlusion.

If topical therapy fails or the infection is severe, consider using oral antifungal agents. Oral azoles can be used for 2 to 6 weeks until symptoms have resolved. In adults, common dosing regimens include: fluconazole, 50 to 100 mg daily or 150 mg weekly; itraconazole, 200 mg twice daily; or ketoconazole, 200 mg daily. Griseofulvin has no activity against candida. The patient should be monitored for drug interactions with oral azoles.

Dermatophyte Infections

Tinea cruris occurs more often in men than in women. As opposed to candidal groin infections, which usually simultaneously involve the thigh and scrotum in men, tinea infections generally start on the inner thigh with a small red patch and then spread outward from the center, first down the leg and then into the pubic region. The scrotum is typically spared in tinea infections, which differs from candidal infections. Moreover, tinea cruris should not have papulopustular satellite lesions. The tinea lesion is usually slightly elevated, with an erythematous and sharply demarcated border and partial central clearing (**Fig. 15**). Using a hand lens may reveal very small vesicles at the

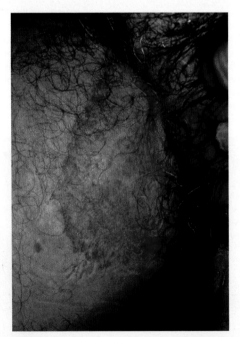

Fig. 15. Tinea cruris. Note the expanding annular red rim with partial central clearing along the inner thigh. (*From* Elewski BE, Hughey LC, Sobera JO, et al. Fungal diseases. In: Bolognia JL, Jorizzo JL, Schaffer JV, editors. Dermatology. 3rd edition. Philadelphia: Elsevier/Saunders; 2012. p. 1251–84; with permission.)

border. If tinea cruris is suspected, look for other sites of tinea infection such as the buttocks, feet, toenails, or hands, as multiple sites are often affected and patients can reinfect the groin area if other sites of infection are not also treated. A KOH prep from the active border of the lesion may show long, filamentous, and segmented hyphae (see **Fig. 13**A). In addition to the azoles already mentioned, allylamines (terbinafine and naftifine), benzylamines (butenafine), and hydroxypyridone (ciclopirox) are highly effective against most dermatophytes, whereas nystatin is not. In general, symptoms will resolve within 2 weeks with treatment. Encouraging patients to apply the creams to at least 3 cm beyond the advancing edge of the lesion, treating for 1 week after clinical clearing, and treating other sites of active infection may help to prevent recurrence. Treatment of onychomycosis may be necessary if patients continue to develop recurrent infection. For cases resistant to topical therapy, and severe or recurrent cases, oral treatment with griseofulvin, 250 mg 3 times daily for 14 days, or any of the previously mentioned oral azoles or terbinafine can be tried.

Erythrasma

Erythrasma is a superficial infection of the skin caused by *Corynebacterium minutissimum,* a gram-positive, non–spore-forming bacillus. Most patients will be asymptomatic and often present for treatment for cosmetic reasons. Some patients may complain of mild itching. The most common site of infection is the web spaces between the toes followed by the groin and axilla. In the interdigital areas, macerated, scaly plaques are common, and closely resemble the findings of tinea pedis. In the groin or axilla, erythrasma may present with well-demarcated red patches or plaques that eventually turn a lighter brownish color. Fine-scale and "cigarette-paper" wrinkles are often apparent (**Fig. 16**A). Assuming that the patient has not recently scrubbed the affected area in an attempt to get it clean, a Wood's lamp examination may reveal a coral-red fluorescence that develops after 5 to 10 seconds, owing to the production of porphyrins by the *C minutissimum* (see **Fig. 16**B). A KOH prep may also be performed because concomitant infection with tinea or candida can occur.

Most cases can be treated with topical antibiotics or antifungals. There are few data available to guide therapy recommendations. Small studies support the use of clindamycin 1% or erythromycin 2%, 2 to 3 times daily for 1 to 2 weeks.[56] Randomized

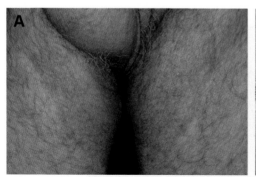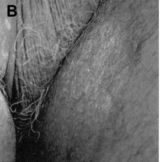

Fig. 16. Erythrasma. (*A*) A slightly brownish, evenly colored patch is often seen without the erythema or annular character of other rashes in this area. (*B*) Porphyrins fluoresce coral-red on Wood's lamp examination. (*From* Millett CR, Halpern AV, Reboli AC, et al. Bacterial diseases. In: Bolognia JL, Jorizzo JL, Schaffer JV, editors. Dermatology. 3rd edition. Philadelphia: Elsevier/Saunders; 2012. p. 1187–220; with permission.)

controlled trials with small numbers of patients have demonstrated benefit with topical azoles twice daily (miconazole, tioconazole, econazole) or once daily (oxiconazole) for 7 to 60 days.[57–60] Although no clinical trials support its use, benzoyl peroxide 5% gel has been reportedly effective based on clinical experience. Small studies show that Whitefield's ointment (containing 12% benzoic acid and 6% salicylic acid) applied twice a day for 1 week is effective.[56]

If patients have multisite disease or interdigital involvement, oral antimicrobials plus topical agents should be considered.[56] One randomized, placebo-controlled trial comparing erythromycin (1 g daily × 14 days), clarithromycin (single dose 1 g), 2% fusidic acid (applied twice a day × 14 days [not available in the United States]), placebo cream, and placebo tablet showed the following complete response rates at 14 days based on a reflection score of 0 on Wood's lamp examination: fusidic acid (97%), clarithromycin (67%), erythromycin (53%), placebo cream (13%), placebo tablet (3%).[61]

Several other small, randomized controlled trials and case reports demonstrate efficacy of oral erythromycin. Erythromycin is usually prescribed at a dose of 250 mg 4 times daily for 14 days, but is associated with gastrointestinal upset and drug interactions. One study of tetracycline, 250 mg 4 times daily showed benefit, although it may be less effective than erythromycin.[62] When considering the diagnosis and treatment of erythrasma multiple sites must be examined, as recurrence may occur if all sites are not treated. Data supporting prophylactic therapy with topical agents to prevent recurrence are not available.

Inverse Psoriasis

Plaque psoriasis is the most common variant of psoriasis, and typically develops in young adulthood. These plaques are generally raised and erythematous with a thick silvery scale, and develop on the extensor surfaces such as elbows and knees, umbilicus, scalp, back, and gluteal fold. Inverse psoriasis is a variant, which presents in flexural and intertriginous areas and is often misdiagnosed as a fungal or bacterial infection. Family history can be helpful because approximately one-third of patients with psoriasis will have a first-degree relative with this condition.[63] Inverse psoriasis plaques are uniformly and evenly erythematous and well demarcated, but generally lack scale in comparison with plaque psoriasis (**Fig. 17**), likely because of the friction in these areas rubbing off the scale or the moist areas where it occurs. It also tends to

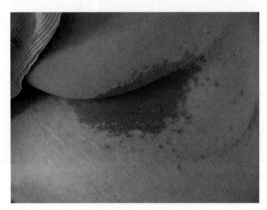

Fig. 17. Inverse psoriasis of the breast in an obese woman. (*From* Berth-Jones J. Psoriasis. Medicine 2009;35:240; with permission.)

be shinier than erythrasma, and should lack the pruritic papulopustular and satellite lesions of candida and the central clearing of a dermatophyte infection. Closely examining the fingernails for pitting, subungual keratosis, the oil-drop sign, and onycholysis can also be helpful, as 80% to 90% of patients with psoriasis will develop nail disease over their lifetime (**Fig. 18**).[63] Negative KOH and Wood's lamp examinations may also point toward inverse psoriasis as the cause. Inverse psoriasis is often diagnosed after multiple failed treatment attempts with antifungals or antibacterials. The condition can usually be diagnosed clinically, but biopsy may be necessary. Short-term therapy (2–4 weeks) with low- to moderate-potency topical steroids can be used to initiate therapy; however, long-term use of daily steroids in intertriginous areas should be avoided to prevent the development of atrophy, striae, and telangiectasias. Tachyphylaxis can also develop with continuous long-term use of topical steroids. If necessary, maintenance therapy can involve the use of topical vitamin D analogues (calcipotriene or calcitriol), topical calcineurin inhibitors (pimecrolimus or tacrolimus) or pulse-dosed topical steroids 1 to 2 times per week.[63] Systemic therapies administered by a dermatologist may be needed for severe or refractory cases, although this is uncommon.[63]

THE RED LEG

Patients often present to primary care providers with red rashes on the lower extremities. Differentiating between diagnostic possibilities is urgently needed to decide how a patient should be treated, as such rashes may require admission to a hospital or merely some compression stockings. This section discusses the clinical presentations of cellulitis and erysipelas, stasis dermatitis, allergic contact dermatitis, and DVT, and pearls for quickly differentiating between these possibilities through history taking and physical examination (**Table 5**).

Although ruling out infection may seem like the most pressing clinical priority, it is estimated that inappropriate treatment of cellulitis may account for more than a billion dollars in the Medicare system alone, in addition to the difficult to capture costs of adverse antibiotic reactions and complications of hospitalization.[64] Key elements to consider in an initial assessment include the acuity of onset, differentiating pain versus pruritus as the sensory complaint, and the distribution of the rash, as well as

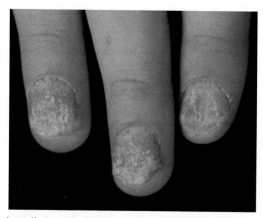

Fig. 18. Nail psoriasis. Nail pits with distal yellowing and subungual debris caused by onycholysis. (*From* van de Kerkhof PC, Nestlé FO. Psoriasis. In: Bolognia JL, Jorizzo JL, Schaffer JV, editors. Dermatology. 3rd edition. Philadelphia: Elsevier/Saunders; 2012. p. 135–56; with permission.)

Table 5
Differential diagnoses for the red leg

Condition	History/Demographics/Risk Factors	Physical Examination Findings
Cellulitis and erysipelas	Abrupt onset (hours to days) Higher risk with older age or obesity or chronic edema Usually a portal of entry can be found	Painful expanding area of redness Unilateral Crosses anatomic boundaries and may be discontinuous in its spread
Stasis dermatitis	Subacute onset (many days to weeks) Pruritic rather than painful Edema is always present	Scaly erythematous patches or plaques nearly continuous from the upper calf and shin to the top of the ankles, but usually not involving the joints or feet Often bilateral
Contact dermatitis	Irritant contact dermatitis is nonimmune mediated and appears in hours Allergic contact dermatitis is idiosyncratic and may take days to appear Exposure history may include metals, topical antibiotics, topical agents with fragrance or preservatives, rubber products, latex, leather	Shape usually matches an external exposure and is geometric rather than following anatomy, suggesting an "outside job" Very pruritic if allergic Marked epidermal change with vesiculation often
Deep vein thrombosis (DVT)	History of injury History of immobility History of prior DVT is a risk factor	Acute unilateral edema and tenderness Erythema is usually absent or localized only to the proximal medial thigh

predisposing factors such as preexisting leg edema, recent hospitalizations, or injuries. Treatments for each are also be briefly discussed.

Infectious entities tend to develop quickly in hours to days, whereas stasis dermatitis has a more insidious onset over the course of weeks. Pruritus is a predominant feature of dermatitis, whether from stasis or contact sensitization, whereas pain is predominant from the tissue destruction of infection or from DVT. Preexisting leg edema might suggest stasis dermatitis as a leading contender, whereas recent prolonged immobilization or surgery would push DVT higher in the differential. If symptoms are rapidly progressing over minutes to hours and are accompanied by pain out of proportion to examination and beyond the obvious area of involvement or a dusky gray to black color centrally, necrotizing fasciitis should be considered. Necrotizing fasciitis is a surgical emergency that is not medically treatable, and is not covered further herein.[65]

Cellulitis and Erysipelas

Already covered in the portion of this article on facial rashes, cellulitis and erysipelas in the lower extremities has some characteristic differences in both history and physical examination. Predisposing factors for both types of lower extremity infections include obesity, older age, edema, venous insufficiency, and greater saphenous vein stripping/harvesting, while lymphedema specifically is a significant risk factor for erysipelas.[66,67]

Most cellulitis and erysipelas occurs from common skin-colonizing bacteria, β-hemolytic streptococci and *Staphylococcus aureus*, which enter through breaks in the integument from abrasions, arthropod bites, or maceration between the toes, the latter being commonly from tinea pedis.[67,68] As a result, a history of such predisposing events or conditions can be helpful in suspecting the diagnosis. Incidence rates nearly double with each 10-year increment of age, with a prevalence of about 200 per 100,000 person-years, although estimates vary widely.[69]

Patients typically present complaining of a painful expanding area of redness on the affected limb, usually over the course of a few days. Occasionally, systemic symptoms may precede the rash, possibly deriving from the significant inflammatory response to invasive bacterial soft tissue infection.[66] Patients with cellulitis present with a localized and sometimes discontinuous area of erythema, edema, warmth, and tenderness, similar to the classic hallmarks of inflammation originally described by Celsus as *rubor*, *tumor*, *calor*, and *dolor* 2000 years ago (**Fig. 19**).[70] Lower extremity cellulitis is nearly always unilateral and 95% occurs below the knee.[69] The erythema usually blanches early in the process, but owing to extravasation of erythrocytes from inflammation and the increased intravascular hydrostatic pressures of the lower extremities, nonblanching erythema will often develop; this is often centered around the site of initiation but may spread proximally along lymphatics as red streaks. Bullae may occur as a result of either production of bacterial toxin or acute edema. Suppuration in the form of pustules or frank abscess may also occur, the latter of which should raise suspicion for *Staphylococcus aureus* and MRSA.

Because of its more superficial location and involvement of lymphatics, erysipelas is typically a bright red erythema that is sharply marginated and has a more defined superficial peau d'orange edema as described previously. Fever and adenopathy of the draining lymph nodes may also be present, although these are probably less common in the outpatient setting. Laboratory studies will show leukocytosis in most cases.[66]

Treatment of cellulitis and erysipelas is usually empiric as most cases are not culturable, most instances being caused by β-hemolytic streptococci, with only about 10% caused by *S aureus*. Whereas MRSA is a common cause of furuncles, it is relatively uncommon in nonsuppurative cellulitis. As a result, empiric treatment need only cover β-hemolytic streptococci and MSSA if suppuration is not present, as illustrated by a study of 179 patients with nonculturable cellulitis, which showed that 96% improved with β-lactam antibiotics despite a high prevalence of MRSA at the institution.[71] Addition of prednisolone to antibiotics can hasten symptom improvement and shorten hospital stays in patients with cellulitis.[72] Antibiotic treatments are generally as those described earlier for facial rashes.

Stasis Dermatitis

Erythema and scale can occur in any area of the body that has acutely worsening edema, although it is by far most common on the lower legs as a result of venous disease. Here, either venous obstruction or loss of venous valve competence commonly results in venous congestion in the leg and resulting edema. When chronic, the veins become more visible with enlargement, such as with varicose veins (bluish veins over 3 mm diameter that protrude from the skin surface) or corona phlebectasia (purplish 1-mm diameter branching vessels around the sides of the ankle and foot, resembling a broad cascading waterfall). The higher intravascular pressure is also associated with erythrocyte extravasation and accumulation of hemosiderin, giving the legs and dorsal foot a speckled, rusty brown color.[65]

When this chronic edema acutely worsens, the skin can become red and scaly, even with serous drainage and crust (dried serum), and can mimic cellulitis or erysipelas,

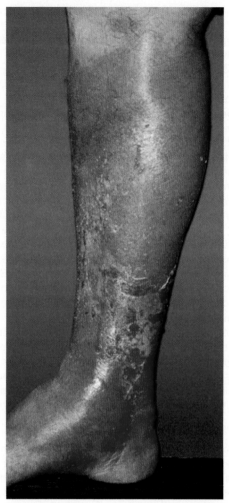

Fig. 19. Lower extremity cellulitis. (*From* James WD, Berger TG, Elston DM. Andrews' diseases of the skin: clinical dermatology. Philadelphia: Elsevier/Saunders; 2011; with permission.)

although there are several distinguishing factors that help differentiate it from infection. The history is typically one of slow development over weeks rather than hours to days. Although there may be some burning pain, pruritus is usually the predominant complaint, as it is a dermatitis rather than pathogen-mediated tissue damage. On examination, scale (white flaky skin) is prominent, unlike in infection. Erythema involves only the leg, respecting the anatomic boundaries of the ankle and knee, typically only on the lower half of the shin and calf (**Fig. 20**).[65] Although infection may also occur here, it is more likely to spread into adjacent anatomic areas. Most importantly, stasis dermatitis is typically bilateral, whereas "bilateral lower extremity cellulitis" is the Sasquatch of Dermatology: believed by many to exist, but rarely actually seen.

Eczema craquelé (asteatotic eczema) is a rash similar to and often concurrent with stasis dermatitis. As its name suggests, it appears as if the skin is cracking apart, showing a pattern reminiscent of sun-baked desert clay or glazed pottery (**Fig. 21**).

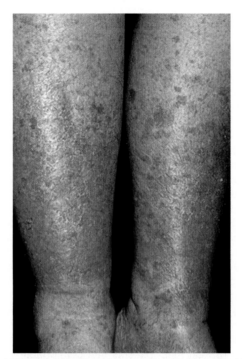

Fig. 20. Stasis dermatitis. Typical distribution from the mid shin and calf to the ankle of both legs. (*From* Habif TP, Campbell JL, Chapman MS, et al. Skin disease: diagnosis and treatment. Philadelphia: Elsevier/Saunders; 2011; with permission.)

In fact, these apparent fissures typically extend only through the stratum corneum. This condition arises from acute edema and is less dependent on presence of venous disease specifically, although a prerequisite is profound xerosis, as seen in the elderly or those abusing their skin with cleaning products in an attempt to disinfect themselves.[73,74]

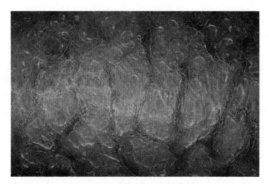

Fig. 21. Asteatotic eczema (eczema craquelé). Note the "dry riverbed" pattern to the superficial cracking of the epidermis. (*From* Norbert Reider N, Fritsch PO. Other eczematous eruptions. In: Bolognia JL, Jorizzo JL, Schaffer JV, editors. Dermatology. 3rd edition. Philadelphia: Elsevier/Saunders; 2012. p. 219–31; with permission.)

Treatment of the acute inflammation is usually achievable with a moderate-potency topical corticosteroid such as triamcinolone 0.1% ointment applied twice daily to the affected areas, although systemic treatment with a short course of prednisone can be helpful in severe cases. Both stasis dermatitis and eczema craquelé require correcting the edema and xerosis for complete resolution and long-term control. Emollients and elevation can be instituted immediately, although in an outpatient setting, elevation of a leg above the level of the heart is impractical for long periods. As a result, external compression is usually desired through compressive wraps such as an Unna boot, a short-stretch bandage, or a multilayer compression device (of which several different brands are available).[75] These devices are typically applied in the office but can be inconvenient and costly for the patient, as they cannot get wet, are too bulky for normal shoes, and require at least weekly changes in a physician's office. As a result, most ambulatory patients transition to a graduated compression stocking or adjustable elastic compression (eg, CircAid) as soon as they are able.

Graduated compression stockings differ from uniformly compressive thromboembolism deterrent (TED) hose used in immobile patients in that they have higher compression around the foot and ankle, which lessens toward the upper calf. Veins with competent valves use the pumping action of leg-muscle contraction during walking to return blood against gravity to the heart. In the absence of valves, graded compression stockings accomplish the same unidirectional movement by being more permissive to venous flow only in the proximal direction.[76] These stockings still rely on muscle use when patients are upright, so patients should be encouraged to be mobile. Treatment of clinically significant edema may require higher levels of compression stockings (>30 mm Hg) than most patients can comfortably wear or even put on, although there is little consensus as to which level of compression may be needed for different conditions.[77] Stockings of 20 to 30 mm Hg are often a compromise in efficacy and patient adherence. Alternatively, wearing 2 lower-level compression stockings on top of one another achieves a roughly additive compression (eg, wearing two 15–20 mm Hg stockings on the same leg is roughly equivalent to a single 30–40 mm Hg stocking), and may be easier for patients to use with a trade-off of increased material bulk and heat.[78] Compression stockings are commonly available at medical supply stores, online stores, and, more recently, at athletic and yoga stores, in more attractive designs for better adherence. Effects of poor arterial perfusion can be compounded by external compression, of course, so compression is ill advised if the ankle-brachial index is less than 0.8.[75]

Contact Dermatitis

An acute dermatitis caused by either an irritation or allergic cause is also common on the legs. Typically, the clue as to a contact dermatitis is that the shape of involvement will be geometric rather than anatomic such that it appears to be an "outside job."

Irritant contact dermatitis develops within hours after exposure to a chemical that has direct toxic effects on the skin. It is not an immunologic response and therefore is an expected reaction in any person exposed to such an environmental stimulus. Common examples include detergents or soaps left in contact with the skin, or adhesives in bandages (which may less commonly cause allergic contact dermatitis as well). Erythema, scale, and crust occur with vesiculation or bullae in more profound responses. The predominant symptom is typically one of pain or burning rather than pruritus.[65]

Allergic contact dermatitis is an immunologic response to an allergen, and therefore is more unique to an individual in that a sensitized person will contract a rash any time they are exposed to this product, whereas a nonsensitized person would have no reaction at all. Common causes include metals such as nickel and cobalt, topical antibiotics such as neomycin or bacitracin, fragrances, lanolin, textile dyes in socks, latex in compression stockings, potassium dichromate used in leather tanning, or numerous chemicals used in the production of rubber or neoprene used in footwear.[79] As with irritant contact dermatitis, erythema, scale and crust, and vesiculation and bullae can occur, but the predominant symptom is primarily one of pruritus.[65] Onset is typically delayed by 1 or 2 days, and relies on a type IV hypersensitivity response rather than the immediate toxic effects seen in irritant dermatitis.

The acute onset, erythema, and pain of either reaction may mimic cellulitis, but the pattern of involvement will stay localized only to the area of contact, and the marked epidermal change (scale and serous exudate and crust) and pruritus help to suggest a dermatitic process. The shape of involvement will also give clues as to the cause (**Fig. 22**).

Treatment is, of course, complete removal of the causative agent, followed by topical corticosteroids. A moderate-potency steroid such as triamcinolone is often sufficient, but a week-long course of an ultrapotent steroid such as clobetasol and even systemic prednisone may be needed for severe cases.

Deep Vein Thrombosis

Though not necessarily a problem of the skin, acute DVT is often in the differential for an edematous painful and red leg. Whereas edema and pain are typical in DVT, erythema is not in fact a typical symptom. Erythema was only one of the minor criteria for DVT in the original Wells score, yet did not hold up after regression analyses and is absent from the currently used Revised Wells score.[80,81] Venous congestion may leave a purplish hue to the leg, but erythema only occurs when overlying a DVT of the proximal medial thigh where the femoral vein is close enough to the skin that the inflammation is visible externally.[65] However, chronic edema of DVT may result in secondary stasis dermatitis or eczema craquelé.

TREATMENT

Although systemic agents are heavily used in dermatology, often patients and providers alike prefer topical management. Whether using corticosteroids, antimicrobials,

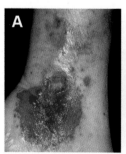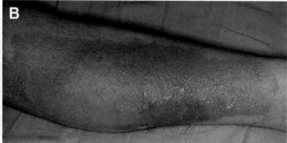

Fig. 22. (A) Allergic contact dermatitis resulting from use of neomycin-containing topical antibiotic to a leg wound. (B) Allergic contact dermatitis resulting from application of benzoin tincture. Note the well-circumscribed boundaries that do not conform to normal anatomy. (*From* [A] Habif TP. Clinical dermatology: a color guide to diagnosis and therapy. 5th edition. Philadelphia: Elsevier; 2010; and [B] *From* Mowad CM, Marks JG. Allergic contact dermatitis. In: Bolognia JL, Jorizzo JL, Schaffer JV, editors. Dermatology. 3rd edition. Philadelphia: Elsevier/Saunders; 2012. p. 233–48; with permission.)

or comedolytics, topical vehicles allow a high concentration of a medication where it is needed while minimizing systemic side effects. The normal epidermis functions as a barrier to these medications, however, and the vehicle can affect not only medication efficacy but also patient adherence. **Fig. 23** shows some of the characteristics of the most common vehicles for which ease of application is in general inversely related to efficacy. All medications containing water require the use of preservatives, which can cause allergic contact dermatitis, so nonaqueous ointments are preferable when this is a concern. Greasier medications such as ointments also penetrate the hydrophobic epidermis more readily and thus are more potent.[82]

All topical agents are most easily applied to moist skin just after showering, although patients may not like the slimy feeling that results on the skin. Advising patients to only apply the minimum necessary to feel something has "just barely" gotten on all the affected area is important, as overapplication is not generally more efficacious but results in excess medicine on clothes and bedsheets, limiting adherence quickly. The concept of the fingertip unit (FTU) of topical medication (a single line of cream or ointment from a standard tube that extends along the distal phalanx of the patient's index finger) can be useful in advising how much to apply. A single FTU is enough for one hand, 2 FTU enough for a foot, 3 FTU for an arm, and 6 FTU for a leg.[83,84]

Corticosteroids are among the most commonly prescribed class of topical medications. In the United States these are grouped by their varying efficacy from class 1 (superpotent) to class 7 (least potent). Because the vehicle can affect efficacy by increasing absorption, any given steroid may belong to more than one class depending on its vehicle; for example, fluticasone 0.005% ointment is class 3, whereas the more concentrated 0.05% cream and lotion are class 5. Similarly, flurandrenolide 0.05% lotion is a class 5, whereas tape impregnated with flurandrenolide is a class 1 owing to its occlusive effects. Concern about side effects from overuse by both clinicians and patients results in ineffective treatment being more of a problem than overuse. Side effects of topical corticosteroids include striae distensae, bruising, telangiectasias, skin fragility, pigmentary changes, and suppression of the hypothalamic-pituitary-adrenal axis (though the latter is not clinically significant without extensive areas of application over long periods).[82] A conservative rule of thumb is that a steroid can be used for as many weeks as its class without concern for side effects; for example, a class 2 could be used for 2 weeks while a class 6 could be used for 6 weeks.

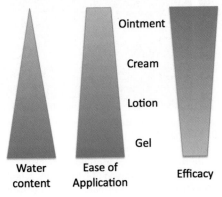

Fig. 23. Characteristics of vehicles.

SUMMARY

When assessing a patient with a new dermatologic condition, developing a differential diagnosis is essential to ensure the condition is not elusive as a workup and potential therapy are considered. Subsequent narrowing of that differential based on history and physical examination can allow a more targeted approach to diagnostic testing and triage, and hasten an effective treatment and resolution.

The authors hope to have provided useful historical and clinical clues to aid in the rapid differentiation of the more common diagnoses for alopecias and rashes of the face, intertriginous areas, and legs.

REFERENCES

1. Fien S, Berman B, Magrane B. Skin disease in a primary care practice. Skinmed 2005;4(6):350–3.
2. Lowell BA, Froelich CW, Federman DG, et al. Dermatology in primary care: prevalence and patient disposition. J Am Acad Dermatol 2001;45(2):250–5.
3. Hamilton JB. Patterned loss of hair in man; types and incidence. Ann N Y Acad Sci 1951;53(3):708–28.
4. Norwood OT. Incidence of female androgenetic alopecia (female pattern alopecia). Dermatol Surg 2001;27(1):53–4.
5. Futterweit W, Dunaif A, Yeh HC, et al. The prevalence of hyperandrogenism in 109 consecutive female patients with diffuse alopecia. J Am Acad Dermatol 1988;19(5 Pt 1):831–6.
6. Karrer-Voegeli S, Rey F, Reymond MJ, et al. Androgen dependence of hirsutism, acne, and alopecia in women: retrospective analysis of 228 patients investigated for hyperandrogenism. Medicine (Baltimore) 2009;88(1):32–45.
7. Ellis JA, Sinclair R, Harrap SB. Androgenetic alopecia: pathogenesis and potential for therapy. Expert Rev Mol Med 2002;4(22):1–11.
8. Camacho-Martinez FM. Hair loss in women. Semin Cutan Med Surg 2009;28(1): 19–32.
9. Arias-Santiago S, Gutierrez-Salmeron MT, Castellote-Caballero L, et al. Androgenetic alopecia and cardiovascular risk factors in men and women: a comparative study. J Am Acad Dermatol 2010;63(3):420–9.
10. Olsen EA, Whiting D, Bergfeld W, et al. A multicenter, randomized, placebo-controlled, double-blind clinical trial of a novel formulation of 5% minoxidil topical foam versus placebo in the treatment of androgenetic alopecia in men. J Am Acad Dermatol 2007;57(5):767–74.
11. Lucky AW, Piacquadio DJ, Ditre CM, et al. A randomized, placebo-controlled trial of 5% and 2% topical minoxidil solutions in the treatment of female pattern hair loss. J Am Acad Dermatol 2004;50(4):541–53.
12. Blume-Peytavi U, Hillmann K, Dietz E, et al. A randomized, single-blind trial of 5% minoxidil foam once daily versus 2% minoxidil solution twice daily in the treatment of androgenetic alopecia in women. J Am Acad Dermatol 2011; 65(6):1126–34.e2.
13. Kaufman KD, Olsen EA, Whiting D, et al. Finasteride in the treatment of men with androgenetic alopecia. Finasteride Male Pattern Hair Loss Study Group. J Am Acad Dermatol 1998;39(4 Pt 1):578–89.
14. Mella JM, Perret MC, Manzotti M, et al. Efficacy and safety of finasteride therapy for androgenetic alopecia: a systematic review. Arch Dermatol 2010;146(10): 1141–50.

15. Irwig MS, Kolukula S. Persistent sexual side effects of finasteride for male pattern hair loss. J Sex Med 2011;8(6):1747–53.

16. Redman MW, Tangen CM, Goodman PJ, et al. Finasteride does not increase the risk of high-grade prostate cancer: a bias-adjusted modeling approach. Cancer Prev Res (Phila) 2008;1(3):174–81.

17. Eun HC, Kwon OS, Yeon JH, et al. Efficacy, safety, and tolerability of dutasteride 0.5 mg once daily in male patients with male pattern hair loss: a randomized, double-blind, placebo-controlled, phase III study. J Am Acad Dermatol 2010; 63(2):252–8.

18. Rathnayake D, Sinclair R. Innovative use of spironolactone as an antiandrogen in the treatment of female pattern hair loss. Dermatol Clin 2010;28(3): 611–8.

19. van Zuuren EJ, Fedorowicz Z, Carter B. Evidence-based treatments for female pattern hair loss: a summary of a Cochrane systematic review. Br J Dermatol 2012;167(5):995–1010.

20. Mackenzie IS, Macdonald TM, Thompson A, et al. Spironolactone and risk of incident breast cancer in women older than 55 years: retrospective, matched cohort study. BMJ 2012;345:e4447.

21. McMichael AJ, Pearce DJ, Wasserman D, et al. Alopecia in the United States: outpatient utilization and common prescribing patterns. J Am Acad Dermatol 2007;57(Suppl 2):S49–51.

22. Gilhar A, Etzioni A, Paus R. Alopecia areata. N Engl J Med 2012;366(16): 1515–25.

23. Alkhalifah A, Alsantali A, Wang E, et al. Alopecia areata update: part I. Clinical picture, histopathology, and pathogenesis. J Am Acad Dermatol 2010;62(2): 177–88 [quiz: 189–90].

24. Goh C, Finkel M, Christos PJ, et al. Profile of 513 patients with alopecia areata: associations of disease subtypes with atopy, autoimmune disease and positive family history. J Eur Acad Dermatol Venereol 2006;20(9):1055–60.

25. Messenger AG, McKillop J, Farrant P, et al. British Association of Dermatologists' guidelines for the management of alopecia areata 2012. Br J Dermatol 2012;166(5):916–26.

26. Whiting DA. Chronic telogen effluvium: increased scalp hair shedding in middle-aged women. J Am Acad Dermatol 1996;35(6):899–906.

27. Kligman AM. Pathologic dynamics of human hair loss. I. Telogen effluvium. Arch Dermatol 1961;83:175–98.

28. Shrivastava SB. Diffuse hair loss in an adult female: approach to diagnosis and management. Indian J Dermatol Venereol Leprol 2009;75(1):20–7 [quiz: 27–8].

29. Harrison S, Sinclair R. Telogen effluvium. Clin Exp Dermatol 2002;27(5). 389–5.

30. O'Connor K, Paauw D. Erysipelas: rare but important cause of malar rash. Am J Med 2010;123(5):414–6.

31. Stathakis V, Kilkenny M, Marks R. Descriptive epidemiology of acne vulgaris in the community. Australas J Dermatol 1997;38(3):115–23.

32. Thiboutot D, Gollnick H, Bettoli V, et al. New insights into the management of acne: an update from the Global Alliance to Improve Outcomes in Acne Group. J Am Acad Dermatol 2009;60(Suppl 5):S1–50.

33. Williams HC, Dellavalle RP, Garner S. Acne vulgaris. Lancet 2012;379(9813): 361–72.

34. Gamble R, Dunn J, Dawson A, et al. Topical antimicrobial treatment of acne vulgaris: an evidence-based review. Am J Clin Dermatol 2012;13(3):141–52.

35. Simonart T. Newer approaches to the treatment of acne vulgaris. Am J Clin Dermatol 2012;13(6):357–64.
36. Mays RM, Gordon RA, Wilson JM, et al. New antibiotic therapies for acne and rosacea. Dermatol Ther 2012;25(1):23–37.
37. Tan J. Dapsone 5% gel: a new option in topical therapy for acne. Skin Therapy Lett 2012;17(8):1–3.
38. Gallo R, Drago F, Paolino S, et al. Rosacea treatments: what's new and what's on the horizon? Am J Clin Dermatol 2010;11(5):299–303.
39. May D, Kelsberg G, Safranek S. Clinical inquiries. What is the most effective treatment for acne rosacea? J Fam Pract 2011;60(2):108a–100c.
40. Altinyazar HC, Koca R, Tekin NS, et al. Adapalene vs. metronidazole gel for the treatment of rosacea. Int J Dermatol 2005;44(3):252–5.
41. Fowler JF Jr. Combined effect of anti-inflammatory dose doxycycline (40-mg doxycycline, usp monohydrate controlled-release capsules) and metronidazole topical gel 1% in the treatment of rosacea. J Drugs Dermatol 2007;6(6): 641–5.
42. Sanchez J, Somolinos AL, Almodovar PI, et al. A randomized, double-blind, placebo-controlled trial of the combined effect of doxycycline hyclate 20-mg tablets and metronidazole 0.75% topical lotion in the treatment of rosacea. J Am Acad Dermatol 2005;53(5):791–7.
43. Bencini PL, Tourlaki A, De Giorgi V, et al. Laser use for cutaneous vascular alterations of cosmetic interest. Dermatol Ther 2012;25(4):340–51.
44. Lipozencic J, Ljubojevic S. Perioral dermatitis. Clin Dermatol 2011;29(2): 157–61.
45. Hafeez ZH. Perioral dermatitis: an update. Int J Dermatol 2003;42(7):514–7.
46. Oppel T, Pavicic T, Kamann S, et al. Pimecrolimus cream (1%) efficacy in perioral dermatitis—results of a randomized, double-blind, vehicle-controlled study in 40 patients. J Eur Acad Dermatol Venereol 2007;21(9):1175–80.
47. Schwarz T, Kreiselmaier I, Bieber T, et al. A randomized, double-blind, vehicle-controlled study of 1% pimecrolimus cream in adult patients with perioral dermatitis. J Am Acad Dermatol 2008;59(1):34–40.
48. Weber K, Thurmay R, Meisinger A. A topical erythromycin preparation and oral tetracycline for the treatment of perioral dermatitis: a placebo controlled trial. J Dermatol Treat 1993;4:57.
49. Veien NK, Munkvad JM, Nielsen AO, et al. Topical metronidazole in the treatment of perioral dermatitis. J Am Acad Dermatol 1991;24(2 Pt 1):258–60.
50. Soeprono FF, Schinella RA, Cockerell CJ, et al. Seborrheic-like dermatitis of acquired immunodeficiency syndrome. A clinicopathologic study. J Am Acad Dermatol 1986;14(2 Pt 1):242–8.
51. Berger RS, Stoner MF, Hobbs ER, et al. Cutaneous manifestations of early human immunodeficiency virus exposure. J Am Acad Dermatol 1988;19(2 Pt 1): 298–303.
52. Wolf R, Oumeish OY, Parish LC. Intertriginous eruption. Clin Dermatol 2011; 29(2):173–9.
53. Janniger CK, Schwartz RA, Szepietowski JC, et al. Intertrigo and common secondary skin infections. Am Fam Physician 2005;72(5):833–8.
54. Cramer DW, Liberman RF, Titus-Ernstoff L, et al. Genital talc exposure and risk of ovarian cancer. Int J Cancer 1999;81(3):351–6.
55. Phillips RM, Rosen T. Topical antifungal agents. In: Wolverton SE, editor. Comprehensive dermatologic drug therapy. 2nd edition. Philadelphia: Saunders Elsevier; 2007. p. 547–68.

56. Holdiness MR. Management of cutaneous erythrasma. Drugs 2002;62(8): 1131–41.
57. Clayton YM, Hay RJ, McGibbon DH, et al. Double blind comparison of the efficacy of tioconazole and miconazole for the treatment of fungal infection of the skin or erythrasma. Clin Exp Dermatol 1982;7(5):543–9.
58. Pitcher DG, Noble WC, Seville RH. Treatment of erythrasma with miconazole. Clin Exp Dermatol 1979;4(4):453–6.
59. Ramelet AA, Walker-Nasir E. One daily application of oxiconazole cream is sufficient for treating dermatomycoses. Dermatologica 1987;175(6):293–5.
60. Grigoriu D, Grigoriu A. Double-blind comparison of the efficacy, toleration and safety of tioconazole base 1% and econazole nitrate 1% creams in the treatment of patients with fungal infections of the skin or erythrasma. Dermatologica 1983; 166(Suppl 1):8–13.
61. Avci O, Tanyildizi T, Kusku E. A comparison between the effectiveness of erythromycin, single-dose clarithromycin and topical fusidic acid in the treatment of erythrasma. J Dermatolog Treat 2013;24(1):70–4.
62. Seville RH, Somerville DA. The treatment of erythrasma in a hospital for the mentally subnormal. Br J Dermatol 1970;82(5):502–6.
63. Weigle N, McBane S. Psoriasis. Am Fam Physician 2013;87(9):626–33.
64. David CV, Chira S, Eells SJ, et al. Diagnostic accuracy in patients admitted to hospitals with cellulitis. Dermatol Online J 2011;17(3):1.
65. Hirschmann JV, Raugi GJ. Lower limb cellulitis and its mimics: part II. Conditions that simulate lower limb cellulitis. J Am Acad Dermatol 2012;67(2):177.e1–9 [quiz: 185–6].
66. Hirschmann JV, Raugi GJ. Lower limb cellulitis and its mimics: part I. Lower limb cellulitis. J Am Acad Dermatol 2012;67(2):163.e1–12 [quiz: 175–6].
67. Roujeau JC, Sigurgeirsson B, Korting HC, et al. Chronic dermatomycoses of the foot as risk factors for acute bacterial cellulitis of the leg: a case-control study. Dermatology 2004;209(4):301–7.
68. Semel JD, Goldin H. Association of athlete's foot with cellulitis of the lower extremities: diagnostic value of bacterial cultures of ipsilateral interdigital space samples. Clin Infect Dis 1996;23(5):1162–4.
69. McNamara DR, Tleyjeh IM, Berbari EF, et al. Incidence of lower-extremity cellulitis: a population-based study in Olmsted county, Minnesota. Mayo Clin Proc 2007;82(7):817–21.
70. Celsus A. De Medicina. Circa 50 AD.
71. Jeng A, Beheshti M, Li J, et al. The role of beta-hemolytic streptococci in causing diffuse, nonculturable cellulitis: a prospective investigation. Medicine (Baltimore) 2010;89(4):217–26.
72. Bergkvist PI, Sjobeck K. Antibiotic and prednisolone therapy of erysipelas: a randomized, double blind, placebo-controlled study. Scand J Infect Dis 1997; 29(4):377–82.
73. Pierard GE, Quatresooz P. What do you mean by eczema craquele? Dermatology 2007;215(1):3–4.
74. Bhushan M, Cox NH, Chalmers RJ. Eczema craquele resulting from acute oedema: a report of seven cases. Br J Dermatol 2001;145(2):355–7.
75. O'Meara S, Cullum N, Nelson EA, et al. Compression for venous leg ulcers. Cochrane Database Syst Rev 2012;(11):CD000265.
76. Shingler S, Robertson L, Boghossian S, et al. Compression stockings for the initial treatment of varicose veins in patients without venous ulceration. Cochrane Database Syst Rev 2011;(11):CD008819.

77. Partsch H, Flour M, Smith PC, et al. Indications for compression therapy in venous and lymphatic disease consensus based on experimental data and scientific evidence. Under the auspices of the IUP. Int Angiol 2008;27(3): 193–219.
78. Cornu-Thenard A, Boivin P, Carpentier PH, et al. Superimposed elastic stockings: pressure measurements. Dermatol Surg 2007;33(3):269–75 [discussion: 275].
79. Smart V, Alavi A, Coutts P, et al. Contact allergens in persons with leg ulcers: a Canadian study in contact sensitization. Int J Low Extrem Wounds 2008;7(3): 120–5.
80. Wells PS, Hirsh J, Anderson DR, et al. Accuracy of clinical assessment of deep-vein thrombosis. Lancet 1995;345(8961):1326–30.
81. Wells PS, Hirsh J, Anderson DR, et al. A simple clinical model for the diagnosis of deep-vein thrombosis combined with impedance plethysmography: potential for an improvement in the diagnostic process. J Intern Med 1998;243(1):15–23.
82. Chowdhury MM. Dermatological pharmacology: topical agents. Medicine 2004; 32(12):16–7.
83. Finlay AY, Edwards PH, Harding KG. "Fingertip unit" in dermatology. Lancet 1989;2(8655):155.
84. Long CC, Finlay AY. The finger-tip unit—a new practical measure. Clin Exp Dermatol 1991;16(6):444–7.

Evaluation and Treatment of Shoulder Pain

Deborah L. Greenberg, MD

KEYWORDS

- Rotator cuff disease • Subacromial impingement syndrome • Adhesive capsulitis
- Painful arc

KEY POINTS

- Shoulder pain can have a significant impact on function.
- A thorough examination of the shoulder is a necessity.
- Most shoulder pain is due to the structure supporting the shoulder joint.
- Pain relief and exercises are the mainstays of therapy.

INTRODUCTION

Shoulder pain is a common presenting concern in outpatient medical practice. Shoulder problems can significantly affect a patient's ability to work and other activities of daily life such as driving, dressing, brushing hair, and even eating. "The shoulder" consists of a complex array of bones, muscles, tendons, and nerves, making the cause of pain seem difficult to decipher. Shoulder pain can be caused by structures within the shoulder or can arise from problems external to the shoulder. Fortunately, most shoulder pain falls into one of several patterns.

The rotator cuff provides stabilization to the glenohumeral joint, and contributes to mobility and strength of the shoulder. Disease of the rotator cuff is the most common cause of shoulder pain seen in clinical practice. The prevalence of rotator cuff disease increases with age, obesity, diabetes, and chronic diseases that affect the strength of the shoulder such as stroke.[1] An experienced practitioner can often recognize the cause of a patient's shoulder pain with a few questions and a focused examination. Treatment of shoulder pain can be successfully managed by a primary care provider in most cases. Referral to a physical therapist can be important to help improve the patient's mechanics and strength. Early use of imaging studies and specialist referrals are overutilized by primary care providers, and should be limited to specific indications.[2] Consultation with an orthopedic surgeon for fractures and tendon tears will be necessary in some cases.

The author declares no financial disclosures or conflict of interest.
Division of General Internal Medicine, University of Washington School of Medicine, 4245 Roosevelt Way Northeast, Seattle, WA 98105, USA
E-mail address: debbiegr@u.washington.edu

When evaluating patients with shoulder pain, it is important to understand the anatomy of the region. The major anatomic structures of interest include (**Fig. 1**)[3]:

- Four main bony structures: proximal humerus, clavicle, scapula, and ribs. The acromion, the superior, anterior extension of the scapula, forms the roof of the shoulder.
- Three main joints: glenohumeral, acromioclavicular (AC), sternoclavicular.
- Four rotator cuff muscles/tendons (SITS): supraspinatus (abduction), infraspinatus (external rotation), teres minor (external rotation, adduction), and subscapularis (adduction, internal rotation). The supraspinatus and infraspinatus tendons pass through the subacromial space to insert on the greater tubercle of the humerus.

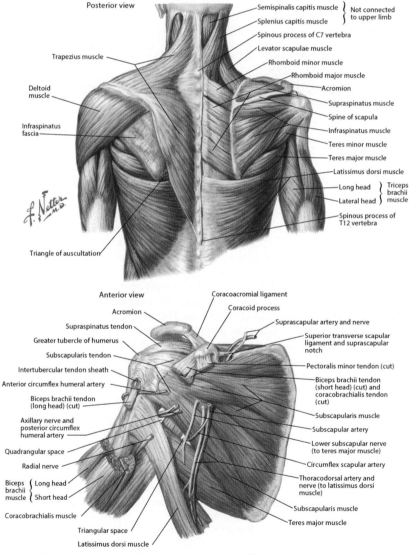

Fig. 1. Muscles: back and scapula region. *From* Netter illustration from www.netterimages.com. © Elsevier Inc. All rights reserved.

- Bursa: the subacromial bursa provides a cushion as the rotator cuff tendons move below the acromion.
- Surrounding musculature: biceps, deltoid, pectoralis, latissimus dorsi, rhomboids.
- Neurovascular: suprascapular nerve and vessels.

Important Terms

Rotator cuff disease

Rotator cuff disease (RCD) is a term encompassing tendinopathy, partial-thickness tear, or complete tear of one or more of the rotator cuff tendons. RCD also includes subacromial bursitis. In general, the term RCD is used synonymously with subacromial impingement syndrome (SIS).

Subacromial impingement syndrome

SIS is an umbrella term that encompasses rotator cuff tendinopathy and partial tears, as well as subacromial bursitis. The term is meant to convey the proposed etiology of these conditions. Inflammation and pain are caused by compression or impingement of the supraspinatus tendon (most common), infraspinatus tendon, subacromial bursa, biceps tendon, or other structures as they pass through the space between the lateral aspect of the acromion and the humeral head. Functional impingement can occur when there are problems with the mobility and stability of the rotator cuff muscles or the position and movement of the scapula.[4] Risk factors for impingement include repetitive activity above the head, increasing age, and conditions such as stroke and Parkinson disease. These risk factors are related to poor mechanics or decreased strength and stability of the rotator cuff and other supporting muscles. The natural history of SIS is often chronic or with recurrent pain and dysfunction.

Adhesive capsulitis (frozen shoulder)

Chronic pain and reduced active and passive mobility in the glenohumeral joint is associated with a variety of shoulder problems or occur as a primary problem of unknown cause. Adhesive capsulitis typically is seen in patients in their 40s to 60s, but is more common in diabetics in whom it is likely to present at a younger age. Adhesive capsulitis may resolve spontaneously over a period of years, but causes significant pain and functional limitations in the meantime.[5]

SYMPTOMS

Symptoms should be evaluated in the context of the patient as a whole. Age, underlying medical conditions, body habitus and overall strength, and smoking status are all important considerations. A systematic approach to history taking is crucial to avoid missing historical information. The most important factors include:

- Prior condition of shoulder
- Location of current pain:
    Localized or diffuse
    Anterior, lateral, or posterior
- Radiation patterns (clue: radiation past the elbow suggests a neurologic component)
- Timing of pain onset: sudden onset or developed gradually? (clue: came on all at once suggests a tear)[6]
- Associated factors: repetitive stress or recent or prior injury
- Duration: acute (<6 weeks), subacute (6–12 weeks), chronic (>3 months)

- Quality of pain: sharp, dull
- Associated symptoms: weakness, stiffness, crepitus, swelling (clue: fear of recurrence suggests shoulder instability)
- Alleviating and exacerbating factors: pain at night, pain worse with overhead activities (pain at night is a classic symptom for tear but likelihood ratios [LRs] are not significant in systematic review)[7]
- Systemic factors: fever, numbness, weight loss, fatigue, dyspnea, chest pain

Common Symptom Patterns

Subacromial impingement: lateral pain, subacute, worse with movement overhead
Rotator cuff tear: sudden onset, weakness, pain at night
Adhesive capsulitis: distant injury or chronic pain, progressive inability to reach over head, decreased mobility

DIAGNOSTIC TESTS AND IMAGING STUDIES
Physical Examination

The physical examination is used to diagnose the cause of the patient's pain but also to assess functional abilities. Elderly patients in particular may not be able to perform activities of daily living and may require assistance at home. A systematic approach to the examination is essential. The initial physical examination for shoulder pain should focus primarily on the musculoskeletal complex. Additional components of the examination can be performed if there is concern about an extrinsic cause of the patient's shoulder pain.

Observing Both Shoulders for Comparison

Further specific testing can be done based on the results of the initial examination. There are many tests for shoulder mobility and strength. None of the maneuvers has been found to be the ideal test for diagnosis of a particular syndrome or lesion.[8] Abduction maneuvers are recommended, given their better performance in systematic reviews in the diagnosis of specific pathologic conditions of the shoulder.

1. General appearance (**Fig. 2**): Symmetry, bulk, deformities, atrophy above or below the scapular spine. Atrophy in the space below the scapular spine suggests RCD (positive LR 2.0, negative LR 0.61)[7] or injury to the suprascapular nerve.[6]
2. Palpation: Sternoclavicular joint, clavicle, acromioclavicular joint, lateral acromion, biceps tendon in the groove between the greater and lesser tubercle of the humerus. Remember: some patients can be tender at many points but you are trying to recreate the pain that they have been experiencing at home. The anterior joint line can be palpated.
3. General range of motion (ROM)/pain provocation testing: ROM testing identifies limitations in ROM and localizes pain. Start with these basic ROM tests with the patient standing. Test active ROM first and add passive ROM if the patient has pain or limited motion. All maneuvers start from the anatomic position with arms at the side and palms facing forward.

Abduction

Ask the patient to raise the arm from the side (0°) to overhead (**Fig. 3**). Normal ROM is 180°. If the patient has limitation in active ROM, assist with passive ROM. Stand behind the patient and place a hand on the unaffected shoulder. With the other hand support the patient's affected arm just above the elbow. The patient's arm

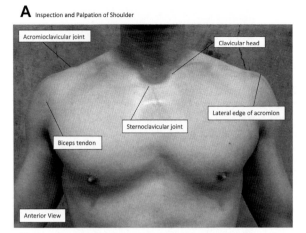

A Inspection and Palpation of Shoulder

Acromioclavicular joint

Clavicular head

Lateral edge of acromion

Sternoclavicular joint

Biceps tendon

Anterior View

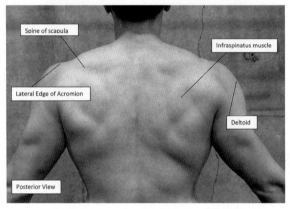

B Inspection and Palpation of Shoulder

Spine of scapula

Infraspinatus muscle

Lateral Edge of Acromion

Deltoid

Posterior View

Fig. 2. General appearance of the shoulder. (*A*) Anterior; (*B*) Posterior.

should remain within the horizontal plane. Raise the arm until limited by pain. If pain occurs with active or passive ROM, specify the location (0°–180°).

Pain in the lateral shoulder between 60° and 120° abduction is known as the painful arc, and suggests disease in the rotator cuff or subacromial bursa,[9-11] also known as subacromial impingement. The painful arc is one of the most helpful physical examination findings when considering RCD (positive LR 3.7, negative LR 0.50).[7]

Pain between 120° and 180° suggests a problem with the AC joint.

External rotation
Stand in front of the patient. Ask the patient to hold the arms in front of the body with elbows bent to 90°, palms facing in; ask the patient to hold the elbows against the sides and move the hands outward, parallel to the floor. Normal external rotation is at least 55° and up to 80°. For passive ROM grasp the affected arm proximal to the wrist and externally rotate. Pain or decreased ROM suggests a problem with the teres minor or infraspinatus muscle.

Internal rotation
Stand in front of the patient. Ask the patient to hold the arms in front of the body with elbows bent to 90°, palms facing in; ask the patient to hold the elbows against the

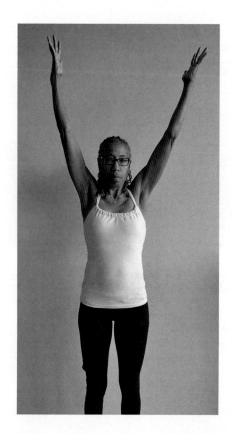

Fig. 3. Abduction.

sides and move the hands inward, parallel to the floor. Normal internal rotation is at least 45°. For passive ROM, grasp the affected arm proximal to the wrist and internally rotate. Pain or decreased ROM suggests a problem with the subscapularis muscle.

Cross-body adduction

Cross-body adduction is also known as the scarf test (**Fig. 4**). The patient reaches the affected arm across the body to the opposite shoulder. Pain in the front of the shoulder suggests AC joint abnormality.

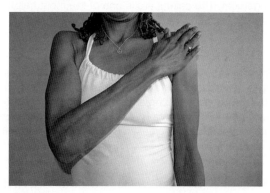

Fig. 4. Cross-body adduction.

- If the basic examination and ROM testing are normal, STOP and consider problems external to the shoulder itself. Pursue more generalized examination: neurovascular examination of the upper extremity, cardiac, pulmonary, abdominal, and neurologic examinations.
- If you are concerned about adhesive capsulitis or glenohumeral arthritis, poorly localized pain, limited range of all active and passive ROM, STOP.
- If you are concerned about AC joint disease, pain over AC joint, pain on abduction, STOP.
- If you are concerned about RCD, further testing for impingement (**Fig. 5**) and strength testing (**Fig. 6**) is required.
- If you are concerned about instability, biceps tendinopathy, or posterior pain, further tests as shown in **Fig. 7** should be considered.

Anteroposterior and Axillary Plain Radiographs of the Shoulder

Radiographs are useful in the setting of trauma, in particular:

- Fall on outstretched arm: fracture of the proximal humerus
- Fall on lateral shoulder: AC joint separation, clavicular or humeral fracture

Radiographs are also useful in evaluating:

- Presence and extent of glenohumeral arthritis, or to differentiate glenohumeral arthritis from adhesive capsulitis in a patient with limited passive ROM
- Presence and extent of AC arthritis
- Shoulder pain in patients with rheumatoid arthritis

Ultrasonography of the Shoulder

Ultrasonography of the shoulder can be used to assess:

- Shoulder dislocation.
- Biceps disorder. Compared with arthroscopy, ultrasonography performs well in the diagnosis of dislocation or subluxation of the long head of the biceps (sensitivity 96%, specificity 100%). Ultrasonography is also reliable for detecting complete tears of the biceps tendon, but may not be adequate for the detection of partial tears (sensitivity 49%, specificity 97%).[12]
- Rotator cuff tears. This modality is operator dependent, but in the hands of a good technician can be as good as magnetic resonance imaging (MRI) for detecting full-thickness tears (sensitivity 92%, specificity 94%) and partial-thickness tears (sensitivity 67%, specificity 94%).[13,14] Summary data for detecting any tear is sensitivity 91% and specificity 85%.[15] Ultrasonography is less expensive than MRI, and is better tolerated and preferred by patients.[16]

Magnetic Resonance Imaging

MRI of the shoulder is indicated for:

- Possible labral tear (trauma, repetitive overhead throwing or playing tennis, catching, or locking)
- Possible rotator cuff tear when quality ultrasonography not available (weakness)

As with ultrasonography, performance characteristics are better for full-thickness tears (sensitivity 84%–96%, specificity 93%–98%) than for partial-thickness tears (sensitivity 35%–44%, specificity 85%–97%).[13] For diagnosing any rotator cuff tear, sensitivity is 98% and sensitivity 79%.[15] MRI allows a better look at the shoulder as a whole, and can be useful if a surgical procedure is planned.

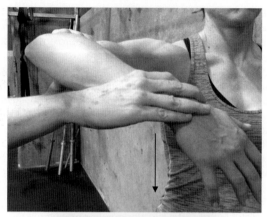

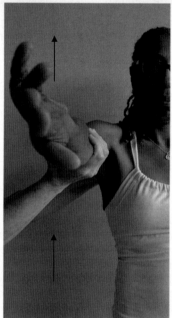

Fig. 5. Additional range of motion/pain provocation tests for suspected impingement. (*A*) Hawkins-Kennedy Impingement Sign:[10] Patient holds arm at 90° flexion with elbow at 90° flexion. Place downward pressure on the forearm and passively internally rotate the arm. (positive LR 1.5, negative LR 0.51).[7] (*B*) Neer's Impingement Sign: The patient internally rotates their hand (thumb toward the ground). Place your hand on the back of the patient's shoulder to stabilize the scapula. Forward flex the patient's straight arm by grasping just below the elbow and lifting. (positive LR 1.3).[7] Full ROM 180°.

Magnetic resonance arthrography (MRA) is better than either ultrasonography or MRI in detecting rotator cuff tears,[17] especially partial-thickness tears. MRA is generally ordered by sports medicine or orthopedic consultants on referral for possible surgical repair in a patient who has not improved with conservative therapy or who has significant strength lost on examination, but in whom a tear was not detected on initial imaging.

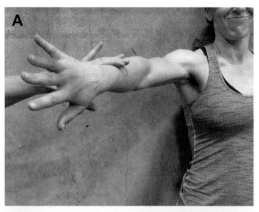

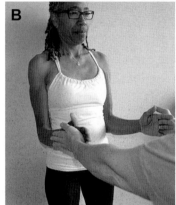
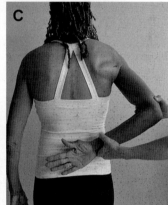

Fig. 6. Strength testing of rotator cuff. (*A*) *Empty Can Test*: Patient starts with a straight arm at 90° abduction. The arm is then brought forward 30° toward center on the horizontal plane and the thumb rotated toward the floor. Apply gentle pressure downward above the elbow while patient attempts to resist this pressure. Pain suggests impingement of the supraspinatus. Weakness suggests a partial- or full-thickness tear.[6] (*B*) *Resisted isometric external rotation*: Patient flexes their arm to 90° and attempts to externally rotate arm against resistance. (positive LR for RCD 2.6, negative LR 0.49).[7] (*C*) *Internal Rotation lag test**: similar to lift-off test. One of the best tests when considering complete tear of subscapularis. Patient places hand on back with elbow at 90°. The examiner lifts the hand off the back. Failure to hold this position is a positive test. (positive LR for full thickness tear 5.6, negative LR 0.04).[7]

Bottom Line

Check radiograph if: trauma or possible arthritis

Check sonogram or MRI if: concern for labral or rotator cuff tear

DIFFERENTIAL DIAGNOSIS

The differential diagnosis is broad and can be aided by the primary location of the pain.

Lateral Shoulder Pain

SIS, rotator cuff tendonitis, subacromial bursitis, full-thickness or partial-thickness tears of the rotator cuff tendons, adhesive capsulitis, multidirectional instability, cervical radiculopathy, proximal humeral fracture, glenohumeral osteoarthritis (**Table 1**).

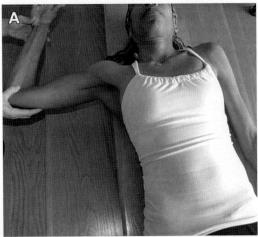

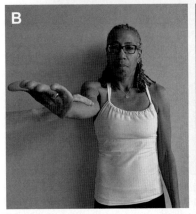
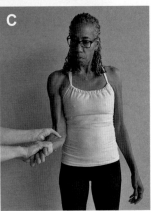

Fig. 7. Further testing if suspecting something other than subacromial impingement syndrome. (*A*) Apprehension Test- patient lies on the table. With their arm positioned off the side of table it is abducted 90° and externally rotated 90° (positive LR 17.2).11 A positive test is patient apprehension in this position. (*B*) Speed's Test: The patient flexes their arm to 90° with palm facing upward. Press downward as the patient resists arm movement. A positive test is pain in area of bicipital groove. (*C*) Yergason's Test: The patient flexes their elbow to 90°. Provide resistance to supination. A positive test is pain in area of bicipital groove.

Anterior Shoulder Pain

RCD, glenohumeral osteoarthritis, AC arthritis, AC separation, biceps tendonitis, adhesive capsulitis, anterior instability, biceps tendon rupture (sudden-onset pain, weakness and swelling), proximal humeral fracture, labral tear (**Table 2**).

Posterior Shoulder Pain

Posterior instability/dislocation, suprascapular nerve entrapment, RCD, labral tear, glenohumeral osteoarthritis, cervical radiculopathy, proximal humeral fracture.

Nonspecific Shoulder Pain

- Polymyalgia rheumatica: older patient, bilateral shoulder pain, full ROM, no weakness, may have hip pain, claudication, fatigue

Table 1
Common causes of lateral shoulder pain

	SIS/RCD	Complete Rotator Cuff Tear	Adhesive Capsulitis
Associated factors	Repetitive movement Stroke Parkinson disease	Long history of shoulder problems Trauma	Diabetes Age
Onset	Subacute to chronic	Acute or chronic with sudden worsening	Subacute to chronic
Other findings	Tenderness below lateral edge of acromion	Pain at night[a] Weakness Catching sensation	Stiffness Significant functional limitations
Range of motion	Full passive ROM	Limited active ROM due to weakness Full passive ROM	Decreased active and passive ROM
Pain with range of motion	[a]Painful arc ± External rotation ± Internal rotation	Often in setting of impingement, thus similar findings possible	Pain with ROM on multiple maneuvers
Weakness	No	Yes Drop-arm test Other tests (see **Fig. 6**)	No
Atrophy	No	Maybe	Maybe

Acute: ≤6 weeks; subacute: 6–12 weeks; chronic: ≥3 months.
Abbreviations: RCD, rotator cuff disease; ROM, range of motion; SIS, subacromial impingement syndrome.
[a] Classic symptom but likelihood ratios not significant in systematic review.[7]

- Cervical radiculopathy: pain below the elbow, numbness or weakness, decreased reflexes
- Glenohumeral osteoarthritis
- Rheumatoid arthritis: stiffness and other joint involvement
- Consider pulmonary, gastrointestinal, and cardiac causes of diaphragm irritation or referred pain

TREATMENT

The goal of treatment is to reduce pain and improve ROM, thus restoring function to the shoulder.

General Measures

- Analgesics: Nonsteroidal anti-inflammatory drugs (NSAIDs) are commonly recommended for the treatment of shoulder pain because of their anti-inflammatory effects. Experience suggests that any commonly used oral analgesics can be used for the treatment of shoulder pain thought to be due to RCD, SIS, AC joint disease, or adhesive capsulitis. There have been no studies comparing oral over-the-counter or prescription acetaminophen with NSAIDs. Thus either can be used, depending on coexistent disease and provider and patient preference.
- Should patients put ice or heat on their shoulder? Ice has traditionally been recommended for painful muscles and joints.[18] There is little evidence to show

Table 2
Differential of anterior shoulder pain

	Biceps Tendonitis	AC Separation	AC Arthritis	Proximal Humeral Fracture	Adhesive Capsulitis	Labral Tear	OA
Associated factors	Age Assoc with SIS	Fall onto lateral shoulder	Repetitive lifting	Age Fall on shoulder or outstretched arm	Chronic progressive pain/stiffness	Repetitive overhead throwing Trauma	Age Prior trauma
Onset	Subacute to chronic	Acute	Chronic	Acute	Subacute to chronic	Acute	Chronic
Specific findings	Tenderness in bicipital groove with internal and external rotation	Unilateral deformity and tenderness of AC joint	Tenderness over AC joint	Bruising	Decreased passive/active ROM	Deep shoulder pain Joint-line tenderness	Stiffness Crepitus Joint-line tenderness
ROM	Normal	Normal except adduction	Normal except adduction	Reluctant to attempt	Decreased passive/active ROM	Normal	Decreased passive/active ROM
Maneuver	Speed Yergason	Cross-arm adduction	Cross-arm adduction	None	Forward flexion reduced	None	None
Initial evaluation	None	Radiograph	Radiograph	Radiograph	None	MRI	Radiograph

Abbreviations: AC, acromioclavicular joint; MRI, magnetic resonance imaging; OA, osteoarthritis; ROM, range of motion; SIS, subacromial impingement syndrome.

whether ice is effective or even counterproductive in the treatment of soft-tissue inflammation. Ice does produce analgesia. Recommend ice for 20 to 30 minutes as often as every 2 hours if it provides relief to the patient. Ice should not be used before vigorous exercise. If ice is not helpful, the patient can try heat.

- Activity and work modification: Patients should limit activities that exacerbate their discomfort, especially overhead movements.

Menu of Additional Therapeutic Options

- Physical therapy: Therapists often use a combination of modalities, which can include manual mobilization, ice, heat, ultrasonography, massage, supervised progressive resistance exercises, electric stimulation, acupuncture, and stretching.
- Exercise therapy: Exercise therapy is generally initiated by a physical therapist. The patient is given instruction on strengthening exercises with movements against gravity and then progressive resistance exercises. The patient then follows a self-management plan at home.
- Manual therapy: Joint and soft-tissue mobilization and manipulation. Manual therapy is thought to break down the adhesions that form between different layers of soft tissue and allow unimpeded movement of the muscle. It can be used alone or in combination with exercises.
- Acupuncture: Needles are placed into specific acupuncture points. Sessions typically last 30 to 60 minutes and are performed 1 to 2 times a week for 4 to 8 weeks. Acupuncture can reduce pain,[19,20] allowing the patient to participate in exercise therapy.
- Subacromial corticosteroid injection: The injection can be guided by ultrasound or by clinical landmarks. There is no difference in safety or efficacy with either approach.[21] The routine use of ultrasound-guided glucocorticoid injection is discouraged, given the excess cost. Patients should not engage in heavy lifting for 2 weeks following an injection.
- Platelet-rich plasma injection: Injection of autologous platelet-rich plasma into the subacromial space. There is no evidence that platelet-rich plasma injections in addition to exercise improve pain or function of the shoulder to a greater extent than exercise alone.[22]
- Immobilization should be avoided unless directed by a surgeon for fracture.
- Botulinum toxin: Intramuscular injection of botulinum toxin A, which may be useful in reducing shoulder pain after stroke and in osteoarthritis of the shoulder.[23]
- Surgical intervention.

Condition-Specific Treatment

SIS/RCD, subacromial bursitis
Bottom Line
1. General measures: ice/heat, oral analgesic, avoid exacerbating activities.
2. Patient should have exercise therapy as part of a home self-management plan or as part of a physical therapist treatment plan.
3. The addition of manual therapy, acupuncture, or a subacromial steroid injection can have added benefit. Consider based on availability, cost, and patient preference.
4. If symptoms fail to improve after 3 months of conservative therapy, referral for surgical intervention can be considered.

The cause of this syndrome is dysfunctional mechanics, primarily of the scapula or rotator cuff muscles, leading to inflammation and pain as tendons and other structure are compressed between the acromion and humeral head. Treatment is designed to reduce pain, allowing sufficient strengthening exercises to correct the mechanical deficiencies.

Exercise therapy is universally recommended for the treatment of SIS and RCD. Exercise can significantly reduce pain and improve function.[24,25] Recommended exercises run the gamut from nonspecific shoulder strengthening to exercises designed to correct the mechanical issues leading to impingement. In one study of patients awaiting surgery for impingement, exercise focusing on eccentric strengthening of the rotator cuff muscles and eccentric/concentric strengthening of the shoulder stabilizers substantially reduced the need to for surgery in comparison with nonspecific shoulder exercises (odds ratio 7.7, 95% confidence interval 3.1–19.4; $P<.001$).[26]

Exercise therapy can be supervised as part of regular visits to a physical therapist, or done independently by the patient at home as part of a self-management plan. Patients willing to participate in self-training typically meet with the therapist initially and then attend 1 to 3 follow-up visits to adjust the exercise plan. Both supervised and independent exercise programs improve symptoms in patients with shoulder pain.[25] Self-management involves fewer visits with the therapist and thus, lower cost. Patients who are willing to adhere to a home program likely have better improvement in pain and function than patients who participate in a more traditional physical therapy program.[27]

Exercise therapy can be combined with manual therapy or acupuncture, or started after a subacromial steroid injection. Manual therapy in addition to exercise may be more effective than exercise alone in reducing pain.[28] Subacromial steroid injection or acupuncture plus home exercise therapy are equally effective at reducing pain and improving function in patients with SIS both short term and after 1 year.[20] Initiation of exercise should be delayed for 2 weeks after a steroid injection.

Surgical decompression, either arthroscopically or as an open procedure, is designed to reduce compression in the subacromial space. Studies have not shown a benefit of surgery over conservative therapy for the reduction of pain or improvement of function in patients with impingement syndrome.[29,30] Given the risks of surgery, this modality should be considered only after conservative therapy has failed.

Rotator cuff tear

Rotator cuff tears can be asymptomatic or can cause significant pain and disability. Patients with a rotator cuff tear who are surgical candidates should be referred to an orthopedic surgeon to discuss the risks and expected benefits of surgical repair. Some patients will recover sufficient pain relief and function without surgery, but the outcome in an individual patient is difficult to predict.[31] Because delayed surgery can cause complications in some patients owing to atrophy and scarring of tissue, patients should be fully informed of their options.

Adhesive capsulitis

Reduction of pain followed by improved ROM is the goal of therapy. Pain reduction can be achieved with a subacromial corticosteroid injection or oral analgesics. Randomized trials have shown that steroid injections and oral NSAIDs, when accompanied by therapeutic exercise, are equally effective in improving pain and function over a period of 6 months.[32] The choice of therapy should be based on patient preference, comorbidities, and availability of treatment options. It is unclear whether manual therapy in addition to other treatments improves outcomes.[28] If the patient is in significant pain, declines injection, and has contraindications to other oral analgesics, oral steroids can reduce pain and improve ROM in the short term, but are unlikely to improve long-term function.[33] Patients should be educated on the time course of recovery. Full recovery can often take as long as 6 to 18 months. Adhesive capsulitis may be self-limited in some patients over a period of months to years.[5] Patients who fail to respond to 3 months of therapy or are unable to participate in therapy because of significant pain can be referred for consideration of imaging-guided capsular distention, manipulation under anesthesia, or other surgical options.

Osteoarthritis of the glenohumeral joint

Initial conservative therapy can include pain relief with analgesics and exercise therapy, although there is limited evidence that these modalities improve function or outcomes. Limited evidence suggests that injectable viscosupplementation can be helpful for some patients.[34] Patients who fail conservative therapy can undergo total arthroplasty of the shoulder joint with hopes of reducing pain and improving function. There are no randomized trials comparing surgical treatment with continued conservative measures in these patients.[35]

Nonspecific shoulder pain/dysfunction

Massage therapy helps improve pain and ROM in short-term studies, especially in patients with posterior shoulder pain and limited internal ROM.[36] There is little evidence that it helps improve function of the shoulder over the long term.[28]

MANAGEMENT
Education

In addition to the specific treatment of shoulder pain, patients should be educated on the cause of their problem and the role of each of the modalities used in treatment. Failure to engage in self-management, particularly rehabilitation exercises, can significantly delay or prevent full return to function.

Prevention

Many shoulder problems are due to repetitive motion with the arms or the lack of strength and mobility. Patients with work-related symptoms should undergo an ergonomic review at work to reduce the risk of persistent problems.[37] All patients should be encouraged to incorporate upper extremity ROM and strengthening to their overall fitness routine.

CASES
Case 1

A 58-year-old man with a history of obesity and diabetes reports pain in his right shoulder over the last several months. He does not remember a specific injury, but is now having difficulty performing his job as a house painter and putting on and taking off his shirt. He has difficulty laying on his right side to sleep. When asked to locate the pain he places his hand over the lateral aspect of his right shoulder. On physical examination he has tenderness below the lateral edge of the acromion. His active ROM is limited to 100° abduction because of the pain, but he has full passive ROM. He has pain with external rotation but no evidence of weakness in his right arm. Hawkins and Neer tests are positive. He has tried ice, a 2-week trial of ibuprofen, and then a 2-week trial of acetaminophen without significant improvement.

Discussion

This patient has a history and examination consistent with SIS. Review his dosing of analgesics to ensure that he tried adequate doses. Further NSAIDs may be contraindicated if he has renal dysfunction. He should be prescribed ice, heat, and then specific exercises with manual therapy, acupuncture, or a subacromial bursa injection.

Case 2

A 63-year-old woman has had pain in her left shoulder for the last 6 months. Pain began while trimming some plum trees in her yard. Initially she had difficulty putting dishes into an overhead cabinet. She has been avoiding all overhead activities for the last 3 months. She finds that her shoulder is stiff and she has difficulty brushing her hair. She is not able to localize her pain to one spot. On examination she has limited active and passive ROM with forward flexion, abduction, internal rotation, and external rotation of her left arm. She does not have weakness.

Discussion

This patient most likely has adhesive capsulitis. If you were concerned about glenohumeral arthritis, a radiograph would be reasonable to exclude this possibility. Oral analgesics and referral to a physical therapist for exercises is the appropriate initial step.

Case 3

A 74-year-old woman lost her balance while boating. She fell and hit her right shoulder against the seat in the boat. She had immediate pain in her right shoulder, and has been holding her arm against her side in the 3 hours since the accident, as any movement is uncomfortable. Her arm is bruised and she is reluctant to move it. Her pulses and neurologic testing in that arm are intact.

Discussion

No further examination is needed at this point. A radiograph to assess for fracture showed a proximal nondisplaced humeral fracture. After discussion with an orthopedist, she was placed in an arm sling and followed up in the clinic.

FUTURE CONSIDERATIONS AND SUMMARY

Shoulder pain is a common symptom in the adult population. The most common cause of shoulder pain is SIS, reflecting a problem with the rotator cuff or subacromial bursa. Determining the cause of a patient's pain is usually a clinical diagnosis based on careful history taking and physical examination. Limited use of imaging studies will be needed in the setting of trauma, possible glenohumeral arthritis, or when a complete tendon tear is suspected. Therapy is based on pain control and therapeutic exercises in almost all cases. Despite the prevalence of shoulder pain, there is no consensus on the best way to achieve pain control or on the type of exercise most likely to achieve speedy recovery.

REFERENCES

1. Rechardt M, Shiri R, Karppinen J, et al. Lifestyle and metabolic factors in relation to shoulder pain and rotator cuff tendinitis: a population-based study. BMC Musculoskelet Disord 2010;11:165.
2. Buchbinder R, Staples MP, Shanahan EM, et al. General practitioner management of shoulder pain in comparison with rheumatologist expectation of care and best evidence: an Australian National Survey. PLoS One 2013;8:e61243.

3. Thompson JC. Netter's concise orthopaedic anatomy. Chapter 3. Saunders, an imprint of Elsevier Inc; 2002. p. P75–107 Copyright © 2010.

4. Arce G, Bak K, Bain G, et al. Management of disorders of the rotator cuff: proceedings ISAKOS upper extremity community consensus meeting. Arthroscopy 2013;29:1–11.

5. Ewald A. Adhesive capsulitis: a review. Am Fam Physician 2011;83:417–22.

6. Jobe FW, Jobe CM. Painful athletic injuries of the shoulder. Clin Orthop Relat Res 1983;(173):117–24.

7. Hermans J, Luime JJ, Meuffles DE, et al. Does this patient with shoulder pain have rotator cuff disease? The rational clinical examination systematic review. JAMA 2013;310(8):837–47.

8. Hanchard NC, Lenza M, Handoll HH, et al. Physical tests for shoulder impingements and local lesions of bursa, tendon or labrum that may accompany impingement. Cochrane Database Syst Rev 2013;(4):CD007427.

9. Kessel L, Watson M. The painful arc syndrome: clinical classification as a guide to management. J Bone Joint Surg Br 1977;59(2):166–72.

10. Hawkins RJ, Kennedy JC. Impingement syndrome in athletes. Am J Sports Med 1980;3:151–8.

11. Hegedus EJ, Goode AP, Cook CE, et al. Which physical examination tests provide clinicians with the most value when examining of the shoulder? Update of a systematic review with analysis of individual tests. Br J Sports Med 2012;46:964–78.

12. Armstrong A, Teefey SA, Wu T, et al. The efficacy of ultrasound in the diagnosis of long head of the biceps tendon pathology. J Shoulder Elbow Surg 2006;15:7–11.

13. Gazzola S, Bleakney RR. Current imaging of the rotator cuff. Sports Med Arthrosc 2011;19:300–9.

14. Teefey SA, Rubin DA, Middleton WD, et al. Detection and quantification of rotator cuff tears. Comparison of ultrasonographic, magnetic resonance imaging, and arthroscopic findings in seventy-one consecutive cases. J Bone Joint Surg Am 2004;86:708–16.

15. Lenza M, Buchbinder R, Takwoingi Y, et al. Magnetic resonance imaging, magnetic resonance arthropathy and ultrasonography for assessing rotator cuff tears in people with shoulder pain for whom surgery is being considered. Cochrane Database Syst Rev 2013;(9):CD009020.

16. Middelton WD, Payne WT, Teefey SA, et al. Sonography and MRI of the shoulder: comparison of patient satisfaction. Am J Roentgenol 2004;183:1449–52.

17. de Jesus JO, Parker L, Frangos AJ, et al. Accuracy of MRI, MR arthropathy, and ultrasound in the diagnosis of rotator cuff tears: a meta-analysis. Am J Roentgenol 2009;192:1701–7.

18. Swenson C, Sward L, Karlsson J. Cryotherapy in sports medicine. Scand J Med Sci Sports 1996;6:193–200.

19. Green S, Buchbinder R, Hetrick S. Acupuncture for shoulder pain. Cochrane Database Syst Rev 2005;(18):CD005319.

20. Johansson K, Bergstrom A, Schröder K, et al. Subacromial corticosteroid injection or acupuncture with home exercises when treating patients with subacromial impingement in primary care—a randomized controlled trial. Fam Pract 2011;4: 355–65.

21. Bloom JE, Rischin A, Johnston RV, et al. Image-guided versus blind glucocorticoids injection for shoulder pain. Cochrane Database Syst Rev 2012;(9):CD009147.

22. Kesikburun S, Tan AK, Yilmaz B, et al. Platelet-rich plasma injections in the treatment of chronic rotator cuff tendinopathy: a randomized controlled trial with one-year follow-up. Am J Sports Med 2013;41(11):2609–16.

23. Singh JA, Fitzgerald PM. Botulinum toxin for shoulder pain. Cochrane Database Syst Rev 2010;(9):CD008271.
24. Hanratty CE, McVeigh JG, Kerr DP, et al. The effectiveness of physiotherapy exercises in subacromial impingement syndrome: a systematic review and meta-analysis. Semin Arthritis Rheum 2012;42:297–316.
25. Littlewood C, Ashton J, Chance-Larsen K, et al. Exercise for rotator cuff tendinopathy: a systematic review. Physiotherapy 2012;98:101–9.
26. Holmgren T, Hallgren H, Öberg E, et al. Effect of specific exercise strategy on need for surgery in patients with subacromial impingement syndrome: randomized controlled study. BMJ 2012;344:e787.
27. Littlewood C, Malliaras P, Mawson S, et al. Self-managed loaded exercises versus usual physiotherapy treatment for rotator cuff tendinopathy: a pilot randomized controlled trial. Physiotherapy 2014;100(1):54–60.
28. Ho CC, Sole G, Munn J. The effectiveness of manual therapy in the management of musculoskeletal disorders of the shoulder: a systematic review. Man Ther 2009;14:463–74.
29. Gebremariam L, Hay EM, Koes BW, et al. Effectiveness of surgical and postsurgical interventions for the subacromial impingement syndrome: a systematic review. Arch Phys Med Rehabil 2011;92:1900–13.
30. Dorrestijn O, Stevens M, Winters JC, et al. Conservative or surgical treatment for subacromial impingement syndrome? A systematic review. J Shoulder Elbow Surg 2009;18:652–60.
31. Pegreffi F, Paladini P, Campi F, et al. Conservative management of rotator cuff tear. Sports Med Arthrosc 2011;19:348–52.
32. Dehghan A, Pishgooei N, Salami MA, et al. Comparison between NSAID and intra-articular corticosteroid injection in frozen shoulder of diabetic patients; a randomized clinical trial. Exp Clin Endocrinol Diabetes 2013;121:75–9.
33. Buchbinder R, Green S, Youd JM, et al. Oral steroids for adhesive capsulitis. Cochrane Database Syst Rev 2006;(4):CD006189.
34. American Academy of Orthopedic Surgeons. The treatment of glenohumeral joint osteoarthritis. Guideline and evidence report [online]. 2009. Available at: http://www.aaos.org/research/guidelines/gloguideline.pdf. Accessed February 25, 2014.
35. Singh JA, Sperling J, Buchbinder R, et al. Surgery for shoulder osteoarthritis. Cochrane Database Syst Rev 2010;(10):CD008089.
36. Yang J, Chen S, Hsieh C, et al. Effects and predictors of shoulder muscle massage for patients with posterior shoulder tightness. BMC Musculoskelet Disord 2012;13:46–53.
37. Hoe VC, Urquhart DM, Kelsall HL, et al. Ergonomic design and training for preventing work-related musculoskeletal disorders of the upper limb and neck in adults. Cochrane Database Syst Rev 2012;(15):CD008570.

Diagnosis and Treatment of Headache in the Ambulatory Care Setting
A Review of Classic Presentations and New Considerations in Diagnosis and Management

Natalie Hale, MPH, MDc[a], Douglas S. Paauw, MD, MACP[b],*

KEYWORDS

- Primary headache • Secondary headache • Tension headache • Migraine headache
- Triptans • Cluster headache • Hypnic headache • Chronic daily headache

KEY POINTS

- The 4 most common headache subtypes are tension, migraine, cluster, and chronic daily headaches.
- Headache diagnoses are generally made on clinical grounds. Imaging is often required if a secondary cause of headache is suspected.
- A number of diagnoses that have caused confusion in the past are now recognized as migrainous disorders. These include abdominal migraine, cyclic vomiting syndrome, and, more often than not, sinus headache.
- Special considerations are necessary when working up and treating headaches in pregnant women and the elderly.
- Addition of metoclopramide can improve the efficacy of oral migraine therapies and reduce nausea.
- A number of new complementary modalities show promise in the treatment of headache disorder. In particular, butterbur, a petasite, is now recognized as a highly effective preventive therapy for migraine sufferers.

INTRODUCTION

Headaches are the most prevalent constellation of neurologic disorders and are among the most common reasons patients present for care.[1] The most important first

The authors have nothing to disclose.
[a] Department of Medicine, University of Washington School of Medicine, Seattle, WA 98195, USA; [b] Medicine Student Programs, University of Washington School of Medicine, Seattle, WA 98195, USA
* Corresponding author.
E-mail address: dpaauw@medicine.washington.edu

step in the diagnosis of headache is determining whether the headache is a primary or secondary disorder. Secondary headaches result from an underlying pathology and are generally very serious in nature and must be worked up and treated in an urgent manner. Common causes of secondary headache include subarachnoid hemorrhage, intraparenchymal bleed, temporal arteritis, mass effect from a tumor or abscess, or intracranial infection.[2] Although this article will touch on the workup of secondary headaches, it will focus on primary headache disorders, which comprise 90% of all headaches.[3]

The 3 most common types of primary headaches include tension, migraine, and cluster headaches, comprising 40%, 10%, and 1% of all headaches, respectively.[1,2] Tension headaches affect approximately half of all individuals at some point in their lifetime and have equal prevalence across genders. Although common, tension headaches are usually mild and are rarely the cause for clinic visits. The lifetime prevalence of migraine headache is 18% and these headaches are particularly common in women.[1] Cluster headaches, on the other hand, are more common in men.[2] Other types of related disorders that are discussed in this article are cyclic vomiting syndrome (CVS) and abdominal migraine. We also consider special populations, including women, who tend to experience a greater number of migraines during their menstrual cycles, and the elderly, whose headache syndromes are markedly different from those in younger age groups and for whom many of the rescue and prophylactic medications prescribed for younger populations may actually be quite harmful. This article will help practitioners differentiate complex headache disorders from one another and provides a review of the latest modalities in treatment, including lifestyle modification, complementary modalities, and nonprescription supplements. A number of case scenarios also are presented to help highlight characteristic presentations of common headache syndromes.

PATIENT HISTORY

In patients presenting with headache, the first objective is determining whether a primary or a more serious secondary headache is present.[2] The patient history is particularly helpful in differentiating between these etiologies. Primary headaches typically develop before the third decade of life and tend to have stereotyped presentations and triggers, whereas secondary headaches more commonly occur at an age older than 55, often for the first time and with a high degree of severity.[4] Secondary headaches are often described as having a "thunderclap" onset, as they appear suddenly and with great intensity. Sudden-onset, excruciatingly painful headaches may indicate several concerning pathologic processes, including hypertensive emergency, acute angle-closure glaucoma, vertebral artery dissection, intraparenchymal hemorrhage, carotid artery dissection, or subarachnoid hemorrhage. Subarachnoid hemorrhage is particularly likely when a patient older than 45 presents with the worst headache of his or her life. Both prescribed medications and drugs of abuse, including methamphetamines, cocaine, nonsteroidal anti-inflammatory drugs (NSAIDs), anticoagulant drugs, and glucocorticoids increase the risk of intracranial bleeding. Fever, altered mental status, and symptoms of infection elsewhere are suggestive of infection, whereas immunosuppression or human immunodeficiency virus (HIV) infection predispose to intracranial abscess, infection, and malignancy, all of which may cause secondary headache.[2]

Primary headache disorders are differentiated by their severity, location, frequency, and the degree of disability they cause. The most common types of primary headaches are tension, migraine, and cluster headaches. A number of tools are available to assist practitioners in the diagnosis of these disorders, including the International Headache Society (IHS) Classification System, the Migraine Disability Assessment (MIDAS) questionnaire, and headache diaries. The MIDAS questionnaire and headache diaries kept over 4 to 6 weeks are helpful in differentiating among headache types and determining patient disability and the impact of headache on patient quality of life.[4,5] This section focuses on the typical patient histories for the 3 most common types of primary headaches and a number of rare, but related diagnoses, including chronic daily headache, CVS, and abdominal migraine. Special attention also is paid to headaches in the elderly, whose histories may differ from those provided by younger individuals (**Table 1**).

Tension Headaches

A 27-year-old computer programmer mentions that he has been having frequent headaches. He describes them as a bandlike discomfort around his scalp to the back of his head. He has found that using 600 mg of ibuprofen helps alleviate the symptoms greatly.

The patient in this case presents with the classic features of tension headache. This most common form of headaches presents with a bilateral feeling of mild-to-moderate tension and pressure.[2] The associated pain can occur anywhere from the neck to the head, but is not typically disabling. Patients will report that headache frequency is related to stress levels and that relief is generally achieved with acetaminophen or NSAIDs.[6] Tension headaches have received little research attention as compared with other primary headache syndromes, likely owing to their association with mental and physical stress and tension, but in more recent years, efforts have been made to better understand potential treatment modalities, as shall be discussed later in this article.[7] The classic features of infrequent episodic tension-type headaches are listed in **Fig. 1** and **Box 1**.[8]

Migraine Headaches

A 22-year-old woman presents for evaluation of headaches. She has had headaches for the past 6 months, occurring 4 to 5 times a month. The headaches are of great intensity, involving the right side of her head with the maximum intensity of pain occurring behind her right eye. Symptoms worsen with exertion. Her headaches last 3 to 6 hours, are sometimes associated with nausea, and, on 2 occasions, have been preceded by a scotoma in her right eye. Neurologic examination is unremarkable.

Table 1 Overview of major headache types	
Headache Type	**Characteristics**
Tension	Bilateral nondebilitating headache, often associated with stress.
Migraine	Unilateral mild-to-severe and often debilitating headache. May be associated with aura.
Cluster	Unilateral retro-orbital headache, often associated with lacrimation, nasal drainage, and erythematous conjunctiva. Untreated, occurs daily in "clusters" of 6–12 wk, often with up to 1 y between each cluster period.
Chronic daily	Daily headaches that develop after heavy use of analgesics, NSAIDs, and migraine-specific therapies. Underlying headache disorder may be mild, but patients can develop severe headaches due to medication overuse.

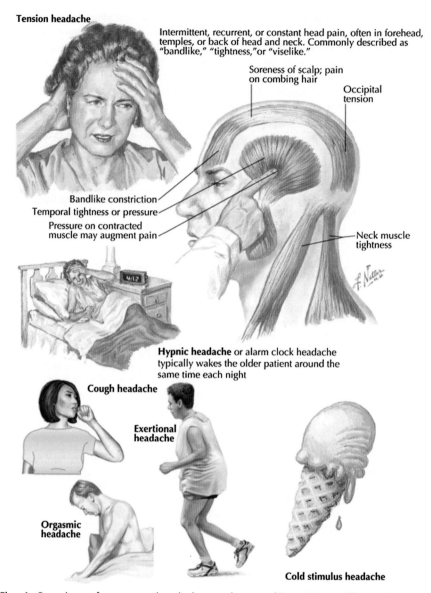

Tension headache

Intermittent, recurrent, or constant head pain, often in forehead, temples, or back of head and neck. Commonly described as "bandlike," "tightness," or "viselike."

Soreness of scalp; pain on combing hair

Occipital tension

Bandlike constriction
Temporal tightness or pressure
Pressure on contracted muscle may augment pain

Neck muscle tightness

Hypnic headache or alarm clock headache typically wakes the older patient around the same time each night

Cough headache

Exertional headache

Orgasmic headache

Cold stimulus headache

Fig. 1. Overview of common headache syndromes. (*From* Netter illustration www. netterimages.com. © Elsevier Inc. All rights reserved.)

This case exemplifies some of the hallmark characteristics of migraine headache. Patients with this condition often complain of disabling unilateral pain with possible photophobia or phonophobia, nausea and vomiting, and/or an aura.[2] Most patients experience a prodrome of symptoms, which may last for hours to days before the migraine.[4] This prodromal period is not to be confused with aura, described in the case scenario as a scotoma in the patient's right eye. The prodromal period may be characterized by mental status change, such as depression, drowsiness, restlessness, or euphoria; neurologic changes, such as photophobia, phonophobia,

---

Box 1
International Headache Society (IHS) tension headache criteria (infrequent episodic)

Infrequent episodes of mild-to-moderate bilateral pain, which is tightening or pressing in nature and lasts for minutes to days.

Diagnostic criteria

A. ≥10 episodes on <1 day per month and fulfilling criteria B–D

B. Duration of 30 minutes to 7 days

C. Characterized by ≥2 of the following: (1) bilaterality, (2) tightening or pressing (nonpulsating), (3) mild-to-moderate intensity, (4) not aggravated by routine physical activity, such as walking

D. Lack of nausea, vomiting, or photo-phonophobia

E. Cannot be attribute to another disorder

---

hypersomnolence, yawning, or decreased concentration; or other symptoms, such as gastrointestinal upset, food cravings, or temperature dysregulation.[4] Auras are seen in 15% to 20% of patients with migraine and typically last between 15 and 60 minutes.[4] Auras are most commonly visual, in which case they often present with a hemifield defect or start centrally and spread outward, but they can have sensory or motor characteristics or involve speech as well.[2–4] Migraine headaches are strongly heritable. First-degree relatives of patients with migraines without aura experience 1.4 and 1.9 times higher risks for developing migraines with and without aura, respectively. Even more strikingly, first-degree relatives of individuals with migraine with aura have a 4 times higher risk of developing migraine with aura, but no increased risk of developing migraine without aura. And twin studies of monozygotic and dizygotic twins suggest an approximately 50% rate of heritability, with the mode of heritability being multifactorial and polygenic.[9] The POUND criteria are particularly helpful in diagnosing migraine:

Pulsatile headache
One-day duration (4–72 hours)
Unilateral location
Nausea or vomiting
Disabling intensity

With 4 of 5 of these symptoms, there is a 92% probability that the patient is suffering from a migraine. If 3 of 5 are present, the probability is 64%.[10] Many patients will complain of migraine triggers. These triggers may be additive and may not always produce migraine with exposure. Examples include stress or recovery from stress, too much or too little sleep, flickering lights, or loud noises. Consumption of a number of foods or preservatives may also be responsible, such as monosodium glutamate; nitrites; the tyramine contained in wine and aged cheese; alcohol; artificial sweeteners; citrus; pickled foods; vinegars; caffeine overuse or withdrawal; or the phenylethylamine in chocolate, garlic, seeds, nuts, or raw onions. Importantly, menses is a trigger in 60% of female migraine sufferers and 14% of women with migraines experience their headaches only during menses.[3] These headaches are thought to be triggered by changing estrogen levels, which may in part explain the decrease in prevalence of migraine after age 50 and in postmenopausal women, unless estrogen replacement therapy is used (**Fig. 2**).[1]

Patients with migraine often have psychiatric comorbidities. This is particularly true in patients with migraine with aura, who are 4 to 7 times more likely to have

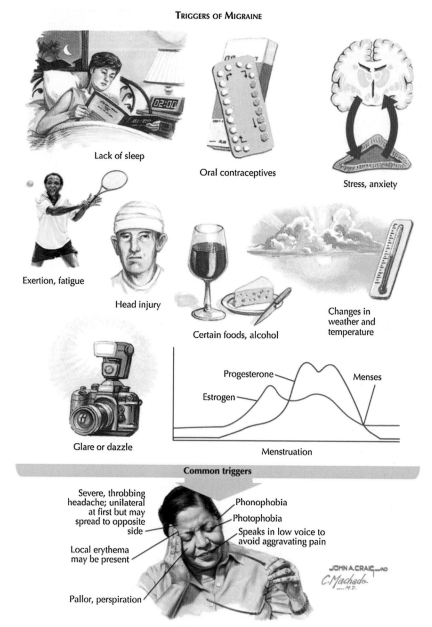

TRIGGERS OF MIGRAINE

Lack of sleep

Oral contraceptives

Stress, anxiety

Exertion, fatigue

Head injury

Certain foods, alcohol

Changes in weather and temperature

Glare or dazzle

Progesterone

Estrogen

Menses

Menstruation

Common triggers

Severe, throbbing headache; unilateral at first but may spread to opposite side

Phonophobia

Photophobia

Speaks in low voice to avoid aggravating pain

Local erythema may be present

Pallor, perspiration

JOHN A.CRAIG—MD
C.Machado—M.D.

Fig. 2. An overview of migraine headache triggers. (*From* Netter illustration www. netterimages.com. © Elsevier Inc. All rights reserved.)

a psychiatric diagnosis and who are more likely to attempt suicide than patients with migraine who do not experience aura.[4] These factors emphasize the importance of collecting a complete psychiatric history in patients who suffer from migraine and screening for depression, suicidality, and anxiety disorders. The IHS guidelines for migraine headache diagnoses are listed in **Boxes 2** and **3**.[8]

Box 2
IHS migraine without aura criteria

Recurrent headache disorder, with attacks lasting between 4 and 72 hours. Headaches are unilateral, pulsating, moderate-to-severe in intensity, aggravated by routine physical activity, and often associated with nausea and photo-phonophobia.

Diagnostic criteria

A. ≥5 attacks, all fulfilling criteria B–D

B. Headache duration of between 4 and 72 hours (untreated or unsuccessfully treated)

C. ≥2 of the following characteristics: (1) unilaterality, (2) pulsating quality, (3) moderate-to-severe intensity, (4) aggravation by or causing avoidance of routine physical activity (i.e., walking)

D. Experience of at least 1 of the following: (1) nausea, (2) vomiting, (3) photophobia, (4) phonophobia

E. Not attributed to another disorder

Cluster Headaches

A 28-year-old man presents to the emergency department at 3:00 AM with severe right-sided retro-orbital pain, lacrimation, sweating, and nasal drainage. He reports that this pain awakened him from sleep and that he had a number of similar episodes, which occurred over a period of 8 weeks last year. He smokes 2 packs of cigarettes a day, as he has for the past 10 years. He is in excruciating pain and requests immediate treatment.

This patient presents with the classic signs and symptoms of cluster headache. This relatively rare condition typically causes severe, sharp, unilateral retro-orbital pain in addition to autonomic symptoms, such as lacrimation, sweating, and nasal drainage on the same side as the pain. Approximately 70% of cluster headache sufferers are younger than 30 years when the headaches begin. This condition can exist in the more common episodic form, which constitutes 80% to 90% of cases, or the more rare, but debilitating chronic form of cluster headaches. Like the headaches seen in the patient in the example, episodic cluster headaches occur every day, and often multiple times per day, for 6 to 12 weeks, followed by periods of remission of up to 12 months. Conversely, in the chronic form, episodes appear without significant periods of remission (**Fig. 3**).[2]

Box 3
IHS migraine with aura criteria

Recurrent headache disorder with associated reversible focal neurologic symptoms that develop over 5–20 minutes and last for <60 minutes. Headache with features of the aforementioned migraine without aura typically ensues following the aura, but, less commonly, headaches may lack some of the features of a typical migraine or migraine symptoms may be altogether absent.

Diagnostic criteria

A. ≥2 attacks fulfilling criterion B (as listed above in **Box 2**)

B. Migraine aura fulfilling criteria of specific aura syndromes (various neurologic symptoms, including visual and tactile disturbances, parasthesias, hemiplasia, and dysarthria)

C. Not attributed to another disorder

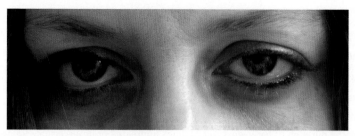

Fig. 3. Miosis, ptosis and increased lacrimation during a left sided cluster headache. (*From* Netter illustration www.netterimages.com. © Elsevier Inc. All rights reserved.)

Cluster headaches often have a strong familial pattern and are frequently misdiagnosed as migraine, sinusitis, or allergies. In fact, only 25% of sufferers receive the correct diagnosis within the first year of onset. A number of serious comorbidities are associated with cluster headaches, including depression in up to 24% of sufferers, sleep apnea, asthma, and restless leg syndrome.[2] Thus, as with migraines, it is important to collect a very complete patient history and screen patients for psychiatric comorbidities. Cluster headaches are more common in men and 87% of sufferers of chronic cluster headaches are cigarette smokers.[11] IHS criteria for cluster headache diagnosis are listed in **Box 4**.[8]

Chronic Daily Headache

Individuals experiencing headache on 15 or more days per month for longer than 3 months are considered to suffer from chronic daily headaches. Chronic daily headache is not a diagnosis itself, but instead encompasses a number of conditions, the most common of which are transformed migraines, chronic tension-type headaches, and medication-overuse headaches.[4,12] These headache subtypes are all related in that preexisting episodic headaches are converted into more severe forms through the overuse of analgesic or other antimigraine medications, including narcotics, barbiturates, triptans, and ergotamines.[4] Medication overuse is defined as the overuse of medications for at least 3 months. Although the amount necessary for each patient may differ, the amount of medication generally needed to induce medication overuse

---

Box 4
IHS cluster headache criteria

Severe attacks of unilateral, orbital, supraorbital, or temporal pain, lasting 15–180 minutes. Attacks occur from once every other day to 8 times per day and are associated with one of the following: conjunctival injection, lacrimation, nasal congestion, rhinorrhea, forehead or facial sweating, miosis, ptosis, or eyelid edema.

Diagnostic criteria

A. ≥5 attacks fulfilling the criteria B–E

B. Severe to very severe unilateral pain lasting for 15–180 minutes if left untreated

C. Accompanied by ≥1 of the following: (1) ipsilateral conjunctival injection and/or lacrimation, (2) ipsilateral nasal congestion and/or rhinorrhea, (3) ipsilateral eye edema, (4) ipsilateral forehead and/or facial sweating, (5) ipsilateral miosis and/or ptosis, (6) sense of restlessness or agitation

D. Attacks occur anywhere from 8 per day to every other day in frequency

E. Not attributed to another disorder

headaches is more than 14 days per month use of simple analgesics, more than 10 days per month use of migraine-specific drugs, or more than 14 days per month use of all headache medications. Risk factors for chronic daily headache includes obesity, caffeine consumption, sleep and psychiatric disorders, and the use of acute antiheadache medications on more than 10 days per month. Most patients with chronic daily headache are women with long-running histories of episodic headache disorders that transform from a more benign to a more severe form over months to years.[12] IHS criteria for the diagnosis of medication overuse headache is listed in **Box 5.**[8]

Headaches in the Elderly

The presentation of headaches in the elderly differs quite significantly from younger populations. Older patients are at significantly higher risk of secondary headache and, instead of traditional migraine symptoms, they tend to experience more aura-like migraine accompaniments. In addition, hypnic headaches, a condition unique to the elderly, cause morbidity in these patients, as do cough headaches and chronic daily headaches. The prevalence of migraines decreases with age, but the rate of chronic daily headaches actually increases, owing to the use of analgesics and other medications for the treatment of various age-related medical conditions. Vasodilators, such as nitroglycerin, nifedipine, and dypiridamole, in addition to selective serotonin reuptake inhibitors (SSRIs), serotonin norepinephrine reuptake inhibitors (SNRIs) and analgesic drugs are commonly prescribed in this population and are well known as contributors to chronic daily headache. Auralike migraine accompaniments are more prominent in this population, consisting of traveling paresthesias, scintillating scotomas, speech disturbances, and homonymous field defects. These symptoms typically demonstrate a buildup and spread of visual scintillations, a spreading of paresthesias from hands to face, or a progression from one accompaniment symptom to another, typically lasting between 15 and 30 minutes. These migraine accompaniments can be distinguished from transient ischemic attacks (TIAs), in that TIAs most commonly last fewer than 15 minutes and migraine accompaniments, unlike TIAs, show normal cerebral blood flow patterns when compared with age-matched controls. Further, visual field defects related to aura typically last between 15 and 60 minutes and involve both fields and feature bright, shimmering lights with moving shapes, whereas those associated with

---

Box 5
IHS medication overuse headache criteria

Headache that develops when susceptible patients use excessive amounts of a therapeutic agent. These headaches present with a mixture of tension and migrainelike qualities and are present on ≥15 days per month. Overuse of ergotamines, triptans, analgesics, opioids, other medications, or a combination of medications will each present with slightly different symptomatology.

Diagnostic criteria

A. Headache present ≥15 days per month with varying symptomatology based on therapeutic modality used

B. Medication in question used on ≥10 days per month on a regular basis for ≥3 months

C. Headache developed or markedly worsened during medication overuse

D. Headache resolves or reverts to previous pattern within 2 months after discontinuation of medication

TIAs most commonly last between 2 and 5 minutes, are usually unilateral, unmoving, and involve a darkening or dimming of the visual field. Further, aura-related paresthesias typically last for 20 to 30 minutes and come on gradually, with the first area affected typically being the last area to clear. Paresthesias related to TIAs, on the other hand, frequently arise suddenly, last for between 5 and 10 minutes, and clear in the same order that they emerged (**Tables 2** and **3**).[13]

Cough headache is typically seen in men older than 40 and is characterized by 1-second to 30-minute bouts of pain in association with episodes of coughing. Although mostly benign, a number of reports exist linking cough headache with Chiari I malformation, so these patients require magnetic resonance imaging (MRI) with sagittal views to rule out this more serious diagnosis. Finally, hypnic headaches are entirely unique to patients older than 60. These headaches awaken patients from their sleep and are almost always benign. The pain is dull and diffuse, typically lasting for 30 to 60 minutes per episode. This condition's lack of autonomic symptoms differentiate it from cluster headaches and its dull, diffuse pain pattern separates it from diagnoses like trigeminal neuralgia.[14]

The risk of secondary causes of headache increases with age. It is important to be able to differentiate potentially life-threatening causes of headache from bothersome, but more benign etiologies in this more aged population. Beyond the aforementioned TIAs, other causes of headache that must be ruled out include temporal arteritis, trigeminal neuralgia, subdural hematoma, herpes zoster, and postherpetic neuralgia. Temporal, or giant cell, arteritis (GCA) is typically seen in individuals older than 50 (mean age of patients with positive temporal artery biopsies is 73) and must be considered as a cause of headache in anyone in this age group, as the risk of vision loss is quite high, occurring in up to 15% to 20% of patients with GCA.[15,16] Patients with temporal arteritis typically complain of a throbbing pain or steady ache in their temples, scalp tenderness, a diminished pulse over a thickened temporal artery, and pain with chewing, known as jaw claudication. The symptoms with the highest likelihood ratios (LR) for GCA are jaw claudication with a LR of 4.2 and diplopia with a LR of 3.4.[15] The workup for temporal arteritis includes an erythrocyte sedimentation rate and a temporal artery biopsy, and treatment involves immediate administration of high-dose steroids.[13]

Table 2 Causes of primary headache in the elderly	
Type	**Description**
Hypnic	Dull, diffuse pain that awakens patients from sleep, typically lasting for 30–60 min. Benign and unique to patients older than 60.
Cough	One-second to 30-min bouts of pain associated with coughing. Generally seen in men older than 40. Mostly benign, but association with Chiari I malformation. Requires MRI with sagittal views as part of workup.
Medication use/overuse	Headaches develop due to use of SSRIs, SNRIs, and vasodilators, such as nitroglycerin, nifedipine, and dypiridamole. Overuse of analgesic medications for other bodily aches and pains also may contribute.
Migraine accompaniments	Migraines decrease in frequency with age, but older patients may experience auralike migraine accompaniments. These consist of traveling paresthesias, scintillating scotomas, speech disturbances, and homonymous field defects, which may build up and spread and typically last between 15 and 30 min.

Table 3
Causes of secondary headache in the elderly

Type	Description
Temporal arteritis	Associated with a throbbing pain in the temples, scalp tenderness, a diminished pulse over a thickened temporal artery, and pain with chewing, known as jaw claudication. The workup for temporal arteritis includes an erythrocyte sedimentation rate and a temporal artery biopsy.
Trigeminal neuralgia	Common in patients older than 40. In this condition, severe, sharp, unilateral, waxing, and waning pain is seen with minor stimulation of the face, such as shaving, brushing teeth, laughing, or chewing.
Subdural hematoma	Common in the elderly after light trauma. Anticoagulant drugs and aspirin use put patients at higher risk. Suspect in older patients experiencing a dull headache in the setting of altered mental status, confusion, or personality changes.
Herpes zoster/postherpetic neuralgia	Can cause severe facial pain, with pain often preceding associated vesicular lesions. Postherpetic neuralgia causes pain that persists for >3 mo after the acute attack of zoster.
Cerebral metastases	Most commonly lung, melanoma, renal, breast, or colorectal (in descending order of prevalence of brain metastases). Melanoma has the highest propensity to metastasize to brain of all malignant tumors.[38]

Subdural hematomas also are much more common in the elderly and may be observed even after very light trauma, such as a minor head injury, or even vigorous sneezing or coughing. Anticoagulant drugs and aspirin use put patients at higher risk as well. Tears in bridging veins are most commonly responsible for subdural hematoma formation and the ensuing bleeding may not cause symptoms for days to weeks after the initial insult. Subdural hematoma should be suspected in older patients experiencing dull headache in the setting of altered mental status, confusion, or personality changes. Patients with this condition can usually just be followed closely with serial computed tomography (CT) scans, but large hematomas require urgent surgical evacuation.[13]

Specific neuropathic pain conditions are more common in the elderly population, and must be considered in any new patient complaining of new-onset headache. Idiopathic trigeminal neuralgia is common in patients older than 40. In this condition, severe, sharp, unilateral, waxing and waning pain is seen with minor stimulation of the face, such as shaving, brushing teeth, laughing, or chewing. Similarly, herpes zoster can cause severe facial pain, depending on the distribution of the reactivated virus, with pain often preceding associated vesicular lesions by several days. Further, postherpetic neuralgia results in as many as 50% of patients older than 60 and causes pain that persists for longer than 3 months following the acute attack of zoster. Thus, providers should inquire as to recent infection history in the consideration of any older patient presenting with new-onset headaches.[13]

Physical Examination

The physical examination, and particularly the neurologic examination, is important in ruling out harmful secondary headache pathologies. Physical examination findings also play a role in making the correct primary headache diagnosis, especially when autonomic symptoms are present. The physical examination for a chief complaint of headache should include vital signs; the cardiopulmonary examination; auscultation of the carotid and vertebral arteries; palpation of the head, neck, and temporal arteries; and a complete neurologic examination focusing on fundoscopic and pupillary assessment, neck stiffness, focal weakness, sensory loss, and gait. Special attention must be given to patients with fever or altered mental status, those with neurologic signs, and older patients presenting with the first or worst headache of their life.[4] Importantly, positive neurologic signs on examination are very important predictors of central nervous system (CNS) pathology and cannot be attributed to migraine unless the patient's headaches have a pattern of presenting with the same neurologic signs.[2] With the exception of rare syndromes, such as hemiplegic migraine, the physical examination is typically negative in the case of primary headaches, making the patient history most important with respect to diagnosis.

IMAGING AND ADDITIONAL TESTING

A 46-year-old woman develops a severe headache this morning while at work. She also has nausea and has had one episode of emesis. She has shoulder and neck stiffness that developed today. She denies any history of migraine headaches or any similar headaches.

Imaging is a very important step in assessing patients with signs and symptoms of secondary headache and the case scenario exemplifies the type of situation when imaging might provide valuable insight into the patient's underlying pathology. Neuroimaging is 98.6% sensitive for serious intracranial pathology if any one of the following risk factors are present: age older than 45 years, abnormal neurologic examination, or sudden onset of headache.[10] Other conditions requiring neuroimaging in patients with new-onset headache include immunosuppression, suspected temporal arteritis, possible meningitis, or severe headache in pregnancy. Of note, HIV-positive patients presenting with headache and CD4 counts less than 300 should receive CT imaging, given the high probability of finding some underlying CNS pathology.[17] A noncontrast CT should be ordered to rule out intracranial bleeding and in the case of head trauma, although MRI is more effective in patients suspected of parenchymal pathology, such as infection, abscess, or tumor. MRI also is more helpful in the diagnosis of subdural hematoma or smaller lesions. Lumbar puncture can help diagnose infection, CNS malignancy, or subarachnoid hemorrhage, and is an appropriate follow-up test in patients with suspected subarachnoid hemorrhage who have a negative CT scan.[2]

If no abnormalities are noted on physical examination or in the patient's history, there is no need for neuroimaging. This concept is exemplified by typical migraine. If a patient has a regular pattern of migraines, no abnormalities on neurologic examination, and no changes in headache characteristics over time, they have only a 0.18% chance of having a clinically significant intracranial lesion.[3] In fact, no diagnostic tests are required to diagnose primary headache. Unnecessary exposure to CT ionizing radiation should be avoided, as it contributes a small lifetime increase in cancer risk and increases the chances of making incidental, but likely benign, findings that require further workup, likely at great cost, both financially and emotionally, to the patient.[5] **Boxes 6** and **7** are helpful in identifying patients in need of neuroimaging and clinical features that may raise one's suspicion for potentially worrisome findings that may be identified through imaging.

DIAGNOSTIC DILEMMAS AND SPECIAL SITUATIONS
The "Sinus" Headache

Recent research has brought to light that many headaches previously considered to be "sinus headaches" may actually be migrainous in nature. This is exemplified in the following case history:

Box 6
Clinical features indicating need for neuroimaging with severe acute headache

Sudden onset

Age >45 with no previous headache history

Onset with vigorous exercise/sexual activity

Altered mental status

Trauma

Neurologic abnormalities

A 29-year-old woman presents with frequent headaches over the past 12 months that include pressure pain on her forehead, under her eyes, and over her cheeks. She has not had any fevers or purulent nasal discharge.

In the past, this woman would likely have been described as a sinus headache sufferer, yet more recent findings have suggested that many headaches previously described as "sinus headaches" are actually migraine headaches. In one 2004 study, it was found that 88% of patients with self-diagnosed or physician-diagnosed sinus headaches actually met IHS criteria for migraine headache. These patients most commonly complained of sinus pressure, sinus pain, and nasal congestion.[18] Further, many patients previously thought to have sinus headache appear to be responsive to typical migraine therapy, with 82% being responsive to triptans and 92% responding to migraine-directed therapy in one study.[19]

Menstrual Migraines and Prescription of Oral Contraceptives in Women with Migraines

Menstrual migraines, or migraines experienced between 2 days before or 3 days after the onset of menstruation, occur in approximately 20% of women between the ages of 17 and 49, with peak prevalence in women in their 30s. It is thought that the declines of estrogen levels in the late luteal phase may be responsible for menstrual migraines. Increased levels of prostaglandins during menstruation may also play a role. Treatment of menstrual migraines is almost identical to treatment of typical migraines, with the notable exception of administration of intermittent prophylaxis, which involves therapy administered prophylactically during the perimenstrual period. NSAIDs, coxib drugs, and triptans are currently used for this purpose, and may be dosed as many as 7 days before and 6 days after the start of menses. Hormonal prophylaxis, such as percutaneous estradiol gel 1.5 mg administered perimenstrually for up to 6 cycles or continuous administration of oral contraceptives,

---

Box 7
Clinical features that suggest higher risks for a positive neuroimaging study

Abnormal neurologic examination

Personality change, cognitive deficit, memory loss

Head trauma (within 4 months)

History of malignancy (excluding basal cell carcinoma)

Chronic anticoagulation

HIV infection with CD4 count <300

---

also may be administered.[20] It is the opinion of these authors that, given the known risks of estrogen therapy, the continuous administration of oral contraceptives or instillation of a levonogestrel-releasing intrauterine device would be preferable to administration of estrogen for the prophylaxis of menstrual migraines. It is particularly important that women with migraines, and particularly those with migraine with aura, be prescribed progestin-only oral contraceptives or some other mode of non–estrogen-containing contraceptive, because of the increased risk of stroke in these individuals.[21]

A recent meta-analysis of 35 studies, including more than 600,000 patients, found a very strong correlation between migraine and an increased risk of stroke, with a relative risk of 2.41 overall. The risk associated with migraine with aura was even higher at 2.51; however, this value was not statistically significant. The data also suggested a stronger association between migraine and stroke in women; however, a direct comparison between genders could not be made, as the studies included did not present data separately based on gender. This increased risk may be related to increased estrogen levels, which in turn increase propensity toward coagulability, endothelial dysfunction, and inflammation.[22]

CVS and Abdominal Migraine

A number of gastrointestinal manifestations of migraine have been identified as potential causes of abdominal discomfort and nausea and vomiting. CVS and abdominal migraine have long been recognized as childhood conditions and are still considered by the IHS to be "childhood periodic syndromes" and common migraine precursors in the pediatric population.[23,24] CVS affects 2% of children, 87% of whom go on to develop migraine headaches later in life.[23] CVS is characterized by severe, recurrent episodes of nausea and vomiting, which may last for hours to days. Like migraine headaches, prodromal symptoms are often present that warn patients of an impending attack and a given patient may experience between 6 and 12 attacks per year.[25] More recently, it has become clear that CVS is a disorder that can have its primary presentation in adulthood. The prevalence is unknown, but recent studies have suggested that as many as 14% of patients in gastrointestinal motility clinics have CVS, with a mean age of onset of 25.4. The prevalence of migraine headaches in these individuals was 56% and 56% also had a family history of migraine headache. And, as with other headache syndromes described thus far, depression is prevalent in approximately 40% of patients with the adult form of CVS.[23]

Also a childhood periodic syndrome, abdominal migraine has only recently been recognized as a disorder that can occur in adult populations. Abdominal migraine is characterized by acute paroxysmal episodes of abdominal pain, with possible concomitant flushing, vomiting, pallor, anorexia, or photo-phonophobia. Headache may or may not be present with these episodes of abdominal pain and the patient is free of abdominal pain between attacks.[10] In children, 52% of patients with abdominal migraine go on to develop migraine within a decade, compared with 20% of their age-matched peers.[24] These pediatric patients are diagnosed based on the International Headache Classification System and Rome III criteria.[26,27] Although abdominal migraine has been recognized as an adult disease only relatively recently, a number of studies have identified similarities between suspected patients and have supported the notion that this condition does occur in adults and should be considered in patients complaining of recurrent abdominal pain.[26] Almost all of these patients have strong family histories of migraine and their abdominal pain tends to be nonradiating in nature, located in the midline epigastric area.[24]

TREATMENT
Tension Headaches

Although self-limiting and nondebilitating, tension headaches can be a nuisance and many patients require treatment. Identifying risk factors and triggers, such as stress and a lack of or too much sleep, is important. The mainstays of therapy are NSAIDs, acetaminophen, and aspirin.[5] With these modalities, it is important to set daily and weekly upper limits of use to prevent the development of chronic daily headache. Two prophylactic therapies have also emerged as potentially useful in decreasing the frequency and severity of tension migraines, namely low-dose amitriptyline and injection of botulinum toxin. Amitriptyline, given in doses between 10 and 75 mg daily, has proven effective in a number of placebo-controlled double-blinded studies, and research on pericranial muscle injection of botulinum toxin is also promising.[7] Other potentially helpful modalities include massage, stretching routines, regular exercise, relaxation training, and stress management.[5]

Migraine Headaches

Migraine headache sufferers require acute therapies for severe flares, in addition to prophylactic treatment aimed at reducing the frequency and severity of headaches experienced. In both scenarios, it is important to consider medical and psychiatric comorbidities and, whenever possible, offer combination therapies that treat multiple conditions with the least number of medications possible.[4] The following section will outline both acute and prophylactic modalities.

Acute therapy

Migraine headaches can be severely debilitating and, in the acute setting, the goals of therapy should be to abort the migraine headache and prevent recurrence.[5] Therapeutic modalities include nonspecific drugs, such as NSAIDs or acetaminophen, or specific therapies, such as triptans or ergotamines.[4] Acute therapy should start with an NSAID early in the onset of the migraine, followed by metoclopramide for individuals with nausea and vomiting or for those who do not respond to analgesics alone.[4] Metoclopramide can help treat the slowed gastric motility that occurs in some patients with migraine, which can promote the absorption of oral migraine therapies. In the emergency department (ED) setting, intravenous (IV) ketorolac can relieve symptoms within 1 hour and antiemetics play a role independent of their antinausea roles.[10] Metoclopramide is considered primary therapy in the ED given its lack of side effects and risk of dependency.[10] If NSAIDs and metoclopramide prove ineffective, a triptan should be used. A single triptan should be used for 3 separate migraines in different doses before trying another triptan or another class of drugs. The 3 most effective triptans in the acute setting include rizatriptan (typically at a 10-mg dose), eletriptan (80 mg), and almotriptan (12.5 mg); rapid dissolving tablets or subcutaneous injections may be used for patients with severe nausea and vomiting.[10] A combination of 900 mg aspirin in conjunction with an antiemetic may actually be as effective at 2 hours as 100 mg of sumatriptan. Further, combination triptan/NSAID drugs, such as Trexima (sumatriptan 85 mg/naproxen 500 mg) are more effective than either drug alone.[4,10] Dexamethasone IV may also be considered in the ED setting to help prevent acute migraine recurrence.[10] Ergotamine and dihydroergotamine (DHE) drugs have largely been replaced by triptans, as there is very little evidence supporting their use and they are typically not well-absorbed.[10] Finally, intranasal lidocaine may be considered as a short-term temporizing step until longer-acting therapies can be administered. This modality works quickly, but recurrence is a common problem.[10] **Table 4** draws on recommendations from the American Academy of Neurology.[28]

Table 4
Recommendations for the treatment of acute migraine

Medication	Comments
Group 1 – medications with a strong evidence base	
Triptans	
Naratriptan PO	*Grade A*. Few adverse effects.
Rizatriptan PO	*Grade A*. Occasional adverse effects.
Sumatriptan SC, PO, intranasal	*Grade A*. Occasional adverse effects; for moderate-to-severe migraines. SC and intranasal forms helpful with nausea and vomiting.
Zolmitriptan PO	*Grade A*. Occasional adverse effects.
Ergotamines	
DHE SC, IM, IV, intranasal	Frequent adverse effects; for moderate-to-severe migraines. Nasal spray and IV forms have a low recurrence rate. Nasal spray is *Grade A*.
DHE IV, plus antiemetic	Frequent adverse effects; for status migrainosus. Strongly consider in treatment of acute headache in the emergency department.
Nonspecific	
Acetaminophen, aspirin, plus caffeine PO	*Grade A*. Few adverse effects; first-line treatment for acute migraine.
Aspirin PO	*Grade A*. Few adverse effects; first-line treatment for mild-to-moderate migraines.
Butorphanol intranasal	*Grade A*. Frequent adverse effects; for moderate-to-severe migraines. Use sparingly.
Ibuprofen PO	*Grade A*. Occasional adverse effects; first-line treatment for mild-to-moderate migraines.
Naproxen sodium PO	*Grade A*. Occasional adverse effects; first-line treatment for mild-to-moderate migraines.
Prochlorperazine IV	Occasional adverse effects. Adjunct first-line therapy in emergency department or outpatient setting.

Abbreviations: DHE, dihydroergotamine; IM, intramuscular; IV, intravenous; PO, oral; SC, subcutaneous.

Data from Silberstein SD. Practice parameter: Evidence-based guidelines for migraine headache (and evidence-based review). American Academy of Neurology Quality Standards Subcommittee Report. Neurology 2000;55(6):754–62.

Pregnancy necessitates important considerations in the treatment of migraine. Migraine frequency typically decreases during pregnancy, but some women continue to experience these debilitating headaches. Many of the standard therapies, such as antiepileptics, opiates, ergotamines, and triptans, must be avoided in this population. However, metoclopramide, pyridoxine, codeine, or, if given before the third trimester, NSAIDs, would all be appropriate choices for the treatment of acute migraine in pregnant patients.[4,10] Acetaminophen, although not typically effective in acute migraine, continues to be recommended in pregnancy, given its benign side-effect profile.[10]

Prophylactic therapy

Prophylactic treatment of migraine headaches aims to decrease the intensity, frequency, and duration of migraine headaches.[4] Typically, prophylactic therapy is considered if abortive therapy is required more than 2 times per week, if the patient cannot tolerate acute therapies, if headaches significantly undermine quality of life despite appropriate abortive therapy, or for uncommon migraine conditions, such as hemiplegic or basilar migraines.[10] Depending on the severity and frequency of migraine attacks, these drugs can be taken on different schedules. For example, if the patient has known triggers, such as exercise or changes in altitude, prophylactic therapy can be taken before these activities. For menstrual migraines, prophylactic treatment can be offered for the 1 to 8 days when the migraines are typically at their worst. Treatment also can be offered on a continuous basis for those who suffer from chronic, frequent migraines.[4] The MIDAS criteria, which assesses the number of work or school days lost during a 3-month period due to migraines, assists physicians in understanding patients' migraine-related disability.[3,4] This tool helps providers determine when chronic, daily therapy is required and, when used in a serial manner, is useful in assessing response to therapy.[3,4] **Box 8** and **Table 5** outline the MIDAS criteria and scoring system.[29,30]

Specific therapies can be derived from a number of drug classes. A large number of drugs from a variety of drug classes may be used to treat migraine headaches. These include anticonvulsants, such as divalproex sodium, gabapentin, and topiramate; antidepressants, such as tricyclic antidepressants (TCAs), SSRIs, and SNRIs, especially venlafaxine; β-blockers, such as atenolol, metoprolol, nadolol, and propranolol; serotonin antagonists, such as methysergide; neuroleptics; NSAIDs; magnesium; angiotensin receptor blockers; angiotensin-converting enzyme inhibitors; and butterbur. It is important to start with the lowest dose possible and to slowly increase dosages until an acceptable therapeutic effect is achieved.[4]

Therapies should be chosen based on the specific patient population served and individual patient comorbidities. For example, divalproex or topiramate would be appropriate for the elderly population, whereas those with comorbid insomnia or depression might be particularly well treated by TCAs or the SNRI venlafaxine. Overweight individuals would likely benefit from treatment with topiramate, and divalproex is a good choice in those with seizure disorders.[4] Menstrual migraine sufferers benefit from sumatriptan, rizatriptan, or the NSAID mefanamic acid (Ponstel) for abortive therapy,

---

Box 8
Migraine Disability Assessment (MIDAS) criteria

1. On how many days in the past 3 months did you miss work or school because of your headaches?

2. How many days in the past 3 months was your productivity at work or school reduced by half or more because of your headache (do not include days you counted in question 1)?

3. On how many days in the past 3 months did you not do household work because of your headaches?

4. How many days in the past 3 months was productivity in household work reduced by half or more because of your headache (do not include days you counted in question 3)?

5. On how many days in the past 3 months did you miss family, social or nonwork activities because of your headache?

Unscored section (used to further inform physician)

A. On how many days in the past 3 months did you have a headache?

B. On a scale of 0–10, how painful were these headaches on average?

Adapted from Stewart W, Lipton R, Downson A, et al. Development and testing of the Migraine Disability Assessment (MIDAS) Questionnaire to assess headache-related disability. Neurology 2001;56(Suppl 1):S20–8.

Table 5
Migraine Disability Assessment (MIDAS) scoring

MIDAS Grade	Definition	MIDAS Score
I	Little or no disability	0–5
II	Mild disability	6–10
III	Moderate disability	11–20
IV	Severe disability	21+

Adapted from Migraine disability assessment test insert. Available at: http://uhs.berkeley.edu/home/healthtopics/pdf/assessment.pdf. Accessed September 9, 2013.

and long-acting triptans, such as fovatriptan and naratriptan taken premenstrually as prophylactic therapy.[10] **Table 6** provides the most evidence-based guidelines regarding prophylactic therapies, both pharmacologic and complementary in nature, from the American Academy of Neurology and the American Headache Society.[31,32]

There is also increasing interest in nonpharmacologic approaches to the treatment of migraine headaches. From biofeedback, to osteopathic manipulative therapy, to vitamin and herbal modalities, such as petasites like butterbur, coenzyme Q10, feverfew, magnesium, and riboflavin, these new treatment options have a growing body of evidence and are increasingly used as prophylactic therapy for migraines.[3] **Table 7** reviews the evidence regarding the use of complementary modalities in the prophylactic treatment of migraine headaches.

Melatonin is another such natural therapy that may be useful not only in migraine prevention, but also the prophylactic management of cluster and tension headaches. An antinociceptive, anxiolytic, analgesic, antiallodynic, and, perhaps as it's best known, a sleep aid, melatonin has recently been proposed as a therapy for multiple types of headaches. Melatonin is found in a number of medicinal plants, including feverfew, which are commonly used in natural migraine therapy, thus raising the question as to whether it is melatonin, some other substance, or a synergism between multiple substances that leads to the headache relief attributed to these products.[33]

Acupuncture is also gaining more acceptance, as recent studies support its usefulness in the treatment of migraine, chronic tension-type, and chronic daily headaches. Acupuncture also has been found to have significant benefit with respect to health care costs, saving approximately $13,000 per quality-adjusted life-year in a recent study. It should be noted, however, that research on acupuncture has natural limitations, as the standardized approach required by research studies differs significantly from the individualized approach generally used in acupuncture practice.[34]

CLUSTER HEADACHES

This rare form of headache is generally seen in men. The rapid onset and short time to peak intensity demand that treatment be delivered quickly. Therapy involves administration of 100% oxygen at 10 to 15 L/min for 10 to 20 minutes or subcutaneous sumatriptan 6 mg. Cluster periods typically last for 6 to 12 weeks, and the goal of treatment is to combine acute and prophylactic therapy, with an emphasis on gaining control of the headaches with the latter. Prophylactic therapy should be started as soon as possible after a new cluster period begins. The calcium channel blocker, verapamil, is the first-line choice for prophylactic therapy and dosing should start at 240 mg, with upward titrations according to efficacy and tolerability. Short-course high-dose prednisone or prednisolone also may be added in the first 2 weeks as a bridging therapy until the verapamil takes full effect. Verapamil therapy should be continued until

Table 6
Traditional Prophylactic Pharmacologic Agents (based on the 2012 recommendations of the Quality Standards Subcommittee of the American Academy of Neurology and the American Headache Society)

Medication	Dose	Side Effects	Comments
Level A			
Divalproex sodium (ER)	500–1000 mg/d	Weight gain with long-term use Potential risk of pancreatitis and liver failure	Contraindicated in pregnancy
Topiramate	25–200 mg/d	Paresthesias, weight loss, gastrointestinal intolerance, somnolence	—
Metoprolol	47.5–200 mg/d	No significant adverse effects	—
Propranolol	80 mg/d	Drowsiness, sleep disturbance, weight gain, fatigue, dry mouth	—
Fovatriptan	2.5 mg twice daily	Similar to placebo	Especially useful in reducing perimenstrual migraine incidence
Level B			
Amitriptyline	10 mg daily for 3 d; 25 mg daily for 3 d; then 75 mg daily[39]	Hypersomnolence, dry mouth, difficulty with concentration	—
Venlafaxine (ER)	150 mg/d	Nausea, vomiting, drowsiness, tachycardia	—
Naratriptan	1 mg twice daily (given for 5 d, starting 2 d before onset menses)	Similar to placebo, with fewer than 10% of patients experiencing dizziness, chest pain, malaise	Useful in reducing perimenstrual migraine incidence
Zolmitriptan	2.5 mg twice or 3 times daily	Asthenia, headache, dizziness, nausea	Useful in reducing perimenstrual migraine incidence
Level C			
Lisinopril	10 mg daily for 1 wk; then 20 mg daily[40]	Cough, dizziness, tendency to faint	—
Candesartan	16 mg daily[27]	Dizziness, musculoskeletal system complaints, fatigue	—

Data from Silberstein S, Holland S, Freitag F, et al. Evidence-based guideline update: pharmacologic treatment for episodic migraine prevention in adults. Neurology 2012;78:1337–45.

Table 7
Complementary and NSAID prophylactic medications (based on the 2012 recommendations of the Quality Standards Subcommittee of the American Academy of Neurology and the American Headache Society)

Medication	Dose	Side Effects	Contraindications
Level A			
Petasites (butterbur)	50–75 mg twice daily	None	Risks of prolonged use not understood
Level B			
NSAIDs (fenoprofen, ibuprofen, ketoprofen, naproxen)	Dose dependent on drug chosen	—	Modest therapeutic benefit is observed with NSAID drugs
Magnesium	300 mg daily	—	—
MIG-99 (feverfew)	6.25 mg 3 times daily	Gastrointestinal or respiratory system disorders	—
Riboflavin	400 mg daily	—	—
Histamine SC	1–10 ng twice weekly	Transient itching at injection site	—
Level C			
Co-Q10	100 mg 3 times daily	—	—
Estrogen	Soy isoflavones 60 mg daily; dong quai 100 mg daily; black cohosh 50 mg daily; estradiol 1.5 mg gel patch	—	Helpful in reducing frequency of menstrually related migraines Limited data available regarding long-term safety
Cyproheptadine	4 mg daily	—	—

Abbreviations: NSAID, nonsteroidal anti-inflammatory drug; SC, subcutaneous.

Data from Silberstein S, Holland S, Freitag F, et al. Evidence-based guideline update: NSAIDs and other complementary treatments for episodic migraine prevention in adults. Neurology 2012;78:1346–53.

headaches have ceased for at least 7 to 14 days, and patients should then slowly be tapered off.[5] Avoidance of potential triggers, such as smoking and alcohol, should also be encouraged.[35]

Chronic Daily Headaches

For patients suffering from chronic daily headaches, providers must structure a guided medication withdrawal plan to help patients discontinue medications causing dependency. Once this has been achieved, both short-term and long-term headache management plans should be developed.[4] Behavioral modifications that may improve chronic daily headache symptoms and frequency include limiting caffeine intake, promoting good sleep hygiene, addressing psychiatric disorders, and providing training in relaxation techniques and biofeedback modalities. Discontinuation of offending drugs also should be undertaken in the case of medication-overuse headaches. Ergotamines, triptans, and NSAIDs may be withdrawn abruptly; however, patients should be tapered off of butalbital-containing analgesics and opioids over the course of

1 month. Preventive medications include tricyclic antidepressants, SSRIs, anticonvulsants, tizandine, and botulinum toxin injection, and these medications should be given at the smallest dose at which therapeutic effect is achieved and should be continued for at least 3 to 6 months once the patient is being effectively treated.[12]

Headaches in the Elderly

Treatment of migraines in the elderly presents special challenges. Given their vasoconstrictive nature, triptans, ergotamines, and DHE pose risks to individuals with cardiovascular disease. Thus, acute management in the ED should involve divalproex sodium, metoclopramide, or IV magnesium; whereas acute treatment at home can include naproxen or hydroxyzine. Some prophylactic medications, such as TCAs, can be dangerous in this population. Instead, prophylactic management should include anticonvulsants, such as divalproex sodium or topiramate, or β-blockers, such as metoprolol or propranolol.[14]

Hypnic headaches can be treated prophylactically with either 1 to 2 cups of coffee or lithium 150 to 600 mg at bedtime. Indomethacin or acetazolamide are effective in the prophylactic treatment of cough headaches. And, from a nonpharmacologic perspective, weight reduction through diet and exercise can be effective in decreasing the rate of migraines, as overweight and obese individuals are at higher risk of developing migraine headaches.[14] Finally, cough headache is most effectively treated by indomethacin, with dosages ranging from 25 to 150 mg per day; however, some patients find that the pain associated with this condition is so benign that prophylactic therapy is not necessary. For patients with Chiari I malformation, suboccipital craniectomy, with or without a C1–C3 laminectomy, generally leads to resolution of headaches.[36]

Treatment of Abdominal Migraine and CVS

Patients suspected of having abdominal migraine should be started on a trial of prophylactic topiramate therapy. Prophylactic therapies, such as divalproex sodium and propranolol, also have been considered useful. Abortive triptan therapy, preferably in a subcutaneous form, also may be used in patients who continue to experience attacks despite administration of prophylactic therapy.[24]

Acute treatment of CVS is mostly supportive, involving hydration, electrolyte management, and placement in a quiet, dark, nonstimulating environment. In combination with ondansetron, benzodiazepines, or diphenhydramine, this approach is effective in as many as 62% of cases. With respect to prophylaxis, many patients respond to traditional antimigraine therapy, such as sumatriptan, and, in one study, 86% of individuals achieved partial or complete response with the TCAs amitriptyline or nortriptyline. As with other headache syndromes, stress and anxiety reduction have proven helpful to management.[23]

FUTURE CONSIDERATIONS AND SUMMARY

Headaches represent the most common constellation of neurologic disorders and are a very common cause of morbidity, lost work time, and decreased quality of life among sufferers. In this article, the diagnostic features, workup, and treatment of common, nuanced, and difficult-to-diagnose headache conditions were addressed. The future will hold a number of changes, with respect to both the diagnosis and treatment of headache disorders. As the aging population continues to grow, primary care providers will need to become increasingly familiar with differentiating between benign primary and more serious secondary headache disorders and will need to be able to treat the headache disorders unique to the elderly. With respect to therapeutic options, the future for treatment of the various headache disorders is promising. With the rise in popularity of complementary medical practices, there is likely to be more research on the roles of acupuncture, herbal and alternative remedies, massage therapy, and mind-body techniques. Further, new research is suggesting that neurostimulation may be useful in certain chronic, intractable headache conditions.[37] Finally, the pathophysiology of headache disorders is still poorly understood and there is great hope that better understanding of the underlying mechanics of headache might contribute to improved treatment modalities and better quality of life for patients.

REFERENCES

1. Epidemiology of headache. Washington, DC: International Association for the Study of Pain; 2011.
2. Hainer B, Matheson E. Approach to acute headache in adults. Am Fam Physician 2013;87(10):682–7.
3. Mueller L. Diagnosing and managing migraine headache. J Am Optom Assoc 2007;107(11):ES10–6.
4. Silberstein S, Merli G, Wender R. Issues in primary care headache management in primary care. Philadelphia: Thomas Jefferson University Medical College; 2003.
5. Zagami A, Singh TH. Headache diagnosis, management and prevention. Surry Hills (Australia): National Prescribing Service; 2012. ISSN 1441–7421.
6. Millea P, Brodie J. Tension-type headache. Am Fam Physician 2002;66(5): 797–805.
7. Jensen R, Olesen J. Tension-type headache: an update on mechanisms and treatment. Curr Opin Neurol 2000;13:285–9.
8. Olesen J. The international classification of headache disorders. Cephalalgia 2004;24(Suppl 1):1–150.
9. Gardner K. Genetics of migraine: an update. Headache 2006;46(Suppl 1): S19–24.
10. Gilmore B, Michael M. Treatment of acute migraine headache. Am Fam Physician 2011;83(3):271–80.
11. Manzoni GC. Cluster headache and lifestyle: remarks on a population of 374 male patients. Cephalalgia 1999;19(2):88.
12. Dodick D. Chronic daily headache. N Engl J Med 2006;354:158–65.
13. Kunkel R. Headaches in older patients: special problems and concerns. Cleve Clin J Med 2006;73(10):922–8.
14. Hershey L, Bednarczyk E. Treatment of headache in the elderly. Curr Treat Options Neurol 2013;15:56–62.
15. Smetana GW, Shmerling RH. Does this patient have temporal arteritis? JAMA 2002;287:92.
16. Aiello PD, Trautmann JC, McPhee TJ, et al. Visual prognosis in giant cell arteritis. Ophthalmology 1993;100:550.
17. Graham C, Wippold F, Pilgram T, et al. Screening CT of the brain determined by CD4 count in HIV-positive patients presenting with headache. AJNR Am J Neuroradiol 2000;21:451–4.
18. Schreiber CP, Hutchinson S, Webster CJ, et al. Prevalence of migraine in patients with a history of self-reported or physician-diagnosed "sinus" headache. Arch Intern Med 2004;164(16):1769–72.
19. Kari E, DelGaudio JM. Treatment of sinus headache as migraine: the diagnostic utility of triptans. Laryngoscope 2008;118(12):2235–9.

20. Mannix L. Menstrual-related pain conditions: dysmenorrheal and migraine. J Womens Health (Larchmt) 2008;17(5):879–89.
21. Allias G, Lorenzo C, Mana O, et al. Oral contraceptives in women with migraine: balancing risks and benefits. Neurol Sci 2004;25:S211–4.
22. Spector J, Kahn S, Jones M, et al. Migraine headache and ischemic stroke risk: an updated meta-analysis. Am J Med 2010;123(7):612–24.
23. Evans R, Whyte C. Cyclic vomiting and abdominal migraine in adults and children. Headache 2013;53:984–93.
24. Woodruff A, Cieri N, Abeles J, et al. Abdominal migraine in adults: a review of pharmacotherapeutic options. Ann Pharmacother 2013;47:e27.
25. Fleisher D, Gornowicz B, Adams K. Cyclic vomiting syndrome in 41 adults: the illness, the patients, and problems of management. BMC Med 2005;3:20.
26. Roberts J, deShazo R. Abdominal migraine, another cause of abdominal pain in adults. Am J Med 2012;125(11):1135–9.
27. Tronvik E, Stovner L, Helde G. Prophylactic treatment of migraine with an angiotensin II receptor blocker. JAMA 2003;289(1):65–9.
28. Silberstein S. Practice parameter: Evidence-based guidelines for migraine headache (an evidence-based review): Report of the Quality Standards Subcommittee of the American Academy of Neurology. Neurology 2000;(55):754–63.
29. Stewart W, Lipton R, Downson A, et al. Development and testing of the Migraine Disability Assessment (MIDAS) Questionnaire to assess headache-related disability. Neurology 2001;56(Suppl 1):S20–8.
30. Migraine disability assessment test insert. Available at: uhs.berkeley.edu/home/healthtopics/pdf/assessment.pdf. Accessed September 9, 2013.
31. Silberstein S, Holland S, Freitag F, et al. Evidence-based guideline update: pharmacologic treatment for episodic migraine prevention in adults. Neurology 2012;78:1337–45.
32. Silberstein S, Holland S, Freitag F, et al. Evidence-based guideline update: NSAIDs and other complementary treatments for episodic migraine prevention in adults. Neurology 2012;78:1346–53.
33. Goncalves A, Ribeiro R, Peres M. Melatonin in headache disorders. Headache Medicine 2012;3(2):61–9.
34. Kelly R. Acupuncture for pain. Am Fam Physician 2009;80(5):481–4.
35. Beck E, Sieber W, Trejo R. Management of cluster headache. Am Fam Physician 2005;71(4):717–24.
36. Cordenier A, De Hertogh W, De Keyser J, et al. Headaches associated with cough: a review. J Headache Pain 2013;14:42.
37. Saper J, Dodick D, Silberstein S, et al. Occipital nerve stimulation for the treatment of intractable chronic migraine headache: ONSTIM feasibility study. Cephalalgia 2010;31(3):271–85.
38. Barnholtz J, Sloan A, Davis F, et al. Incidence proportions of brain metastases in patients diagnosed (1973 to 2001) in the Metropolitan Detroit Cancer Surveillance System. J Clin Oncol 2004;22(14):2865–72.
39. Bulut S, Berilgen M, Baran A, et al. Venlafaxine versus amytriptyline in the prophylactic treatment of migraine: randomized, double-blind, crossover study. Clin Neurol Neurosurg 2004;107:44–8.
40. Schrader H, Stovner L, Helde G, et al. Prophylactic treatment of migraine with angiotensin converting enzyme inhibitor (lisinopril): randomized, placebo controlled, crossover study. BMJ 2001;322:19.

Evaluation and Treatment of Colonic Symptoms

Mark E. Pasanen, MD

KEYWORDS

- Diarrhea • Constipation • Irritable bowel syndrome • Laxatives • Antidiarrheals

KEY POINTS

- Most acute diarrhea is infectious, with empiric antibiotics reserved for patients with high fever, blood diarrhea, or other worrisome features.
- Irritable bowel syndrome (IBS) and functional diarrhea are the most common causes of chronic diarrhea.
- In chronic diarrhea, fecal calprotectin may help differentiate IBS from an inflammatory disorder.
- Determine if constipation is due to a defecatory disorder by history (excessive straining, need for perineal pressure, and/or manual disimpaction) because treatment with pelvic floor training is superior to laxatives.
- For idiopathic chronic constipation, initial treatment should include fiber and polyethylene glycol with stimulants and new secretagogues as secondary options.

DIARRHEA

In the past, the definition of diarrhea relied on increased stool weight (>200–300 g/d) and increased frequency of stools (>3/day). However, most definitions now focus on loose or watery stool consistency and urgency because these are most consistent with patient self-reports of diarrhea.[1] Probably the best description is that the stool takes the shape of the container in which it is collected. Diarrhea is considered acute if duration is less than 2 weeks, persistent if 2 to 4 weeks, and chronic if more than 4 weeks. Often, it is classified by the underlying pathologic process: inflammatory, watery, or malabsorptive.

Prevention

Although the focus of this article is the evaluation and management of bowel symptoms, several strategies may be effective in prevention of diarrhea. Clearly, careful

Disclosures: None.
Department of Medicine, University of Vermont College of Medicine, 1234 Spear Street, 111 Colchester Avenue, South Burlington, VT 05403, USA
E-mail address: mark.pasanen@yahoo.com

Med Clin N Am 98 (2014) 529–547
http://dx.doi.org/10.1016/j.mcna.2014.01.009
0025-7125/14/$ – see front matter

hygiene and attention to food and water safety is critical. In addition, inappropriate antibiotic use should be minimized. However, when antibiotics are indicated, there may be a role for probiotic use to prevent both antibiotic-associated and *Clostridium difficile*-associated diarrhea. The most commonly studied probiotics include *Lactobacillus*, *Bifidobacterium*, and *Saccharomyces*. A systematic review of 63 randomized trials of probiotics, in which a broad range of antibiotics were used, found a 32% reduction in antibiotic-associated diarrhea. Therefore, a physician would need to treat 13 patients on antibiotics with probiotics to prevent one episode of diarrhea.[2] In addition, a systematic review has shown an approximately 66% decrease in the number of cases of *C difficile*-associated diarrhea for those patients treated with probiotics (number needed to treat [NNT] 26).[3]

ACUTE DIARRHEA
Epidemiology

In the United States, there are more than 300 million cases of diarrhea per year. However, accurate estimates of incidence are difficult because most patients do not present for evaluation. In addition, the yield of stool culture has been quite low, with historically only 1.5% to 5.8% returning a positive result.[4] Most cases of acute diarrhea are due to infection, including viruses (norovirus or rotavirus), bacteria (*Staphylococcus*, *Salmonella*, *Shigella*, *Campylobacter*, *Escherichia coli*, and *C difficile*), and parasites (*Giardia*, *Blastocystis*, and *Cryptosporidium*). In a recent study, adult subjects presenting to emergency departments with acute gastroenteritis were evaluated with extensive testing. Pathogens were identified in 25%, with yields up to nearly 50% when a whole stool specimen was submitted (compared with only rectal swabs). The most common pathogens identified were norovirus (26%), rotavirus (18%), salmonella (5.3%), clostridium (5.3%), campylobacter (3%), and parasites (3%).[5]

Patient History or Examination

When evaluating a patient presenting with acute diarrhea, the important historical items help determine cause and assesses severity. Therefore, it is critical to get a detailed history of recent travel, antibiotic use, medication changes, ingestions (including raw or undercooked meats), ill contacts (including children), and underlying immune status. Further questions should concern the frequency and consistency of bowel movements, including the presence of blood or pus, as well as whether there is concomitant fever or abdominal pain. The physical examination is primarily focused on volume status and severity of illness. It should include, along with other modalities, orthostatic blood pressure measurement.[4]

DIAGNOSTIC TESTS

In the immune-competent patient who presents in the first 2 to 3 days with acute diarrhea and no worrisome symptoms, no specific diagnostic testing is indicated. Evidence of a more inflammatory or invasive infection includes fever, severe abdominal pain, and blood and/or pus in the stool. If any of these are present, diagnostic testing is indicated. In addition, patients who are immunocompromised, elderly, generally unwell, or having severe symptoms are candidates for testing.

Markers of Inflammation

For years, various investigations have been performed in an attempt to better define cases of inflammatory diarrhea, including stool leukocytes and lactoferrin, a product of leukocytes. Existing guidelines recommend either performing or considering inflammatory testing.[4,6] The data on the usefulness of stool leukocytes have been inconsistent, with sensitivities ranging from 40% to 75% and specificity 50% to 88%.[7,8] A meta-analysis focusing on data from developed countries found a sensitivity of 73% and specificity of 84%. Lactoferrin performed somewhat better, with sensitivity of 78% to 92% and specificity 54% to 79%, making it a reasonable test for ruling out an inflammatory cause.[8]

Stool Culture

When done in a generalized population of patients with diarrhea, stool culture has limited usefulness. However, there is not consistent agreement on when or in whom to order stool cultures. Therefore, typically, cultures are performed in patients who have more significant underlying medical illness and in patients with severe cases (and at times of widespread involvement). The usefulness of routine stool culture in patients hospitalized for 3 days is extremely low and should not be routinely performed. Unless there is a clinical rationale, routine use of ova and parasite testing in patients with acute diarrhea should be discouraged. Possible indications include suspicious travel or exposure, immune-comprised state, or persistent symptoms (**Box 1**).

Stool Toxin

In certain patient populations, it is important to test stool directly for toxin. In a food-borne toxin-related illness (such as *Staphylococcus aureus*), there is not typically a need for testing because the course is self-limited. However, in patients recently treated with antibiotics, recently hospitalized, or residing in skilled-nursing facilities (include hospital staff in this group if they have taken antibiotics), checking for *C difficile* toxin is critical. In addition, Shiga toxin should be checked for in patients in whom the physician suspects possible enterohemorrhagic *E coli*, typically patients with bloody diarrhea but no fever.

GENERAL TREATMENT
Supportive

In severe diarrhea, the initial priority should be to assure adequate hydration. In the United States, this is often done intravenously. However, because most patients with diarrhea can tolerate oral intake, oral rehydration is possible with products such as Pedialyte (which has half the sugar and more than twice the sodium of Gatorade). Although the data are mixed, minimizing dairy intake given possible transient lactase deficiency is reasonable. Otherwise, a regular diet should be maintained because diets such as the BRAT (banana, rice, applesauce, and toast) are likely to be too nutritionally restrictive.

| Box 1 |
Indications for stool culture
Severe illness
Bloody diarrhea
Abdominal pain (not just cramping-type pain)
High fever
Immune-compromised state
Multiple comorbidities

Antidiarrheals

Loperamide, which binds gut wall receptors leading to decreased peristalsis and increased anal sphincter tone, is approved for use in both acute and chronic diarrhea. In acute diarrhea, most data are in patients with traveler's diarrhea, in whom it has been tried in conjunction with antibiotics. In a systematic review, loperamide, when added to antibiotic therapy, was superior to antibiotic alone resulting in decreased illness duration, especially in subjects with increased pretreatment frequency of diarrhea.[9] However, it should be avoided in severe or inflammatory cases. There are limited data on the usefulness of diphenoxylate-atropine in acute diarrhea.

Probiotics

As noted, probiotics may have a role in the prevention of diarrhea in patients on antibiotics. However, there may also be a role in the treatment of acute infectious diarrhea, although most studies have focused on infants and children. A Cochrane review found an approximately 24-hour reduction in duration of diarrhea, decreased stool frequency on day 2, and a lower risk of having diarrhea for 4 or more days (relative risk 0.41).[10]

TRAVELER'S DIARRHEA

For patients who travel to resource-poor regions, the incidence of traveler's diarrhea is 20% to 60%.[11] For acute diarrhea in the traveler, bacterial pathogens are usually the cause. E coli (enterotoxigenic and enteroaggregative) is most commonly identified. In travelers with acute diarrhea, empiric antibiotic treatment for 3 to 5 days, usually with a quinolone, is recommended. For travelers with persistent diarrhea, Giardia, Entamoeba, Strongyloides, and Schistosoma should be considered.[12]

FOOD-BORNE DIARRHEA

For food-borne illness, development of symptoms within 6 to 24 hours is most likely due to preformed toxin, as seen in Staphylococcus, Bacillus, and Clostridium perfringens. In addition, vomiting is frequently present as an initial symptom given upper gastrointestinal involvement. Typically, these patients only require supportive care.

WATERY DIARRHEA

Most watery diarrhea is due to viral gastroenteritis, such as norovirus or rotavirus. However, because there are no specific treatments, care is supportive. Diagnostic testing is not indicated unless there is either epidemiologic concern or history is inconclusive.

INFLAMMATORY DIARRHEA

Bloody diarrhea, fever, and abdominal pain are concerning for an invasive infection such as Shigella, Salmonella, Campylobacter, C difficile, or Yersinia. However, bloody diarrhea without fever is particularly worrisome for enterohemorrhagic E coli (including serotype 0157:H7). It is important to identify this variant of E coli because antibiotics should be avoided and the chance of developing hemolytic uremic syndrome is significant—up to 10% according to the World Health Organization. Antibiotics are also typically not needed in cases of salmonella and yersinia. However, in severe cases, and in cases of shigella and campylobacter, early antibiotics for 3 to 5 days can decrease duration of illness (norfloxacin 400 mg twice a day or, alternatively, quinolone or azithromycin 500 mg daily if quinolone-resistant campylobacter is suspected due to presumed a poultry source outside of the United States).

CHRONIC DIARRHEA

Chronic diarrhea is defined as the presence of loose stools with or without increased stool frequency for at least 4 weeks. As the definition has varied significantly, best estimates are that roughly 3% to 5% of the population suffers from chronic diarrhea. In these patients, the differential diagnosis is much longer than for those with an acute onset.[13] In addition, initially it is important to determine exactly what the patient means by "diarrhea" because the term can be used in describing increased stool frequency, loosened stool consistency, a sense of incomplete emptying, or leakage. For instance, fecal incontinence, which might be reported as diarrhea, is quite common, affecting 8.3% of noninstitutionalized adults and up to 15% of those aged 70 or older. Many of these patients do not have true diarrhea (**Box 2**).[14]

Patient History

Once it has been determined that a patient does have chronic diarrhea, history plays a major role in determining cause and subsequent diagnostic and therapeutic steps. Initially much of this rests on determining the presence of worrisome symptoms, such as weight loss or hematochezia. In addition, identification of medications that

---

Box 2
Differential for chronic diarrhea

Osmotic

- Carbohydrate malabsorption (ie, lactose intolerance)
- Laxative or antacid use
- Sugar alcohol intake (ie sorbitol)

Secretory

- Medications (including nonosmotic laxative use)
- Non- inflammatory bowel disease (IBD) colitis (lymphocytic, collagenous)
- Motility issues (IBS, diabetic enteropathy)
- Neuroendocrine tumors (VIPoma, mastocytosis, carcinoid)

Inflammatory

- IBD
- Infection (C difficile, invasive viral, bacterial, or parasitic infection)
- Ischemic colitis
- Malignancy (colon cancer or villous adenoma)

Fatty or malabsorption

- Celiac disease
- Small intestine bacterial overgrowth
- Giardia
- Pancreatic insufficiency
- Bile acid malabsorption

Data from Fine KD, Schiller LR. AGA technical review on the evaluation and management of chronic diarrhea. Gastroenterology 1999;116:1464–86.

might be contributing to diarrhea and diagnosing irritable bowel syndrome (IBS) are key early in the evaluation. After that, the goal of obtaining a detailed history is to categorize the diarrhea as watery, inflammatory, or fatty, realizing many patients have overlapping features. Common medications associated with diarrhea and the Rome III criteria are shown in **Boxes 3** and **4**.

DIAGNOSTIC TESTS

In patients with chronic diarrhea, it is reasonable to check a complete blood count (to evaluate for anemia and leukocytosis) and electrolytes. In appropriate situations, other testing may include autoantibodies for celiac disease, thyroid function, and protein levels. Although frequently checked, systemic inflammatory markers, such as erythrocyte sedimentation rate and C-reactive protein, have limited data in the diagnostic work-up of chronic diarrhea. If a likely diagnosis is not immediately recognized, stool testing might be of benefit. Although osmotic diarrhea should usually be obvious by history, fecal osmotic gap can help differentiate osmotic from secretory diarrhea (especially when there is concern for factitious cause). In patients with watery diarrhea, a low stool pH (<5.6) suggests carbohydrate malabsorption (**Box 5**).[13]

The role of stool inflammatory markers, such as lactoferrin and calprotectin, to differentiate an inflammatory process from noninflammatory remains unclear. Fecal lactoferrin has been shown to have a sensitivity of approximately 80% and specificity 85% to 100% for abnormal endoscopy findings.[15] More recently, there has been increased interest in calprotectin, a calcium-binding protein in white blood cells with both negative and positive predictive values of approximately 80% for histologic inflammation on colonoscopy.[16,17]

Testing for parasites, especially *Giardia* and *Cryptosporidium*, is appropriate in patients who may have been exposed. Stool antigen testing is more sensitive than routine ova and parasite examination for those organisms. Although bacteria other than *C difficile* are uncommon causes of chronic diarrhea, *Aeromonas*, *Plesiomonas*, and *Klebsiella oxytoca* have all been implicated. Other chronic infections to be aware of are the ulcerating viruses, most commonly in immunosuppressed patients. Stool statins for fat, such as the Sudan stain, and quantitative fat studies can be helpful in the diagnosis of malabsorption but may not add substantial information beyond visible fat in stool. Indications for colonoscopy are listed. There may be roles for other testing, including small bowel follow-through, abdominal-pelvic CT scan, and upper endoscopy (with small bowel biopsies) (**Box 6**).

Box 3
Common medications associated with diarrhea

Antidepressants (selective serotonin reuptake inhibitors)

Diabetic medications (metformin, GLP-1 agonist exenatide, liraglutide)

Antibiotics

Laxatives (osmotic and stimulant)

Nonsteroidal antiinflammatories

Proton pump inhibitors

Colchicine

Box 4
Rome III criteria

- All require onset of symptoms at least 6 months before and ongoing over the last 3 months

IBS

1. Recurrent abdominal pain or discomfort ≥3 d/mo
2. At least two of the following:
   a. Improvement in pain with defecation
   b. Change in frequency of stools at onset of pain
   c. Change in appearance of stools at onset of pain

IBS subtypes (must meet definition of IBS)

- IBS with constipation—hard or lumpy stools ≥25% and loose (mushy) or watery stools ≤25% of bowel movements
- IBS with diarrhea—loose (mushy) or watery stools ≥25% and hard or lumpy stool ≤25% of bowel movements

Functional diarrhea

1. Mushy, loose, or watery stools at least 75% of the time without pain

Functional constipation:

1. Loose stools rare without laxatives
2. Criteria for IBS not met
3. At least two of the following:
   a. <3 bowel movements/wk
   b. Straining during ≥25% of bowel movements
   c. Lumpy or hard stools ≥25 of bowel movements
   d. Sensation of incomplete evacuation for ≥25 of bowel movements
   e. Sensation of blockage for ≥25 of bowel movements
   f. Manual maneuvers to assist defecation in ≥25 of bowel movements

Adapted from Longstreth GF, Thompson WG, Chey WD, et al. Functional bowel disorders. Gastroenterology 2006;130:1480–91.

WATERY DIARRHEA
Osmotic

There are only a few disorders that are consistently osmotic and make evaluation straightforward. Use of fecal osmotic gap is rarely necessary. If history is compatible,

---

Box 5
Fecal osmotic gap

Gap = 290–2 (stool Na^+ + stool K^+)

If gap:

>125, osmotic

<50, secretory or functional

Box 6
Indications for colonoscopy in chronic diarrhea

a. Routine colorectal screening is already indicated

b. Concern for either inflammatory process or microscopic colitis (in which random biopsies necessary)

c. Diagnosis remains unclear

d. Worrisome features such as weight loss, hematochezia

---

the physician can try eliminating lactose from the diet. If there is continued clinical concern for lactose intolerance, hydrogen breath testing can be performed. Otherwise, the most likely diagnosis is intentional or accidental ingestion of an osmotically active agent (or a mixed disorder). Some patients ingest a significant amount of sorbitol in candy and gum and can have diarrhea due to its ingestion.

SECRETORY

IBS or Functional Diarrhea

IBS is characterized by the presence of abdominal pain or discomfort in the setting of irregular bowel function. Functional diarrhea describes frequent loose stool but without the associated abdominal pain or other symptoms. Mucus is a common complaint. Features making IBS less likely include bloody or nocturnal diarrhea and weight loss. Testing on patients with IBS can show abnormal hydrogen and some patients respond to rifaximin, which suggests alteration in bacterial distribution.[18,19] Treatments found to be effective in symptom management include exercise, antispasmodics, rifaximin, and probiotics.[20] In patients with diarrhea, loperamide can decrease stool frequency but has limited effect on pain.

MICROSCOPIC COLITIS

Microscopic colitis is an increasingly recognized cause of chronic diarrhea, especially in older adults. Because diagnosis requires colonic biopsy in the setting of normal-appearing mucosa, it is a challenging and likely underreported diagnosis. Biopsy can show lymphocytic and/or collagenous infiltration, although there are newer reports of both eosinophilic and mast cell populations. The typical presentation is diffuse watery diarrhea, occasionally severe. Associated medications include nonsteroidal antiinflammatory drugs (NSAIDs), proton-pump inhibitors, selective serotonin reuptake inhibitors (SSRIs), ticlopidine, and possibly statins.[21] There also seems to be an association with celiac disease. Treatment is antidiarrheals such as loperamide for mild disease, bismuth subsalicylate for moderate disease, and budesonide for more severe symptoms.[22]

Neuroendocrine

There are no clear guidelines on when testing for these very uncommon causes of diarrhea should be performed. Testing for plasma peptides (gastrin, vasoactive intestinal peptide, somatostatin, and calcitonin) and urine metabolites (5-hydroxyindoleacetic acid, metanephrine, and histamine) are most commonly ordered in atypical presentations or when radiographic studies suggest a cause.

INFLAMMATORY
Inflammatory Bowel Disease

One of the challenges is determining when colonoscopy is indicated to rule out inflammatory bowel disease (IBD) versus irritable bowel syndrome. Fecal calprotectin may aid in this decision. In a meta-analysis of subjects referred for colonoscopy for suspected IBD, calprotectin had a sensitivity of 93% and specificity of 96% in diagnosing IBD. A subsequent study, in which 41% of subjects had histologically confirmed inflammation, sensitivity and specificity were 75% and 88%, respectively.[17] In a lower risk primary care population, a negative calprotectin would be reassuring that inflammation was very unlikely.

FATTY OR MALABSORPTION
Celiac Disease

Although not specifically outlined in the 1999 American Gastroenterological Association (AGA) guidelines, testing for celiac disease should be performed if the diagnosis is not immediately obvious. This is especially true if there is weight loss, steatorrhea, bloating, anemia, abnormal liver enzymes, or bone loss. Both IgA antiendomysial and IgA antitissue transglutaminase have excellent sensitivity in patients with abdominal symptoms (sensitivity 89%–90%, specificity 98%–99%). Gliadin antibodies should not be used for screening because it is inferior.[23] Once diagnosed, if diarrhea persists, consider microscopic colitis (see previous discussion), pancreatic exocrine deficiency, or gastrointestinal lymphoma.[24]

Small Intestine Bacterial Overgrowth

Typically, presentations of small intestine bacterial overgrowth include abdominal pain or cramping, bloating, diarrhea, and steatorrhea. However, because the standard for diagnosis is jejunal aspirate, the diagnosis is often not easily made. Hydrogen breath testing, often with lactulose, is used to help determine likelihood of bacterial overgrowth. If testing is positive, a trial of antibiotics is appropriate (rifaximin, amoxicillin-clavulanate, and norfloxacin). Because some patients with IBS respond to rifaximin, this is an attractive, albeit expensive, option.

Other malabsorptive causes of chronic diarrhea include pancreatic exocrine insufficiency and bile acid malabsorption. Fatty stools, either clinically or by testing, should suggest possible pancreatic or biliary cause of diarrhea. Patients in whom chronic pancreatitis or pancreatic insufficiency is a clinical concern may respond to treatment with pancreatic enzymes. Bile acid malabsorption is an underrecognized cause of chronic diarrhea in which bile is not resorbed properly in the distal ileum. Diarrhea due to increased colonic delivery of bile acids is common in patients who have had a cholecystectomy, causing persistent symptoms in 6% of patients.[25]

Testing for bile issues is challenging and an empiric trial of cholestyramine, a bile acid sequestrant, is reasonable in persistent diarrhea of no other clear cause.[26]

DIARRHEA SUMMARY

Important considerations for diarrhea include:

1. Chronic diarrhea can be due to a large number of underlying diagnoses but irritable bowel or functional disorders are the most common
2. History and examination help determine osmotic, secretory, inflammatory, or malabsorptive causes

3. Testing with fecal calprotectin may help differentiate inflammatory from noninflammatory causes
4. Treatment of chronic diarrhea is driven by diagnosis (**Figs. 1** and **2**)

CONSTIPATION

Chronic constipation is characterized by infrequent and/or difficult bowel movements that persist for at least 3 months.[27] Associated symptoms can include hard or firm stool, incomplete evacuation, bloating, and abdominal discomfort. Although many studies and guidelines use fewer than three bowel movements per week as a criterion, this applies to a marked minority of patients who consider themselves constipated. As many as 50% of patients who report constipation actually have a daily bowel movement.[28] Given variation in definition, precise prevalence is difficult. However, this is an extremely common condition, likely affecting 15% to 20% of adults in their lifetime and up to 33% of those older than 60 years of age.[29] Women are affected more than

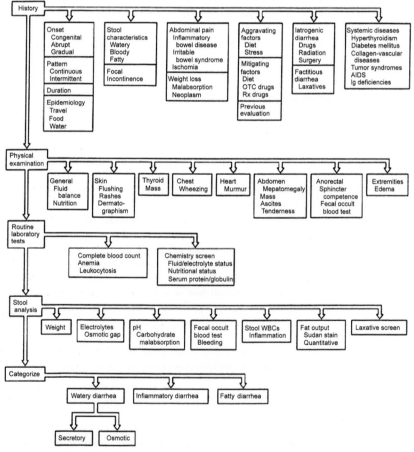

Fig. 1. Initial evaluation for chronic diarrhea. WBC, white blood count. (*From* Fine KD, Schiller LR. AGA technical review on the evaluation and management of chronic diarrhea. Gastroenterology 1999;116:1464–86.)

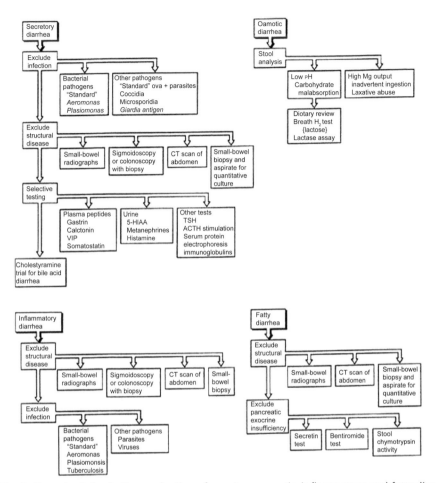

Fig. 2. Flow charts for further evaluation of secretory, osmotic, inflammatory, and fatty diarrhea. (*From* Fine KD, Schiller LR. AGA technical review on the evaluation and management of chronic diarrhea. Gastroenterology 1999;116:1464–86.)

men and prevalence increases with age. In addition, quality of life is aversely affected, with associated loss of work productivity, activity impairment, and increased health-care resource use (**Box 7**).[30]

Evaluation

History should include a detailed review of bowel habits, including frequency and consistency of bowel movements, the need to strain or use manual maneuvers, and sense of incomplete evacuation. It is important to identify the most bothersome symptom because it focuses the evaluation and treatment. Other abdominal symptoms, such as gastrointestinal bleeding, abdominal pain, and bloating, should also be ascertained. Relevant past history such as abdominal surgery, neurologic disorders (Parkinson disease and multiple sclerosis) and hypothyroidism should be collected. A complete medication history, including over-the-counter bulk agents and laxatives, along with other supplements, such as calcium and iron, should be obtained.

> **Box 7**
> **Differential for constipation**
>
> Functional problems
> - IBS with constipation
> - Functional constipation
>
> Defecatory
> - Pelvic floor dysfunction
> - Dyssynergic defecation
> - Rectocele
>
> Diseases of the colon:
> - Stricture
> - Colorectal cancer
>
> Metabolic
> - Hypercalcemia
> - Hypothyroidism
> - Diabetes mellitus
>
> Neurologic
> - Parkinson
> - Multiple sclerosis
> - Spinal cord lesions
>
> *Adapted from* Bharucha AE, Pemberton JH, Locke GR 3rd. American Gastroenterological Association technical review on constipation. Gastroenterology 2013;144:218–38.

Adverse effect of medications can be a reversible cause of constipation. Common offenders include opioids, calcium and iron supplements, calcium channel blockers, anticholinergics (including inhaled agents such as tiotropium), and NSAIDs.

Physical Examination

Physical examination should include:

1. Careful abdominal examination with special attention to surgical scars and masses
2. Examination of the perianal region with attention to fissures and hemorrhoids
3. Perineal inspection during simulated evacuation
4. Rectal examination of sphincter tone, both at rest and with simulated bowel evacuation
5. In women, a pelvic examination may been needed to rule out rectocele

Laboratory Testing

In most patients, complete blood count should be checked.[27] Blood sugar, calcium, and thyroid stimulating hormone can also be considered, although evidence of such an approach is lacking and this approach is not endorsed by AGA.

DEFECATORY DISORDERS

The initial goal of history, examination, and basic testing is to identify concerning symptoms as well as relevant medical or pharmacologic issues. After that, it is important to determine if there is a defecatory disorder in which evacuation is the primary problem. Normal defecation requires relaxation of the puborectalis muscles, pelvic floor descent, abdominal wall muscle contraction, and, finally, relaxation of the anal sphincter.[31] Issues with any of these actions can lead to difficulty with evacuation. In patients with pelvic floor dysfunction, there is a decrease in the strength of the pelvic floor muscles, impaired rectal sensation, and a subsequent decrease in rectal tone. Dyssynergic defecation refers to a lack of coordination of muscle relaxation and contraction. The precise cause of such disorders remains unclear. Other issues that can lead to defecatory difficulty are rectoceles, hemorrhoids, and anal fissure or stricture. Importantly, laxatives have limited effect on these disorders, making it critical to identify these patients (**Box 8**).

Nonpharmacologic Therapy

Constipation has been noted to be more prevalent in patients with limited physical activity and low dietary fiber. However, studies looking at dietary modifications with increased fiber intake (such as bran) have been conflicting. In at least one trial, abdominal pain and bloating actually worsened with added fiber. There have been some data supporting the benefit of prunes.[32] However, soluble fiber (such as psyllium) led to improvements in global symptoms (86.5% vs 47.4%), straining (55.6% vs 28.6%), pain on defecation, and stool consistency compared with placebo.[33] Biofeedback is an effective treatment in defecatory disorders with pelvic floor dysfunction, improving symptoms in up to 70% of affected subjects.[34]

PHARMACOLOGIC THERAPY
Laxatives

The mainstay of treatment over the years has been laxatives. Laxatives are either osmotic (polyethylene glycol, lactulose, and magnesium) or stimulatory (bisacodyl, senna, and cascara). Pooled data on osmotic laxatives reveal a significant effect with only 38% failing to improve compared with 69% for placebo, resulting in an

---

Box 8
Diagnostic tests

1. Anorectal manometry or balloon expulsion test:
   a. Balloon test involves expulsion of a water-filled balloon, with expectation it will be completed within 1 to 5 minutes
   b. Indicated for suspected defecatory disorder or those with poor response to laxatives
2. Defecography
   a. Evacuation of barium is monitored by fluoroscopy
   b. Reserved for inconclusive testing but concern for defecatory issue
3. Colon transit time
   a. Performed with radiopaque makers, with slow transit time defined as multiple retained markers on day 6; wireless motility capsules can also be used (more expensive)
   b. Indicated if defecatory disorder ruled out, laboratory testing unremarkable and poor response to laxatives (or if symptoms persist after treatment of defecatory disorder)
4. Colonoscopy
   a. Indicated if due for routine screening, blood in stools, anemia, weight loss, or severe, persistent symptoms

NNT of 3.[35] In direct comparisons, polyethylene glycol has been found to be more effective than lactulose in improving stool frequency and form, relief of abdominal pain, and need for other agents[36] and, therefore, should be considered the preferred osmotic agent. Stimulant laxatives such as bisacodyl are also effective with 42% failing to improve versus 78% on placebo (NNT 3).[35] Although there have been concerns regarding the long-term safety of stimulant laxatives, there is no convincing evidence of increased risk of cancer or worsening bowel function.

SECRETAGOGUES

There are two relatively new agents approved for use in patients with chronic constipation. Linaclotide is a peptide that stimulates cyclic guanosine monophosphate

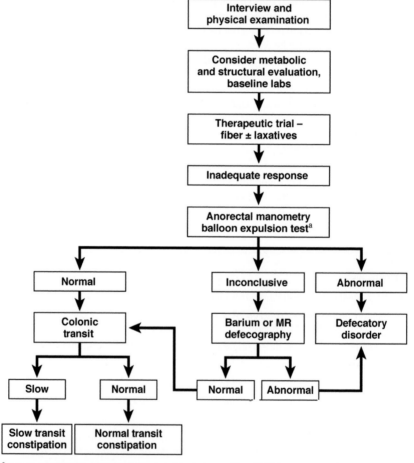

[a]Because anorectal manometry, rectal balloon expulsion test may not be available in all practice settings, it is acceptable, in such circumstances, to proceed to assessing colonic transit with the understanding that delayed colonic transit does not exclude a defecatory disorder.

Fig. 3. American Gastroenterological Association (AGA) 2013 guidelines for initial evaluation and treatment algorithm for chronic constipation. (*From* American Gastroenterological Association, Bharucha AE, Dorn SD, Lembo A, et al. American Gastroenterological Association medical position statement on constipation. Gastroenterology 2013;144:211–17.)

through the guanylate cyclase receptor. This results in chloride-rich fluid secretion into the intestinal lumen. Subjects with chronic constipation (average of 0.3 complete spontaneous bowel movements per week) were studied for 12 weeks with daily linaclotide or placebo. A return to normal bowel function (at least 3 complete spontaneous bowel movements per week in 75% of weeks) occurred in approximately 20% of treated subjects versus 5% with placebo (NNT~6). Diarrhea led to discontinuation in approximately 4% of subjects.[37] In addition, linaclotide has shown promise in subjects with IBS with constipation, with improvements in both spontaneous bowel movements and abdominal pain.[38]

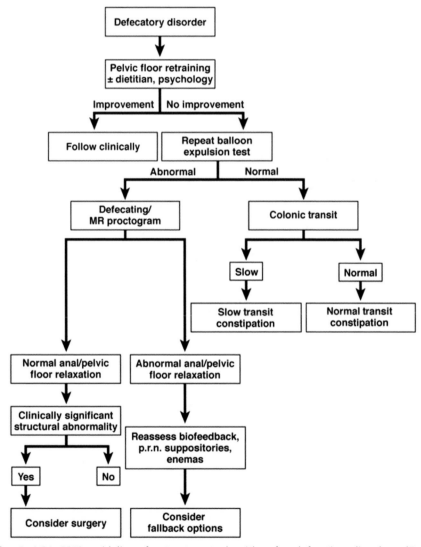

Fig. 4. AGA 2013 guidelines for treatment algorithm for defecating disorders. (*From* American Gastroenterological Association, Bharucha AE, Dorn SD, Lembo A, et al. American Gastroenterological Association medical position statement on constipation. Gastroenterology 2013;144:211–17.)

Lubiprostone, which activates chloride channels leading to increased intestinal fluid secretion, has also been shown to increase the number of spontaneous bowel movements. A meta-analysis of three studies found an NNT of 4 to increase spontaneous bowel movement to at least 3 to 4 per week. The most common adverse effects were nausea and diarrhea.[35]

PROKINETICS

Cisapride and tegaserod, 5-HT$_4$ agonists used for constipation, have been removed from the US market due to concerns of excess cardiovascular events and QT prolongation. Prucalopride, a more selective 5-HT$_4$ agent, is now available in Canada and

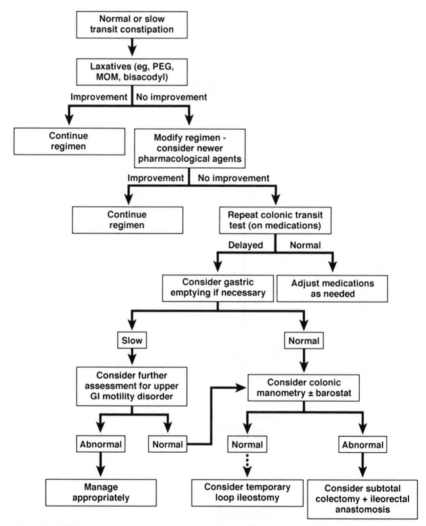

Fig. 5. AGA 2013 guidelines for treatment algorithm for normal or slow transit constipation. GI, gastrointestinal. (*From* American Gastroenterological Association, Bharucha AE, Dorn SD, Lembo A, et al. American Gastroenterological Association medical position statement on constipation. Gastroenterology 2013;144:211–17.)

Europe but has not been approved for use in the United States. In a meta-analysis, the NNT was 6 to return to normal bowel function. Thus far, there has been no significant effect on QT length or increase in adverse cardiovascular events.[35]

OTHERS

Probiotics may have a benefit in patients with functional constipation, with data suggesting improvement in defecation frequency and stool consistency.[39] There are no convincing data on the efficacy of stool softeners such as docusate, although there may be a role in patients with hard stools.

SURGICAL TREATMENT

If slow transit constipation is documented, and a patient fails an aggressive trial of fiber, laxatives, and prokinetics, total colectomy is an option. Obviously, this needs to have been very carefully considered.

SUMMARY

Important considerations for constipation include:

1. Initial evaluation should evaluate for fecal incontinence, fecal impaction, medication side effects, concerning symptoms, underlying medical or metabolic issues and irritable bowel syndrome
2. History and examination should be used to determine if a defecatory disorder is most likely
   a. If defecatory disorder is likely, testing with balloon expulsion or anal manometry can be considered and, if confirmed, treatment with biofeedback (if testing not available, it is reasonable to trial fiber and laxatives because many patients have a mixed disorder)
   b. If it is unlikely, proceed with trial of fiber and/or osmotic laxatives
3. If continued symptoms, consider trial of newer agent (lubiprostone or linaclotide)
4. If ineffective, consider testing for colon transit time and referral to gastroenterology (**Figs. 3–5**)

REFERENCES

1. Talley NJ, Weaver AL, Zinmeister AR, et al. Self-reported diarrhea: what does it mean? Am J Gastroenterol 1994;89:1160–4.
2. Hempel S, Newberry SJ, Maher AR, et al. Probiotics for the prevention and treatment of antibiotic-associated diarrhea. JAMA 2012;207(18):1959–69.
3. Johnston BC, Ma SS, Goldenberg JZ, et al. Probiotics for the prevention of Clostridium difficile-associated diarrhea: a systematic review and meta-analysis. Ann Intern Med 2012;157(12):878–88.
4. Guerrant RL, Van Gilder T, Steiner TS, et al. Practice guidelines for the management of infectious diarrhea. Clin Infect Dis 2001;32:321–51.
5. Bresee JS, Marcus R, Venezia RA, et al. The etiology of severe acute gastroenteritis among adults visiting emergency departments in the United States. J Infect Dis 2012;205(9):1374–81.
6. Dupont HL. Clinical guidelines: acute infectious diarrhea in adults. Am J Gastroenterol 1997;92:1962–75.

7. Chitkara YK, McCasland KA, Kenefic L. Development and implantation of cost-effective guidelines in the laboratory investigation of diarrhea in a community hospital. Arch Intern Med 1996;156:1445–8.

8. Gill CJ, Lau J, Gorback SL, et al. Diagnostic accuracy of stool assays for inflammatory bacterial gastroenteritis in developed and resource-poor countries. Clin Infect Dis 2003;37(3):365–75.

9. Riddle MS, Arnold S, Tribble DR. Effect of adjunctive loperamide in combination with antibiotics on treatment outcomes in traveler's diarrhea: a systematic review and meta-analysis. Clin Infect Dis 2008;47(8):1007–14.

10. Allen SJ, Martinez EG, Gregorio GV, et al. Probiotics for treating acute infectious diarrhea. Cochrane Database Syst Rev 2010;(11):CD003048.

11. Hill DR. The burden of illness in international travelers. N Engl J Med 2006;354:115–7.

12. Ross AG, Olds GR, Cripps AW, et al. Enteropathogens and chronic illness in returning travelers. N Engl J Med 2013;368(19):1817–25.

13. American Gastroenterological Association medical position statement: guidelines for the evaluation and management of chronic diarrhea. Gastroenterology 1999;116:1461–3.

14. Whitehead WE, Borrud L, Goode PS, et al. Fecal incontinence in US adults: epidemiology and risk factors. Gastroenterology 2009;137(2):512–7.

15. Sherwood RA. Faecal markers of gastrointestinal inflammation. J Clin Pathol 2012;65(11):981–5.

16. Licata A, Randazzo LA, Cappello M, et al. Fecal calprotectin in clinical practice: a noninvasive screening tool for patients with chronic diarrhea. J Clin Gastroenterol 2012;46(6):504–8.

17. van Rheenen PF, Van de Vijver E, Fidler V. Faecal calprotectin for screening of patients with suspected inflammatory bowel disease: diagnostic meta-analysis. BMJ 2010;341:c3369.

18. Shah ED, Basseri RJ, Chong K, et al. Abnormal breath testing in IBS: a meta-analysis. Dig Dis Sci 2010;55(9):2441–9.

19. Pimentel M, Lembo A, Chey WD, et al. Rifaximin therapy for patients with irritable bowel syndrome without constipation. N Engl J Med 2011;364(1):22–32.

20. Moayyedi P, Ford AC, Talley NJ, et al. The efficacy of probiotics in the treatment of irritable bowel syndrome: a systematic review. Gut 2010;59(3):325–32.

21. Pardi DS, Kelly CP. Microscopic colitis. Gastroenterology 2011;140(4):1155–65.

22. Yen EF, Pardi DS. Review article: Microscopic colitis—lymphocytic, collagenous and 'mast cell' colitis. Aliment Pharmacol Ther 2011;34:21–32.

23. van der Windt DA, Jellema P, Mulder CJ, et al. Diagnostic testing for celiac disease among patients with abdominal symptoms: a systematic review. JAMA 2010;303(17):1738–46.

24. Rubio-Tapia A, Hill ID, Kelly CP, et al. ACG clinical guidelines: diagnosis and management of celiac disease. Am J Gastroenterol 2013;108(5):656–76.

25. Sauter GH, Moussavian AC, Meyer G, et al. Bowel habits and bile acid malabsorption in the months after cholecystectomy. Am J Gastroenterol 2002;97(7):1732–6.

26. Money ME, Camilleri M. Review: management of postprandial diarrhea syndrome. Am J Med 2012;125:538–44.

27. Bharucha AE, Pemberton JH, Locke GR 3rd. American Gastroenterological Association technical review on constipation. Gastroenterology 2013;144:218–38.

28. Ashraf W, Park F, Lof J, et al. An examination of the reliability of reported stool frequency in the diagnosis of idiopathic constipation. Am J Gastroenterol 1996;91(1):26–32.

29. American Gastroenterological Association, Bharucha AE, Dorn SD, Lembo A, et al. American gastroenterological association medical position statement on constipation. Gastroenterology 2013;144:211–7.

30. Sun SX, Dibonaventura M, Purayidathil FW, et al. Impact of chronic constipation on health-related quality of life, work productivity, and healthcare resource use: and analysis of the National Health and Wellness Survey. Dig Dis Sci 2011; 56(9):2688–95.

31. Leung L, Riutta T, Kotecha J, et al. Chronic constipation: an evidence-based review. J Am Board Fam Med 2011;24:436–51.

32. Gallegos-Orozco JF, Foxx-Orenstein AE, Serler SM, et al. Chronic constipation in the elderly. Am J Gastroenterol 2012;107:18–25.

33. Suares NC, Ford AC. Systematic review: the effects of fibre in the management of chronic idiopathic constipation. Aliment Pharmacol Ther 2011;33:895–901.

34. Koh CE, Young CJ, Young JM, et al. Systematic review of randomized controlled trials of the effectiveness of biofeedback for pelvic floor dysfunction. Br J Surg 2008;95(9):1079–87.

35. Ford AD, Suarez ND. Effect of laxatives and pharmacological therapies in chronic idiopathic constipations: systematic review and meta-analysis. Gut 2011;60: 209–18.

36. Lee-Robichaud H, Thomas K, Morgan J, et al. Lactulose vs polyethylene glycol for chronic constipation. Cochrane Database Syst Rev 2010;(7):CD007570.

37. Lembo AJ, Schneier HA, Shiff SJ, et al. Two randomized trials of linaclotide for chronic constipation. N Engl J Med 2011;365:527–36.

38. Chey WD, Lembo AJ, Lavins BL, et al. Linaclotide for irritable bowel syndrome with constipation: a 26-week randomized, double-blind, placebo-controlled trial to evaluate the efficacy and safety. Am J Gastroenterol 2012;107:1701–12.

39. Chmielewska A, Szajeewska H. Systematic review of randomized controlled trials: probiotics for functional constipation. World J Gastroenterol 2010;16(1): 69–75.

FURTHER READINGS

Brandt LJ, Chey WD, Foxx-Orenstein AE, et al. American College of Gastroenterology Task Force on Irritable Bowel Syndrome. An evidence-based position statement on the management of irritable bowel syndrome. Am J Gastroenterol 2009; 104(Suppl 1):S1–35.

Farthing M, Salam MA, Lindberg G, et al. Acute diarrhea in adults and children: a global perspective. J Clin Gastroenterol 2013;47(1):12–20.

Sandler RS, Everhart JE, Donowitz M, et al. The burden of selected digestive diseases in the United States. Gastroenterology 2002;122:1500–11.

Savola KL, Varon EJ, Tompkins LS, et al. Fecal leukocyte stain has diagnostic value for outpatients but not inpatients. J Clin Microbiol 2001;39(1):266–9.

Shastri YM, Bergis D, Pyse N, et al. Prospective multicenter study evaluating fecal calprotectin in adult acute bacterial diarrhea. Am J Med 2008;121(12):1099–106.

Tack J. Functional diarrhea. Gastroenterol Clin North Am 2012;41:629–37.

Thielman NM, Guerrant RL. Clinical practice. Acute infectious diarrhea. N Engl J Med 2004;350:38–47.

Dyspepsia

Maryann Katherine Overland, MD

KEYWORDS

- Functional dyspepsia • *Helicobacter pylori* test and treat • Peptic ulcer disease
- Gastroesophageal reflux disease

KEY POINTS

- Dyspepsia is a complex disease with multiple potential pathophysiologic mechanisms including abnormal gut motility, visceral hypersensitivity, genetic, infectious/postinfectious, and psychosocial factors.
- Although serious pathology is rare in patients presenting with dyspepsia, physicians should be aware of alarm features and refer those patients promptly for endoscopy or subspecialty care.
- A trial of antisecretory therapy, such as a proton pump inhibitor or histamine-2 receptor antagonist, should be provided to patients without alarm features, especially if their primary symptom is epigastric burning.
- A test-and-treat strategy for *Helicobacter pylori* infection is a cost-effective intervention and provides symptomatic relief for some patients with dyspepsia.
- Patients with depression, anxiety, or a history of abuse should be offered antidepressant therapy and psychotherapy.

INTRODUCTION

Dyspepsia is not a single disease, but rather a complex of symptoms that often overlap with other disease entities.[1] The investigation of undifferentiated dyspepsia poses a diagnostic dilemma for primary care physicians. Because evidence to guide best practices is sparse, it is challenging for the primary care physician to decide the optimal diagnostic and therapeutic plan. Although life-threatening conditions are rare in this setting, a missed diagnosis of esophageal cancer or other serious upper gastrointestinal pathology could be devastating. For this reason, invasive diagnostic tests, including endoscopies, are common in the evaluation of uninvestigated dyspepsia. Given the high prevalence of dyspepsia around the world, developing a prudent and evidence-based method of investigation and treatment of dyspepsia is of the utmost importance to prevent potential harm and unnecessary medical expense.

Division of General Internal Medicine, Primary Care Clinic, VA Puget Sound Health Care System, University of Washington, 1660 South Columbian Way, Seattle, WA 98108, USA
E-mail address: Maryann.Overland@va.gov

Med Clin N Am 98 (2014) 549–564
http://dx.doi.org/10.1016/j.mcna.2014.01.007
0025-7125/14/$ – see front matter Published by Elsevier Inc.

medical.theclinics.com

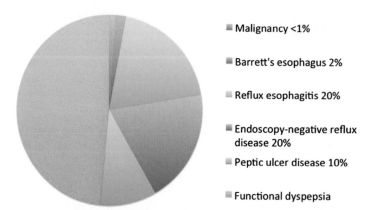

Fig. 1. Causes of dyspepsia. (*Data from* Zagari RM, Fuccio L, Bazzoli F. Investigating dyspepsia. BMJ 2008;337:1–5.)

Dyspepsia affects 25% to 40% of the population over a lifetime and accounts for 3% to 5% of all primary care clinic visits,[2] estimated at 4 million primary care visits a year in the United States alone.[3] One study found that 50% of European and North American patients with dyspepsia are on medication for it, and more than 30% report ever missing work or school because of burdensome symptoms.[4] Another study reported 12.4% of patients with dyspepsia missed work because of their symptoms over a 1-year period.[5] Among active workers with dyspepsia, more than 32% reported their symptoms caused them to be absent from work, and 78% reported reduced productivity because of dyspepsia (presenteeism). That study did not find a difference in lost productivity between those with organic versus those with functional dyspepsia (FD).[6] Nearly 62% of the patients in one study had consulted a physician for their dyspeptic symptoms, and 74% of those went more than once. More than two-thirds of those patients who had consulted

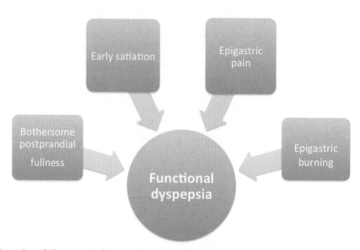

Fig. 2. Functional dyspepsia diagnostic criteria. One or more of the listed symptoms, in the absence of structural disease. Criteria must be fulfilled for the last 3 months with symptom onset at least 6 months before diagnosis.

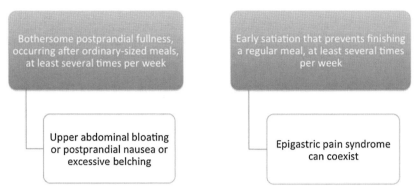

Fig. 3. Postprandial distress syndrome.

a physician were taking medications for their dyspepsia, and 36% underwent endoscopy.[5]

Of patients presenting with dyspepsia symptoms, 50% to 60% have no biochemical or structural lesion to explain their symptoms (**Fig. 1**). FD, previously referred to as "nonulcer dyspepsia," describes these symptoms in the absence of an identifiable organic, systemic, or metabolic etiology (**Fig. 2**).[2,7–9] FD is divided into two categories by the Rome III criteria, although there is considerable overlap between the two. The first is postprandial distress syndrome (**Fig. 3**), characterized by bothersome postprandial fullness and early satiation; the second is epigastric pain syndrome (**Fig. 4**), characterized by epigastric pain and burning, with onset of at

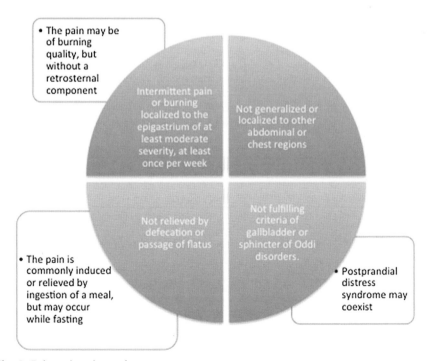

Fig. 4. Epigastric pain syndrome.

least 6 months ago, and present during the last 3 months.[9] The symptoms are usually aggravated by meals. Some older definitions of FD include symptoms of gastroesophageal reflux, such as heartburn and belching, whereas the newer Rome III definition does not include these symptoms. However, there is a great degree of overlap between FD and coexisting reflux disease. One study revealed 37% of patients complaining of symptoms that could be characterized as FD actually had esophageal acid reflux proved by pH monitoring.[10] The exact causes of FD remain unknown[9] but symptoms are more common in women,[5] smokers, aspirin users,[11] and those with a history of acute gastroenteritis.[12] Coffee and alcohol are not definitively associated with FD, and the role of *Helicobacter pylori* infection in FD is still up for debate.

PATHOPHYSIOLOGY

The pathophysiology of FD is not completely understood, with abnormal gut motility, visceral hypersensitivity, genetic, infectious/postinfectious, and psychosocial factors playing a role.

Delayed gastric emptying occurs in 20% to 50% of patients with FD.[13] Up to two-thirds may have abnormalities of either antral or duodenal motility.[14] Those patients with delayed gastric emptying predominantly have symptoms of postprandial fullness, nausea, and vomiting.[15] Up to 40% of patients with symptoms of early satiety and weight loss have impaired gastric accommodation, which suggests those patients' dyspeptic symptoms could be caused by increased intragastric pressure after ingestion of a meal.[16–18] Studies using capsaicin have shown increased sensitivity to visceral stimulation in patients with FD.[19,20] Several genetic polymorphisms are associated with visceral hypersensitivity and other upper abdominal symptoms in FD.[21]

FD occurs at higher rates in people with a history of acute infectious gastroenteritis (IGE), suggesting a role for gut immune dysregulation.[22] After an episode of IGE, patients with FD are noted to have focal T-cell aggregation with elevated CD8+ cells and macrophages and decreased CD4+ cells in and around the crypts and villi of the duodenum. This suggest that patients with FD are slower, or unable, to terminate the inflammatory response.[23] A meta-analysis investigating the risk of developing FD after an episode of acute IGE found an odds ratio of 4.76 in the first year after a self-reported episode of IGE and 1.97 thereafter, with an overall odds ratio of nearly 2.2.[12] Several studies have also linked eradication of *H pylori* to improvement in FD.

Table 1	
Differential diagnosis of dyspepsia	
Upper Gastrointestinal Tract	**Other Sources**
Gastroesophageal reflux with or without esophagitis	Gallbladder: cholelithiasis or cholecystitis
Peptic ulcer disease: gastric or duodenal	Pancreas: pancreatitis or pancreatic malignancy
Esophageal malignancy	Vascular: ischemic heart disease, mesenteric ischemia
Gastric malignancy	Medications: NSAIDS, aspirin, steroids, antibiotics, calcium channel blockers, bisphosphonates, SNRIs, theophylline
Functional dyspepsia	Hepatobiliary: hepatitis and hepatic malignancy

Abbreviations: NSAIDS, nonsteroidal antiinflammatory drugs; SNRIs, serotonin-norepinephrine reuptake inhibitors.

FD is more common in patients with concomitant depression or anxiety, and those with a history of abuse. A recent prospective cohort study of nearly 1200 patients demonstrated that high baseline levels of anxiety were an independent predictor of developing FD in the future.[24] Patients with anxiety and depression are more likely to seek treatment of their dyspepsia,[25] and are also more likely to experience their symptoms as more severe than those without a comorbid psychiatric condition.[26] As with any functional gastrointestinal disorder, somatization is a potential cause (**Table 1**).[27]

GASTROESOPHAGEAL REFLUX DISEASE

Gastroesophageal reflux disease (GERD) is one of the most common upper gastrointestinal disorders in the developed world. It is caused by prolonged gastric acid exposure in the esophagus due to poor esophageal motility, decreased lower esophageal sphincter tone, and impairments in gastroesophageal junctions. Obesity, smoking, alcohol, pregnancy, certain foods, and a recumbent position shortly after eating can all cause GERD or make it worse.[28] There is a great deal of overlap between GERD and FD. A study of prevalence of pathologic esophageal acid reflux in patients with FD found that nearly 32% of patients with FD had pathologic esophageal acid reflux. The prevalence is approximately 50% in patients who complained predominantly of epigastric burning.[10]

The hallmark of GERD is heartburn and regurgitation, particularly after meals. Patients may also have extraesophageal symptoms, such as cough or laryngitis. Endoscopy is 90% to 100% specific for diagnosing esophagitis in reflux disease. However, 50% to 70% of patients with the classic heartburn and regurgitation symptoms of GERD have no esophagitis on endoscopy,[29] making it a rather insensitive screening tool. When typical heartburn and regurgitation occur together, a diagnosis of GERD can be made without further testing with greater than 90% accuracy.[30] A study comparing a 2-week course of high-dose omeprazole versus 24-hour esophageal pH monitoring found the two interventions to be equally sensitive in diagnosing GERD in patients with erosive esophagitis.[31,32] Thus, for those patients presenting with heartburn and regurgitation, an empiric therapeutic trial of a standard-dose proton pump inhibitor (PPI) for 2 weeks or a double-dose of PPI therapy for 1 week is appropriate. If patients respond to an appropriate trial of antisecretory therapy, a diagnosis can be made and no further testing is warranted. However, if patients do not respond to empiric therapy, have chronic symptoms, or have alarm symptoms, endoscopy should be considered to evaluate for Barrett esophagus, stricture, ulcers, or malignancy.[30]

Dietary and lifestyle modifications are often recommended as first-line treatment of GERD. Suggested dietary changes include avoiding foods and drinks that decrease lower esophageal sphincter pressure, delay gastric emptying, or provoke reflux symptoms. These foods include chocolate, mint, alcohol, tomato, citrus juice, carbonated beverages, garlic, onions, and fatty meals. Additionally, instituting behavioral modifications might also decrease reflux symptoms. These modifications include elevating the head of the bed while sleeping, avoiding a recumbent position for 3 hours after meals, sleeping in the left lateral position, smoking cessation, and avoidance of alcohol.[28] Although these recommendations are almost universally accepted, the evidence to support their effectiveness is not strong.

After the diagnosis of GERD is made, patients and providers can engage in shared decision making to determine if a step-up or a step-down approach to therapy is appropriate. A step-up approach starts with over-the-counter therapy with an H_2-receptor antagonist (H_2RA) and steps up therapy to medications with a

Table 2
Standard-dose and high-dose PPIs

Drug	Standard Dose	High Dose
Dexlansoprazole	30 mg daily	30 mg twice daily
Esomeprazole	20 mg daily	40 mg daily
Lansoprazole	15–30 mg daily	30 mg twice daily
Omeprazole	20–40 mg daily	20–40 mg twice daily
Pantoprazole	20–40 mg daily	40 mg twice daily
Rabeprazole	20 mg daily	20 mg twice daily

Data from Wolfe MM, Sachs G. Acid suppression: optimizing therapy for gastroduodenal ulcer healing, gastroesophageal reflux disease, and stress-related erosive syndrome. Gastroenterology 2000;118:S9–31.

higher degree of efficacy (standard-dose PPI, then high-dose PPI) if symptoms persist (**Table 2**). A step-down approach to therapy starts with daily or twice-daily PPI therapy and steps down to therapies with lower degree of efficacy as symptoms allow. With each model, the therapy is maintained at the lowest level that completely controls symptoms.[28] Clinicians should choose the most cost-effective medication at the lowest effective dose for the shortest amount of time possible.

HELICOBACTER PYLORI AND PEPTIC ULCER DISEASE

Helicobacter pylori infection is associated with 90% to 95% of duodenal ulcers and 60% to 80% of gastric ulcers. The prevalence of *H pylori* ranges from 20% in North America and western Europe to more than 80% in eastern Europe, Asia, and most of the developing world.[33] *H pylori* can progress rapidly in high-prevalence areas or slowly in low-prevalence areas toward atrophic gastritis. A fast rate of progression toward gastritis is associated with a higher incidence of gastric cancer, whereas a slower rate of progression is more closely associated with peptic (duodenal) ulcer disease.[34] *H pylori* are a known carcinogen. The International Agency for Research on Cancer estimates 43% of the global burden of gastric cancer to be related to *H pylori*,[35] and this is likely an underestimation.

There is, however, some uncertainty as to whether chronic *H pylori* infection plays a role in dyspepsia in the absence of peptic ulcer disease or gastric cancer. Indeed, multiple systematic reviews and meta-analyses have looked into this question with conflicting results. One trial of *H pylori* eradication found that patients with complete or satisfactory response to a proton pump–based eradication therapy had decreased gastritis and improvement of dyspepsia symptoms at 1 year.[36] Some randomized controlled trials have shown a test-and-treat strategy is equally as effective as prompt endoscopy in reducing the severity of dyspepsia symptoms but with much lower medical costs. Recently, the HEROES trial identified *H pylori*–positive adults with FD by Rome III criteria, and randomized them to *H pylori* triple therapy or omeprazole plus placebo. The main outcome was at least 50% symptomatic improvement at 12 months. Forty-nine percent of the patients in the antibiotics group reached the primary outcome, as opposed to 36.5% in the PPI plus placebo group.[37] Overall, 78% in the antibiotics group and 67.5% in the control group reported some symptomatic improvement. Based on a large Cochrane review, the number needed to treat to achieve a complete symptomatic response in one patient is 14.[38] Some studies suggest a trend toward higher symptom response by *H pylori* eradication treatment in high-prevalence populations.[39] However, a recent meta-analysis of randomized

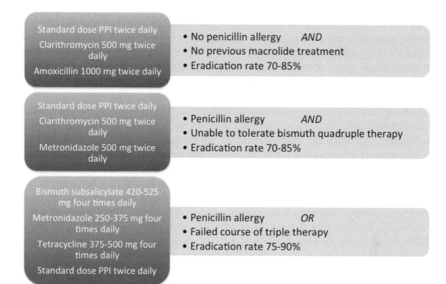

Fig. 5. *Helicobacter pylori* treatment regimens. (*Data from* Chey WD, Wong BC. American College of Gastroenterology Guideline on the Management of *Helicobacter pylori* Infection. Am J Gastroenterol 2007;102:1808–25.)

controlled trials of *H pylori* eradication therapy on symptoms of FD demonstrated improvement in symptoms and a similar rate of response across Asian, European, and American populations.[40] Test-and-treat will cure most cases of underlying peptic ulcer disease, and will prevent most cases of gastric cancer. Although it does not resolve most cases of FD, at least a significant minority of patients will have significant improvements in their dyspepsia symptoms with this intervention. A test-and-treat strategy for *H pylori*, especially in populations with a high prevalence of the disease, is a reasonable approach (**Fig. 5**).

The ^{13}C-urea breath test is 95% sensitive and specific for *H pylori*; however, it is not universally available. The *H pylori* stool antigen test has similar sensitivity (91%) and specificity (93%), but patients have to remain off their PPI therapy for 2 weeks, and antibiotics for 4 weeks, before performing either of these tests. *H pylori* serology is widely available but is considerably less sensitive and specific (85% and 79%, respectively) than the other testing (**Table 3**).[2] However, patients do not need to be off therapies to obtain serology, and the ease with which it is administered (a simple blood draw) makes for improved adherence. In populations with a high prevalence of *H pylori* and challenges with follow through, *H pylori* serology is a reasonable compromise.

Table 3 Sensitivity and specificity of *Helicobacter pylori* tests		
Test	**Sensitivity (%)**	**Specificity (%)**
^{13}C-urea breath test	95	95
Stool antigen test	91	93
Serology	85	79

From Zagari RM, Fuccio L, Bazzoli F. Investigating dyspepsia. BMJ 2008;337:1–5.

NON–UPPER GASTROINTESTINAL MIMICS

Diseases that can mimic symptoms of dyspepsia include cholelithiasis and cholecystitis, chronic pancreatitis, cardiac and mesenteric ischemia, irritable bowel syndrome, and medication side effects. These alternate diagnoses should be considered throughout the work-up of dyspepsia, especially if patients are not reporting symptom improvement with the prescribed therapies.

There are five key decision points in investigating dyspepsia (**Fig. 6**). The first, and most important, is to identify any alarm signs and symptoms. They include bleeding, iron-deficiency anemia, persistent vomiting, an epigastric mass, unexplained weight loss, and persistent dysphagia (**Fig. 7**). Age older than 55 years at the time of onset should also be considered an alarm feature. Patients who present with dysphagia and one or more of these clinical features should be referred for emergent (in the case of hemorrhage) or urgent endoscopy.

For those patients without alarm signs and symptoms, the other key questions are as follows: (1) Are there other possible mimics of the dyspepsia, such as cardiac, hepatobiliary, pancreatic, or vascular? (2) Is the patient on any potentially offending medications? (3) Does the patient have predominant symptoms of heartburn and regurgitation? (4) Has the patient been tested for *H pylori*? Those who are determined to have an alternative source of their dyspepsia should be treated accordingly. If a patient is found to be taking a potentially offending medication, all efforts should be made to find alternative therapies. If this is not possible, then antisecretory therapy, such as a PPI, should be added to the patient's therapy.

Those who have symptoms of heartburn or regurgitation, even if they also have symptoms of epigastric pain and postprandial fullness, deserve a 4- to 6-week trial of a PPI. All others should be tested, and treated if positive, for *H pylori* with the

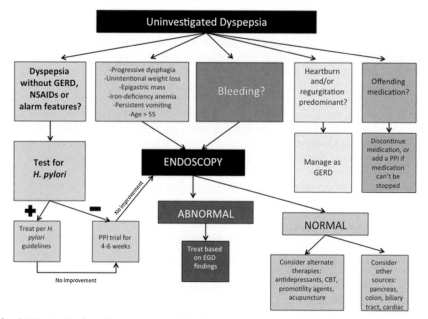

Fig. 6. Diagnosis algorithm. CBT, cognitive behavioral therapy; EGD, esophagastroduodenoscopy; GERD, gastroesophageal reflux disease; *H. pylori, Helicobacter pylori*; NSAIDs, nonsteroidal antiinflammatory drugs; PPI, proton pump inhibitor.

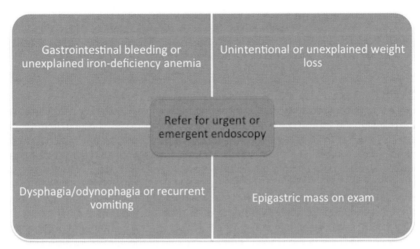

Fig. 7. Dyspepsia alarm signs and symptoms. (*Data from* Zagari RM, Fuccio L, Bazzoli F. Investigating dyspepsia. BMJ 2008;337:1–5.)

most sensitive and specific test available. Those who are negative for *H pylori* should be given a 4- to 6-week trial of antisecretory therapy. If patients fail to respond to these measures, endoscopy is an appropriate next step, and if the endoscopy is negative, gastric emptying studies can be considered. A gastric emptying study can help guide therapy if it demonstrates rapid or delayed emptying. After that, alternate therapies can be explored, including antidepressants, psychotherapy, cognitive behavioral therapy, hypnosis, and acupuncture.

TREATMENT OF FD

Fewer than 60% of patients with FD improve with medication alone.[41]

Acid-suppression Therapy

Various forms of acid-suppression therapy are available, including over-the-counter antacids, H_2RAs, and PPIs. Antacids are commonly used but have the least compelling evidence for effectiveness, and PPIs have the strongest evidence of effectiveness.

The evidence to support the use of H_2RAs for FD is conflicting. Some trials have demonstrated superiority of H_2RAs over placebo, whereas others have not. In a small crossover study, nizatidine was shown to improve postprandial fullness and early satiation over placebo (70% response vs 10% response). The treatment also improved gastroesophageal reflux symptoms over placebo (53% vs 0%). This study evaluated gastric motility and ghrelin levels, and found that the H_2RA improved gastric emptying but had no impact on ghrelin levels.[42] A Cochrane review from 2006 showed H_2RAs improved dyspepsia symptoms in 54% of patients, compared with 40% for placebo. However, some of the studies included in this meta-analysis were of poor quality.[43]

PPIs have been shown to be effective in the treatment of FD in several placebo-controlled, randomized controlled trials. Symptom improvement ranges from 32% in one study[44] to 68% in another.[45] Notably, the response to PPIs tends to be higher in patients with reflux-like dyspepsia, epigastric pain, or burning.[46] The subset of patients with postprandial distress symptoms did not tend to respond to PPI therapy.[47]

Interestingly, the response rate to placebo across several studies ranged from 19% to 49%, which overlaps considerably with the range of responders to PPI therapy.[43–48] A Cochrane review demonstrated overall symptom relief rates of 34% in patients receiving PPI therapy, compared with 25% in patients receiving placebo.[43]

Prokinetics

A brief randomized controlled trial comparing efficacy of PPIs versus prokinetic therapy in relieving the symptoms of patients with FD did not demonstrate a difference between the two, with 50.6% of the PPI group and 47.85% of the prokinetic group achieving meaningful symptom relief. The therapeutic response did not differ in subgroup analyses of patients fulfilling criteria of either epigastric pain syndrome or postprandial distress syndrome.[49] A meta-analysis of 27 randomized, controlled trials of prokinetic agents for treatment of FD symptoms found the prokinetics were significantly more likely to improve symptoms over placebo. However, most of the trials included in this analysis studied cisapride, which is off the market, and domperidone, which is not available in the United States. Only one of the studies included metoclopramide.[50] Thus, although prokinetic agents are likely equally efficacious to PPIs for the treatment of FD, given the risk of tardive dyskinesia with use of metoclopramide, this medication is not generally recommended for prolonged use.

Acotiamide, an acetylcholinesterase inhibitor that works by accelerating gastric motility,[51] has been shown in several placebo-controlled trials to improve FD symptoms and gastric emptying. The number need to treat to improve symptoms was six, and the number needed to treat to eliminate symptoms was 16.[52–54] This medication is still undergoing investigation and has not yet been approved by the Food and Drug Administration.

Anxiolytics and Antidepressants

Several studies have shown possible efficacy of anxiolytics and antidepressants for treatment of FD. A systematic review of studies comparing antidepressants and anxiolytics with placebo in the treatment of FD found benefit with the study drugs. Although there were limitations to the studies included in the review, the therapies (which included tricyclic antidepressant agents, levosulpiride [a dopamine-2 receptor agonist], and anticholinergic and anxiolytic medications) were approximately equivalent to studies of antisecretory agents and prokinetic agents (overall relative risk reduction of 0.45).[55] A more recent review again showed that antidepressants and anxiolytics are associated with significant pain reduction in patients with FD, and are as effective as classic antisecretory and prokinetic agents.[56] Several randomized controlled trials have demonstrated modest efficacy of tricyclic antidepressants in treating FD.[57,58]

Theoretically, serotonin-norepinephrine reuptake inhibitors and tricyclic antidepressants should decrease neuropathic pain and address underlying psychiatric issues, which would address at least two of the potential pathophysiologic mechanisms of FD. Furthermore, selective serotonin reuptake inhibitors may enhance gut transit and alter gastric accommodation.[59] However, study data to support the use of newer antidepressants for FD have been mixed. A randomized clinical trial of venlafaxine, a serotonin-norepinephrine reuptake inhibitor, failed to demonstrate improvement over placebo.[60] The Functional Dyspepsia Treatment Trial, an international multicenter, parallel group, randomized, double-blind, placebo-controlled trial, is ongoing to evaluate whether 12 weeks of treatment with escitalopram or amitriptyline improves FD symptoms compared with treatment with placebo.[61]

Buspirone, an anxiolytic medication with fundus-relaxing properties, was compared with placebo in a small double-blind, randomized, controlled crossover trial. Patients were given the study drug 15 minutes before meals. Buspirone significantly reduced the overall severity of dyspepsia symptoms, including postprandial fullness, early satiation, and upper abdominal bloating. Buspirone increased gastric accommodation but did not alter the rate of gastric emptying.[62]

Other Medications

An industry-sponsored study out of France of 276 general practice patients with dyspepsia compared a combination pill (simethicone, activated charcoal, and magnesium oxide) with placebo. Those receiving the study drug had decreased postprandial fullness, epigastric pain, epigastric burning, and abdominal bloating compared with placebo. The number needed to treat to achieve a 70% decrease in overall dyspeptic symptoms was seven.[63] Although this combination pill is not commercially available in the United States, an interested patient or practitioner could conceivably prescribe the components separately.

Psychotherapy

A recent study out of Japan randomized patients with FD to medical therapy alone or medical therapy with brief psychodynamic therapy. The results demonstrated brief psychodynamic therapy improved all gastrointestinal symptoms, including heartburn, nausea, postprandial fullness, bloating, and upper and lower abdominal pain, over medical therapy alone.[64] Another randomized, controlled trial compared cognitive psychotherapy with usual care and found the intervention group had fewer days of epigastric pain, and less nausea, heartburn, and diarrhea.[65] A randomized controlled trial of psychodynamic-interpersonal therapy versus supportive therapy demonstrated significant improvement with psychodynamic-interpersonal therapy over supportive therapy. However, the differences had disappeared at 1-year poststudy, unless the group with severe heartburn was excluded, in which case the psychodynamic-interpersonal group still did better.[66] However, a systematic review of psychological therapies for FD found insufficient evidence on the efficacy of psychological therapies for FD, noting that the sample sizes were small and the study designs variable. All of the included studies in that review had to adjust for baseline differences to achieve statistical significance.[67]

Acupuncture

Some research has suggested that acupuncture might improve gastric emptying and accommodation.[68] A Cochrane review is underway to survey the available evidence on the effectiveness and safety of this intervention for FD.

SUMMARY

Dyspepsia is a complex disorder with several distinct pathophysiologic mechanisms that are still poorly understood (**Fig. 8**). Patients who experience dyspepsia have a high burden of disease, with significant personal and economic costs. Although serious pathology presenting as dyspepsia is rare, clinicians need to be aware of alarm features that should trigger prompt referral for subspecialty care. Those without alarm features can be managed in a rational way with either empiric antisecretory therapy, test-and-treat for *H pylori* eradication, antidepressants, and psychotherapy, or a combination of these. Given the heterogeneity of symptoms and large variability in

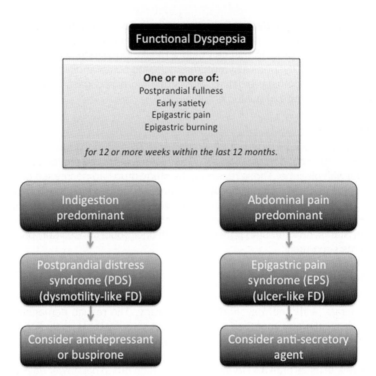

Fig. 8. Functional dyspepsia.

response to different treatments, more research into specific pathophysiologic mechanisms will likely help guide diagnosis and treatment choices in the future.

REFERENCES

1. Van Zanten S, Flook N, Chiba N. An evidence-based approach to the management of uninvestigated dyspepsia in the era of *Helicobacter pylori*. CMAJ 2000; 162(Suppl 12):S3–23.
2. Zagari R, Fuccio L, Bazzoli F. Investigating dyspepsia. BMJ 2008;337:11400.
3. Peery AF, Dellon ES, Lund J, et al. Burden of gastrointestinal disease in the United States: 2012 update. Gastroenterology 2012;143:1179–87.
4. Haycox A, Einarson T, Eggleston A. The health economic impact of upper gastrointestinal symptoms in the general population: results from the Domestic/International Gastroenterology Surveillance Study (DIGEST). Scand J Gastroenterol Suppl 1999;231(Suppl):38–47.
5. Piessevaux H, De Winter B, Louis E, et al. Dyspeptic symptoms in the general population: a factor and cluster analysis of symptom groupings. Neurogastroenterol Motil 2009;21:378–88.
6. Sander GB, Mazzoleni LE, Francesconi CF, et al. Influence of organic and functional dyspepsia on work productivity: the HEROES-DIP study. Value Health 2011;14:S126–9.
7. Talley NJ, American Gastroenterological Association. American Gastroenterological Association medical position statement: evaluation of dyspepsia. Gastroenterology 2005;129(5):1753–5.

8. National Institute for Health and Clinical Excellence (NICE). Dyspepsia: managing dyspepsia in adults in primary care. London: National Institute for Health and Clinical Excellence (NICE); 2004.

9. Tack J, Talley NJ, Camilleri M, et al. Functional gastroduodenal disorders. Gastroenterology 2006;130(5):1466–79.

10. Xiao YL, Peng S, Tao J, et al. Prevalence and symptom pattern of pathologic esophageal acid reflux in patients with functional dyspepsia based on the Rome III criteria. Am J Gastroenterol 2010;105:2626–31.

11. Nandurkar S, Talley NJ, Xia H, et al. Dyspepsia in the community is linked to smoking and aspirin use but not to *Helicobacter pylori* infection. Arch Intern Med 1998;158:1427–33.

12. Pike B, Porter C, Sorrell T, et al. Acute gastroenteritis and the risk of functional dyspepsia: a systemic review and meta-analysis. Am J Gastroenterol 2013; 108(10):1558–63.

13. Talley NJ, Locke GR III, Lahr BD, et al. Functional dyspepsia, delayed gastric emptying and impaired quality of life. Gut 2006;55:933–9.

14. Sha W, Pasricha PJ, Chen JD. Correlations among electrogastrogram, gastric dysmotility, and duodenal dysmotility in patients with functional dyspepsia. J Clin Gastroenterol 2009;43:716–22.

15. Perri F, Clemente R, Festa V, et al. Patterns of symptoms in functional dyspepsia: role of *Helicobacter pylori* infection and delayed gastric emptying. Am J Gastroenterol 1998;93:2082–8.

16. Kindt S, Tack J. Impaired gastric accommodation and its role in dyspepsia. Gut 2006;55(12):1685–91.

17. Quartero AO, de Wit NJ, Lodder AC, et al. Disturbed solid phase gastric emptying in functional dydpepsia: a meta-analysis. Dig Dis Sci 1998;43:2028–32.

18. Stanghellini V, Tossetti C, Paternico A, et al. Risk indicators of delayed gastric emptying of solids in patients with functional dyspepsia. Gastroenterology 1996;110:1036–42.

19. Führer M, Vogelsang H, Hammer J. A placebo-controlled trial of an oral capsaicin load in patients with functional dyspepsia. Neurogastroenterol Motil 2011; 23(10):918–28.

20. Li X, Cao Y, Wong RK, et al. Visceral and somatic sensory function in functional dyspepsia. Neurogastroenterol Motil 2013;25(3):246–53.

21. Holtmann G, Siffert W, Haag S, et al. G-protein beta 3 subunit 825 CC genotype is associated with unexplained (functional) dyspepsia. Gastroenterology 2004; 126:971–9.

22. Mearin F, Perez-Oliveras M, Perello A, et al. Dyspepsia and irritable bowel syndrome after a *Salmonella* gastroenteritis outbreak: one-year follow up cohort study. Gastroenterology 2005;129:98–104.

23. Kindt S, Tertychnyy A, de Hertogh G, et al. Intestinal immune activation in presumed post-infectious functional dyspepsia. Neurogastroenterol Motil 2009;21: 832–8.

24. Koloski NA, Jones M, Kalantar J, et al. The brain-gut pathway in functional gastrointestinal disorders is bidirectional: a 12-year prospective population-based study. Gut 2012;61:1284–90.

25. Talley NJ, Zinmeister AR, Schleck CD, et al. Dyspepsia and dyspepsia subgroups: a population-based study. Gastroenterology 1992;102:1259–68.

26. Konekes K, Jackson JL, Chamberlin J. Depressive and anxiety disorders in patients presenting with physical complaints: clinical predictors and outcomes. Am J Med 1997;103:339–47.

27. Clauwaert N, Jones MP, Holvoet L, et al. Associations between gastric sensori-motor function, depression, somatization, and symptom-based subgroups in functional gastroduodenal disorders: are all symptoms equal? Neurogastroenterol Motil 2012;24:1088–95.

28. Wilson J. Gastroesophageal reflux disease. Ann Intern Med 2008;149(3):ITC(2) 1–15.

29. Tefera L, Fein M, Ritter MP, et al. Can the combination of symptoms and endoscopy confirm the presence of gastroesophageal reflux disease? Am Surg 1997; 63:933–6.

30. DeVault KR, Castell DO. Updated guidelines for the diagnosis and treatment of gastroesophageal reflux disease. Am J Gastroenterol 2005;100:190–200.

31. Fass P, Ofman IJ, Samplinter RE, et al. The omeprazole test is as sensitive as 24-h oesophageal pH monitoring in diagnosing gastrooesophageal reflux disease in symptomatic patients with erosive esophagitis. Aliment Pharmacol Ther 2000;14:389–96.

32. Schenk BE, Kuipers EJ, Klinkenberg-Knol EC, et al. Omeprazole as a diagnostic tool in gastroesophageal reflux disease. Am J Gastroenterol 1997;92: 1997–2000.

33. Breuer T, Halaty HM, Graham DY. The epidemiology of *H. pylori*-associated gastroduodenal disease. In: Ernst P, Michetti P, Smith PD, editors. The immunobiology of *H. pylori* from pathogenesis to prevention. Philadelphia: Lippincott-Raven; 1997. p. 1–14.

34. Forman D, Graham DY. Review article: impact of *Helicobacter pylori* on society: role for a strategy of 'search and eradicate. Aliment Pharmacol Ther 2004; 19(Suppl 1):17–21.

35. Parkin DM, Pisani P, Munoz N. The global burden of cancer. Cancer Surv 1999; 33:5–33.

36. Kim S, Park Y, Kim N, et al. Effect of *Helicobacter pylori* eradication on functional dyspepsia. J Neurogastroenterol Motil 2013;19:233–43.

37. Mazzoleni L, Sander G, Francesconi C, et al. *Helicobacter pylori* eradication in functional dyspepsia. Arch Intern Med 2011;171:1929–35.

38. Moayyedi P, Soo S, Deeks J, et al. Eradication of *Helicobacter pylori* for non-ulcer dyspepsia. Cochrane Database Syst Rev 2006;(2):CD002096.

39. Den Hollander W, Sostres C, Kuipers E, et al. *Helicobacter pylori* and nonmalignant disease. Helicobacter 2013;18(Suppl 1):24–7.

40. Zhao B, Zhao J, Cheng WF, et al. Efficacy of *Helicobacter pylori* eradication therapy on functional dyspepsia: a meta-analysis of randomized controlled studies with 12-month follow up. J Clin Gastroenterol 2014;48(3):241–7.

41. Mönkemüller K, Malfertheiner P. Drug treatment of functional dyspepsia. World J Gastroenterol 2006;12(17):2694–700.

42. Futagami S, Shimpuku M, Song JM, et al. Nizatidine improves clinical symptoms and gastric emptying in patients with functional dyspepsia accompanied by impaired gastric emptying. Digestion 2012;86(2):114–21.

43. Moayyedi P, Shelly S, Deeks JJ, et al. WITHDRAWN: pharmacological interventions for non-ulcer dyspepsia. Cochrane Database Syst Rev 2011;(2): CD001960.

44. Van Zanten SV, Armstrong D, Chiba N, et al. Esomeprazole 40 mg once a day in patients with functional dyspepsia: the randomized, placebo-controlled "ENTER" trial. Am J Gastroenterol 2006;101:2096–106.

45. Meineche-Schmidt V, Christensen E, Bytzer P. Randomised clinical trial: identification of responders to short-term treatment with esomeprazole for dyspepsia

in primary care: a randomized, placebo-controlled study. Aliment Pharmacol Ther 2011;33:41–9.

46. Talley NJ, Meineche-Schmidt V, Pare P, et al. Efficacy of omeprazole in functional dyspepsia: double-blind, randomized, placebo-controlled trials (the Bond and Opera studies). Aliment Pharmacol Ther 1998;12:1055–65.

47. Bolling-Sternevald E, Lauritsen K, Talley NJ, et al. Is it possible to predict treatment response to a proton pump inhibitor in functional dyspepsia? Aliment Pharmacol Ther 2003;18:117–24.

48. Peura DA, Kovacs TO, Metz DC, et al. Lansoprazole in the treatment of functional dyspepsia: two double-blind, randomized, placebo-controlled trials. Am J Med 2004;116:740–8.

49. Hsu YC, Liou JM, Yang TH, et al. Proton pump inhibitor therapy versus prokinetic therapy in patients with functional dyspepsia: is therapeutic response predicted by Rome III subgroups? J Gastroenterol 2011;46(2):183–90.

50. Hiyama T, Yoshihara M, Matsuo K, et al. Meta-analysis of the effects of prokinetic agents in patients with functional dyspepsia. J Gastroenterol Hepatol 2007;22: 304–10.

51. Yoshii K, Hirayami M, Nakamura T, et al. Mechanism for distribution of acotiamide, a novel gastroprokinetic agent for the treatment of functional dyspepsia, in rat stomach. J Pharm Sci 2011;100:4965–73.

52. Matsueda K, Hongo M, Tack J, et al. A placebo-controlled trial of acotiamide for meal-related symptoms of functional dyspepsia. Gut 2012;61(6):821–8.

53. Kusunoki H, Haruma K, Manabe N, et al. Therapeutic efficacy of acotiamide in patients with functional dyspepsia based on enhanced postprandial gastric accommodation and emptying: randomized controlled study evaluation by real-time ultrasonography. Neurogastroenterol Motil 2012;24(6):540–5.

54. Altan E, Masaoka T, Farré R, et al. Acotiamide, a novel gastroprokinetic for the treatment of patients with functional dyspepsia: postprandial distress syndrome. Expert Rev Gastroenterol Hepatol 2012;6(5):533–44.

55. Hojo M, Miwa H, Yokoyama T, et al. Treatment of functional dyspepsia with anti-anxiety or antidepressive agents: systematic review. J Gastroenterol 2005; 40(11):1036–42.

56. Passos MC, Duro D, Fregni F. CNS or classic drugs for the treatment of pain in functional dyspepsia? A systematic review and meta-analysis of the literature. Pain Physician 2008;11:597–609.

57. Grover M, Drossman DA. Psychotropic agents in functional gastrointestinal disorders. Curr Opin Pharmacol 2008;8:715–23.

58. Braak B, Klooker TK, Wouters MM, et al. Randomized clinical trial: the effects of amitriptyline on drinking capacity and symptoms in patients with functional dyspepsia, a double-blind placebo-controlled study. Aliment Pharmacol Ther 2011;34:638–48.

59. Moshiree B, Barboza J, Talley NJ. An update on current pharmacotherapy options for dyspepsia. Expert Opin Pharmacother 2013;14:1737–53.

60. Van Kerkhoven LA, Laheij RJ, Aparicio N, et al. Effect of the antidepressant venlafaxine in functional dyspepsia: a randomized, double-blind, placebo-controlled trial. Clin Gastroenterol Hepatol 2008;6:746–52.

61. Talley NJ, Locke GR III, Herrick LM, et al. Functional Dyspepsia Treatment Trial (FDTT): a double-blind, randomized, placebo-controlled trial of antidepressants in functional dyspepsia, evaluating symptoms, psychopathology, pathophysiology and pharmacogenetics. Contemp Clin Trials 2012;33(3): 523–33.

62. Tack J, Janssen P, Masaoka T. Efficacy of buspirone, a fundus-relaxing drug, in patients with functional dyspepsia. Clin Gastroenterol Hepatol 2012;10(11): 1239–45.

63. Coffin B, Bortolloti C, Bourgeois O, et al. Efficacy of a smiethicone, activated charcoal and magnesium oxide combination (Carbosymag) in functional dyspepsia: results of a general practice-based randomized trial. Clin Res Hepatol Gastroenterol 2011;35(6–7):494–9.

64. Faramarzi M, Azadfallah P, Book HE, et al. A randomized controlled trial of brief psychoanalytic psychotherapy in patients with functional dyspepsia. Asian J Psychiatr 2013;6(3):228–34.

65. Haug T, Wilhelmsen I, Svebak S, et al. Psychotherapy in functional dyspepsia. J Psychosom Res 1994;38:735–44.

66. Hamilton J, Guthrie E, Creed F, et al. A randomized controlled trial of psychotherapy in patients with chronic functional dyspepsia. Gastroenterology 2000; 119:662–9.

67. Soo S, Forman D, Delaney B, et al. A systematic review of psychological therapies for nonulcer dyspepsia. Am J Gastroenterol 2004;99:1817–22.

68. Xu S, Zha H, Hou X, et al. Electroacupuncture accelerates solid gastric emptying in patients with functional dyspepsia. Gastroenterology 2004;126: A-437.

Insomnia

Eliza L. Sutton, MD

KEYWORDS

- Chronotype • Cognitive behavioral therapy for insomnia (CBT-I) • Hyperarousal
- Primary insomnia • Restless legs syndrome • Short sleeper
- Sleep restriction therapy • Stimulus control

KEY POINTS

- To the general public and in primary care, "insomnia" refers to the symptom of difficulty sleeping; to sleep specialists and researchers, it refers to a subset in which common specific causes have been ruled out.
- Acute insomnia should be treated by addressing the underlying cause (if possible) and with safe, effective sleep medication, in part to prevent the development of chronic insomnia.
- Chronic insomnia is best approached via history and/or questionnaires to identify common specific causes that have specific treatments.
- Restless legs syndrome, sleep apnea, and circadian rhythm disorders such as delayed sleep phase syndrome (night owl) are common causes of insomnia presenting in primary care.
- Cognitive behavioral therapy for insomnia is considered first-line therapy for chronic insomnia that is otherwise unexplained (primary insomnia) or is associated with chronic psychological or medical conditions.

EVALUATION AND TREATMENT OF INSOMNIA
Definitions and Presentation

Insomnia as experienced by people and reported to physicians is, simply, difficulty sleeping. Insomnia is typically described in terms of dissatisfaction with, and distress from, the quality or quantity of sleep obtained, despite attempts to obtain sleep. Insomnia is common, affecting most people at some point in a year and 10% to 20% of people chronically, and is commonly associated with a wide range of psychosocial, psychiatric, medical, and underlying sleep disorders. Both short-term and long-term insomnia can impair daytime functioning, and chronic insomnia is associated bidirectionally with adverse health and social outcomes. As with other symptoms such as dizziness or pain, treatment of the symptom without consideration of the underlying condition can be ineffective and misdirected.

Department of Medicine, University of Washington, 4245 Roosevelt Way Northeast, Box 354765, Seattle, WA 98105, USA
E-mail address: esutton@u.washington.edu

Med Clin N Am 98 (2014) 565–581
http://dx.doi.org/10.1016/j.mcna.2014.01.008
0025-7125/14/$ – see front matter © 2014 Elsevier Inc. All rights reserved.
medical.theclinics.com

This article focuses on evaluation and treatment of the symptom insomnia as self-reported by patients in primary care settings. History is the key to uncovering underlying patterns and associated symptoms to determine factors contributing to the insomnia (**Table 1**). In sleep medicine practices, this typically includes a sleep diary and validated questionnaires, but with a framework in mind one can obtain a useful direct history from the patient (**Fig. 1**). Nocturnal polysomnography (PSG) does not diagnose insomnia, and it does not distinguish between satisfied sleepers and those with chronic unexplained insomnia.[1] However, when sleep is described as fragmented or

Table 1				
Causes of insomnia				
	Exogenous Factors (Environment/ Medications)	**Medical Symptoms and Conditions**	**Psychiatric**	**Sleep Disorder**
Acute	Change in environment (new sleep environment) Jet lag Clock change Sunday night insomnia	Acute physical symptoms: Pain Urinary frequency Cough Nasal congestion	Hypomania, mania Anxiety Stress	—
Acute or chronic	Environment Noise Temperature Disruptive presence Discomfort Substances—licit or illicit Alcohol (hours after ingestion) Stimulants Caffeine Nicotine Medications—systemic Armodafinil, modafinil β-Agonists Bupropion Ciprofloxacin Corticosteroids Decongestants Diuretics Stimulants Thyroid hormones (in excessive doses)	Dyspnea (lung disease, heart failure) Gastroesophageal reflux disease Nocturia (consider OSA) Menopause, particularly with vasomotor symptoms	Anxiety Stress Grief Depression	See list below
Chronic	See list above	Chronic pain Chronic renal failure (associated with OSA, RLS)	Depression Bipolar disorder Anxiety Posttraumatic stress disorder ADHD Conditioned insomnia	RLS Sleep apnea (obstructive or central) Primary insomnia Circadian rhythm disorder

1) Is frustration with insomnia (rather than impaired daytime functioning) the primary concern?

2) If yes: The person seems to be attempting to get more sleep than needed and may be a "short sleeper".

- Advise Sleep Restriction Therapy (see Figure 2)

3) If no, is the primary concern:

a) Difficulty falling asleep at desired bedtime?

Pursue history for:

- Restless legs syndrome (urge to move limbs, at night, worse with rest)
- Delayed sleep phase syndrome (chronic "night owl")
- Anxiety, stress
- Conditioned insomnia (stays in bed awake trying to sleep, may watch clock) – advise Stimulus Control and Sleep Restriction Therapy (see Figure 2)
- Use of stimulating medications or substances in evening

b) Waking frequently but briefly, or having restless sleep?

Pursue history for:

- Sleep apnea (gasping or choking at night, witnessed apneas)
- PLMs (kicking or thrashing during sleep)
- Use of stimulating medications or substances, especially in PM
- Menopause (particularly with hot flashes and night sweats)
- Medical symptoms including pain, dyspnea, GERD

c) Waking during the night, then difficulty getting back to sleep?

Pursue history for:

- Alcohol withdrawal (alcohol use before bed, even without dependence)
- Anxiety, stress, post-traumatic stress disorder
- Conditioned insomnia (stays in bed awake trying to sleep, may watch clock) – advise Stimulus Control and Sleep Restriction Therapy (see Figure 2)

d) Waking up too early, then can't get back to sleep?

Pursue history for:

- Depression
- Advanced sleep phase syndrome (longstanding "early bird")
- Conditioned insomnia (stays in bed awake trying to sleep, may watch clock) – advise Stimulus Control and Sleep Restriction Therapy (see Figure 2)

e) Chronic insomnia with 1 or more of above patterns, otherwise unexplained:

- Primary insomnia

Fig. 1. An evaluation approach for chronic insomnia.

shallow, PSG can be helpful in determining whether sleep apnea or periodic limb movements (PLMS, also called nocturnal myoclonus) might be causing frequent brief awakenings.

Insomnia differs from purposeful sleep deprivation in that the person with insomnia not only wants to sleep but is allowing opportunities for sleep to occur. In fact, people suffering from insomnia may try to force sleep, which backfires in contributing further to arousal and alertness.

"Insomnia" has specific definitions in sleep medicine research and practice, in which certain common conditions presenting as the symptom insomnia have been ruled out and certain diagnostic criteria have been met. The distinction between lay use and specialty use of the term is crucial to keep in mind when interpreting medical literature, because interventional studies on "insomnia" typically seek to enroll subjects who have otherwise-unexplained insomnia ("primary insomnia"), sometimes also including people with insomnia related to depression or anxiety.

Research criteria for "insomnia disorder" require not only some pattern of difficulty sleeping but also allowance of adequate opportunity for sleep and any of several daytime symptoms stemming from the sleep problem.[2] Research criteria for "primary insomnia" (chronic otherwise-unexplained insomnia) add that the person is not taking psychoactive substances that would affect sleep, nor that the insomnia can be ascribed primarily to a medical or psychiatric condition or to an underlying sleep disorder such as sleep apnea.[2] On the other hand, the American Psychiatric Association has recategorized "primary insomnia" and other types of insomnia from the Diagnostic and Statistical Manual of Mental Disorders (DSM)-IV all into "insomnia disorder" in DSM-5, aiming to focus on the need to address insomnia regardless of whether it is idiopathic or related to a psychiatric or medical disorder.[3]

Conditions for which people experiencing insomnia would be excluded on first screening from a research study on insomnia include several conditions prevalent in the general population and particularly in primary care practices, such as restless legs syndrome (RLS), circadian rhythm disorders, and suspected obstructive sleep apnea (OSA), which are described further later.

Patterns of Insomnia

Insomnia is commonly divided into several different categories, by duration and by pattern during the night.

Duration is "acute" (or "transient") versus "chronic" (or "persistent"). The research definitions of these timeframes do not assist in the primary care evaluation and management of patients seeking help for insomnia. In acute insomnia, the cause may be readily apparent (for example, a stressful situation, new medication, or uncomfortable new medical symptom) and/or the person may be able to anticipate it in advance (for example, travel across multiple time zones). Acute insomnia should be treated with sedative-hypnotic medication and/or the inciting factor promptly addressed, where possible, to reduce daytime impairment from sleepiness, nighttime suffering, and the likelihood of development of chronic insomnia.

Chronic insomnia can develop when acute insomnia occurs and becomes perpetuated, or it may be longstanding without a clear event or time of onset. It may be multifactorial, becoming (or including a component of) psychophysiologic (also called "conditioned" or "learned") insomnia. Chronic insomnia is associated with dysfunctional beliefs about sleep, including hopelessness, helplessness, and fear about the consequences of sleep loss,[4] or, essentially, performance anxiety regarding one's sleep.

The timing of the difficulty with sleeping during the allotted sleep time is also an important pattern to elucidate:

- Difficulty falling asleep (described medically as "difficulty initiating sleep" and called sleep-onset insomnia)
- Difficulty staying asleep (described medically as "difficulty maintaining sleep" and called sleep-maintenance insomnia)
- Early morning awakening (called terminal insomnia)

Difficulty maintaining sleep can be one or more long awakenings during the night, or poor sleep quality consisting of frequent but brief awakenings or an awareness during the night of being partially awake. This latter pattern may be due to sleep-state misperception (in which states demonstrated on PSG to be "sleep" are experienced as "wake") or may be due to frequent partial awakenings due to an underlying sleep disorder (most commonly OSA, central sleep apnea [CSA], or PLMS).

The symptom of awakening unrefreshed in the morning is called "unrefreshing sleep" and had been considered in the past to qualify as "insomnia," but is now recognized to warrant specific evaluation and treatment, typically including PSG.

Physiology of Sleep and Pathophysiology of Insomnia

Sleep and wake are different but not mutually exclusive states of the brain, and in fact, "sleep" is itself 2 distinct physiologic states, rapid eye movement (REM) and non-REM (NREM) sleep, during each of which the brain and body behave in specific ways. NREM comprises stages 1 through 4; stages 3 and 4 are deeper and known as "slow-wave" sleep. Sleep disorders in which a person is partially roused from deep sleep or REM sleep to a lighter stage of sleep, or to brief awakening, can present as disrupted sleep (insomnia) or unrefreshing sleep.

Sleep and wake are under circadian and homeostatic control, with contributions from volitional behavior. The circadian biologic rhythm of wake and sleep is governed by the internal clock in the suprachiasmatic nucleus, influenced by genetics as well as by environmental cues (light exposure and daily routines). The homeostatic drive to sleep increases as the time since last sleep increases and declines when sleep of refreshing quality is obtained.

The normal human circadian cycle is closer to 25 hours than 24 hours. There are normal developmental changes to circadian sleep-wake patterns in childhood and adolescence before one's "chronotype," the typical daily pattern of alertness and sleepiness for that person, becomes apparent by around age 25. The chronotype is determined by several genes with several polymorphisms, giving an essentially normal distribution of chrono-phenotypes in the adult population, skewed to the right, toward a preference for later sleep times. In people with sleep phase "delay" (those who prefer later sleep and wake times than most of the population), the melatonin peak is delayed. Circadian rhythm disorders manifesting as insomnia due to a mismatch between an individual's chronotype and expectations of normal sleep-wake times are discussed later.

Humans have a unique and notable ability to stay awake despite the homeostatic drive for sleep and the circadian cycle of sleepiness and wakefulness. A person can purposefully avoid behaviors conducive to sleep and instead pursue those conducive to wakefulness, including upright body position, bright light exposure, engagement in a mentally stimulating activity, and consumption of caffeine or other wake-promoting substances. "Insomnia" requires some attempt to sleep (lying down in a darkened place) but in many cases insomnia can be caused or perpetuated by the persistent influence of wake-conducive factors in the hours before sleep. Ironically, although humans can force the wake state, attempting to force sleep can backfire and cause arousal. Sleep has to be "allowed" to occur, which can be very difficult for people who are trying desperately to enter that state. People vary in their susceptibility to hyperarousal and to insomnia. Twin studies demonstrate a genetic component to susceptibility, particularly for sleep maintenance insomnia.[5] "Primary" insomnia, the sleep medicine diagnosis for otherwise-unexplained chronic insomnia, is not just a sleep problem but is characterized by 24-hour hyperarousal.[6]

An important early step in the approach to insomnia is clarifying through history whether the problem is a mismatch of the *timing* of sleep attempted versus achievable for that person, or whether internal and/or external factors cause *hyperarousal* to defeat attempts to sleep at a time that otherwise should work for the person to sleep.

Epidemiology of Specific Sleep Disorders Presenting as Insomnia

Despite the common process of screening potential research subjects to weed out those with insomnia as a symptom but not a research diagnosis, the distribution of different underlying causes for the symptom of insomnia has not been well described. One study in New Zealand[7] using a validated questionnaire found 41% of family practice patients reported insomnia, with multiple overlapping contributing factors: depression in 50%, anxiety in 48%, physical health problems in 43%, primary insomnia in 12%, symptoms of OSA in 9%, and delayed sleep phase "disorder" in 2% (with determination of that disorder requiring substance use and depression in addition to "night owl" phenotype). This study did not comment on the prevalence of delayed sleep phase "syndrome" (the term for someone who is an extreme "night owl") or RLS.

RLS

RLS is common, with a prevalence of roughly 10% overall (5% to 14% in multiple studies using international research criteria), but the severity and frequency vary.[8] It is more common in older patients, occurring in up to 19% of patients greater than the age of 80.[9] People with RLS report 2- to 3-fold higher rates of difficulty falling asleep and difficulty staying asleep than the general population, with 28% to 69% having difficulty initiating sleep and 24% to 51% having difficulty maintaining sleep.[10]

Two to 3% of people qualify as "RLS sufferers," experiencing RLS of moderate severity or worse at least twice a week.[10,11] Among RLS sufferers in the general population, 75.5% report difficulty with sleep: 48% endorsing an inability to fall asleep, 39% endorsing an inability to stay asleep, 61% endorsing disturbed or interrupted sleep, and 40% endorsing insufficient sleep.[11] In primary care practices, the rate of RLS is higher, with 11% to 24% meeting diagnostic criteria and 3.4% to 9% suffering at moderate severity or worse twice a week or more.[10] Among RLS sufferers followed in primary care practices, 88% reported sleep difficulty, with 69% reporting taking 30 minutes or more to fall asleep and 60% reporting waking 3 or more times per night.[12]

PLMS can also cause difficulty maintaining sleep. The prevalence seems to be roughly similar to RLS with significant but not universal overlap in the affected populations. However, PLMS can also be associated with other conditions such as OSA, in which identification and treatment of the specific triggering condition are advised.

RLS can be primary (familial or idiopathic) or secondary to another medical condition. Some studies, but not all, find higher prevalence in women and with increasing age. RLS occurs commonly in pregnancy, is also associated with low iron stores (ferritin <50 μg/L), chronic renal failure, and chronic neurologic conditions, and has been increasingly associated with many chronic medical conditions of varied types. It can be triggered by multiple medications including tramadol, neuroleptics, and most antidepressants,[13] with the exception of bupropion.[14]

Circadian rhythm disorders

The hallmark of circadian rhythm disorders is that the person is sleepy at some time of the 24-hour day and overly awake at other times, in a (typically) regular pattern than does not match the social norm. The distribution of preferred sleep times (chronotypes) in the adult population is essentially a normal distribution skewed toward later sleep-wake times. The most common time to be asleep on non-work days, preferred by 15% of people in a large European study, centers around 4 AM (eg, falling asleep at midnight and waking at 8 AM).[15] However, 35% report sleep centered around an earlier time and 50% report sleep centered around a later time. The later tail extends far, with 8% of people preferring to fall asleep at 3 AM. On work days, the later skewing is not as pronounced, but people who normally go to sleep late and wake up late can have significant sleep loss on work days[15] or school days, and/or be out-of-sync with "normal" sleepers, a phenomenon that has been called "social jet lag."[16]

Delayed sleep phase syndrome (DSPS) describes a chronotype, extreme "night owls", with late bedtime and late wake time compared with the "normal." DSPS was initially reported in 7% of patients referred for specialty evaluation of unexplained insomnia; those with DSPS were younger on average than the rest of the group.[17] Delayed sleep phase is associated with attention-deficit/hyperactivity disorder (ADHD)[18] and with higher rates of smoking, alcohol use, caffeine use, and depression, attributed at least in part to the mismatch between social expectations and achievable wake times.[16] Having one's preferred sleep time not occur until hours later than the social norm is a chronic (lifelong) pattern that can have potentially long-term social consequences.

Other chronic circadian rhythm disorders, less common than DSPS, include advanced phase sleep syndrome (ASPS) and non-24-hour circadian rhythm disorder (or free-running disorder).

People with ASPS have a longstanding pattern of going to sleep earlier than the social norm, but also waking early; these are extreme "early birds," who may enjoy their morning time as productive or may complain of terminal insomnia. Early morning awakening, plus the social isolation that can result from a routine early bedtime, can also be seen in depression. ASPS can occur in an autosomal-dominant inheritance pattern.

Non-24-hour circadian rhythm disorder is seen most commonly in people who lack light perception, thus whose circadian rhythm is not synchronized with the light-dark cycle of daylight.

Shift work sleep disorder results from working during what would normally be one's sleep time and being off work (and expected to sleep) during what would normally be one's wake time. It manifests as insomnia during time off work and/or sleepiness at work. Shift work sleep disorder can be acute, subacute, or chronic depending on the person's schedule at work and on days off.

A short-term mismatch between one's circadian rhythm and local time, causing insomnia and/or excessive daytime sleepiness, commonly occurs in the following 3 situations:

- Jet lag from travel across multiple time zones
- Adjustment to the clock change when daylight savings time takes effect in springtime (where applicable), heralded by a 23-hour day
- "Sunday night insomnia," in which staying up later on non-work or non-school days than on work or school days, typically meaning Friday and Saturday nights, allows one's circadian phase to drift later in relation to clock time, leaving the person not feeling sleepy at the earlier, usual weekday bedtime on Sunday night.

Sleep apnea

OSA can present as insomnia from sleep fragmentation due to frequent brief awakenings. It can also coexist with insomnia of other types, including psychophysiologic insomnia; this complicates treatment. Coexisting insomnia with sleep apnea has been well-described in PSG referral populations, where up to 67% of patients referred for sleep apnea evaluation are also found via sleep questionnaires to have insomnia.[19] The distribution of difficulty initiating sleep and difficulty maintaining sleep in this population is similar to that seen in people with insomnia but no sleep apnea.[19]

OSA is common in the general population, and particularly so among primary care patients and those with various chronic conditions including, particularly, hypertension and obesity. OSA is part of the metabolic syndrome. The likelihood that a person has OSA increases with body mass index and with age,[20] but young people and slender people can have OSA. Using the Berlin Questionnaire, one study at 26 primary care sites in the United States found that 36% of patients had a high pretest probability (86% likelihood) of OSA, with the patient endorsing excessive daytime sleepiness the best marker, and reporting either body mass index in the obese range or known hypertension the second best marker for risk.[21] Tonsillar hypertrophy and certain craniofacial features also increase the risk for OSA.

CSA can also present as insomnia with sleep fragmentation, but may be less commonly suspected in the primary care setting. The prevalence of CSA has not been well-described in the general population. It increases with age, after a stroke or with heart failure, with Cheyne-Stokes respiration, and with opioid use. CSA and OSA can coexist in the same patient, and CSA can emerge as a problem after initiation of continuous positive airway pressure (CPAP) therapy for OSA.

Evaluation

History

History is crucial in the evaluation of insomnia. Validated questionnaires exist to probe different history relevant to insomnia including its severity, RLS, OSA risk, and chronotype; these are used in sleep medicine research and practice, but are unwieldy for most primary care practices to keep on hand. This section discusses aspects of history focused on the features of the patient's insomnia.

Acuity of insomnia should be apparent early on in discussion. For acute insomnia, ask about new stressors, new medications, and new symptoms. If no cause is apparent, consider blood loss (for RLS), nasal congestion (as it causes difficulty breathing), and any new medication or over-the-counter medication or supplement.

For chronic insomnia, probe the pattern (see **Fig. 1**). If the patient is more focused on his or her frustration with having insomnia, rather than feeling tired or having difficulty functioning during the day, consider sleep restriction therapy (discussed in Treatment below and in **Box 1**) as a major focus of therapy. Probe further for a description of the pattern—is it difficulty initiating sleep or maintaining sleep? If difficulty initiating sleep, ask particularly about RLS, DSPS, conditioned insomnia, use of stimulating medications or substances, and anxiety or stress. If the patient describes difficulty maintaining sleep, probe whether it is fragmented sleep, long periods of wakefulness during the night, or early morning awakening and pursue further as appropriate (see **Fig. 1**).

Look for hallmark features, described below.

The diagnostic features of RLS are as follows:

- Compelling urge to move the legs, typically associated with an uncomfortable sensation

> **Box 1**
> **Key components of CBT-I**
>
> Advice for physicians and patients are described here for the 2 most effective elements of CBT-I, Sleep Restriction Therapy and Stimulus Control.
>
> When advising either of these approaches, explicitly acknowledge to the patient that some of these measures will sound counterintuitive and that the insomnia experienced will probably seem worse for the first few days, then should improve.
>
> 1. Sleep restriction therapy: To improve the "sleep efficiency" of time in bed
>   - Have the patient estimate actual time spent asleep each night (average times if they span a range)
>   - Have the patient choose a time to get up each morning, without fail
>   - Have the patient purposefully delay bedtime to only allow the time spent in bed to match his/her estimated time spent asleep plus a 20- to 30-minute cushion (but not less than 5 hours, in case of sleep-state misperception)
>   - Counsel the patient to get up at the planned morning time, no matter how tired he/she is
>   - Counsel the patient to expect to continue to have insomnia and to feel more tired for the first several days, until increased drive for sleep improves the "efficiency" of sleep during the allowed time in bed
>   - After sleep efficiency improves, if daytime tiredness suggests more sleep is needed, the time in bed can be gradually lengthened until efficiency begins to decrease
> 2. Stimulus control: To overcome behavioral conditioning in which the person expects to be awake when attempting sleep.
>   - Only go to bed when sleepy.
>   - Use the bed only for sleep and sex.
>   - Do not watch the clock.
>   - Do not lie awake in bed for more than 20 minutes (estimated). If awake in bed, get up, go to a different room, do some quiet nonstimulating activity in low light, then return to bed when sleepy again. Repeat as many times as necessary.
>   - Keep a regular daily wake time.
>   - Avoid napping.
> 3. Cognitive therapy to address dysfunctional, maladaptive beliefs about sleep
> 4. Relaxation exercises
> 5. Sleep education and hygiene, including advice to avoid caffeine in the afternoon and evening and to get regular exercise

- Occurs in the evening or at night
- Worse with inactivity
- Relieved by movement

The key features of a circadian rhythm disorder are that the person has difficulty being asleep at one end of the day (when sleep is desired) and also has difficulty being awake at another end of the day (when wakefulness is desired). Ask about bedtime and wake time in 3 situations: those that are preferred but do not seem achievable, those that are achieved when aiming for the preferred times, and those achieved when the person can set his or her own schedule (for example, when on vacation). Ask about the circumstances under which a different sleep/wake pattern is required than is readily achievable (for example, work, sleep, child care duties within the family).

For OSA, ask about the following, each associated with increased risk[20–23]: breathing difficulties during sleep (history of nocturnal gasping or choking, witnessed apneas, and/or disruptive snoring), excessive daytime sleepiness, hypertension, nasal congestion, smoking, and male gender. Nocturia has similar sensitivity as snoring (85% vs 82%) but neither is specific (22% and 43%, respectively).[24]

If sleep is described as shallow or fragmented, but OSA seems low likelihood, ask whether the person is known to move or kick a lot during the night, and whether the sheets are torn off the bed in the morning, suggesting PLMS. A suspicion for OSA or PLMS suggests a polysomnogram may be warranted.

Physical Examination, Laboratory Work, and Sleep Studies

Physical examination is of limited utility in evaluating insomnia. Certain features may suggest OSA: obesity,[21] large neck circumference (>40 cm),[22] crowded oropharynx or craniofacial anatomy such as retrognathia.[23]

Laboratory work is of limited utility in evaluating insomnia, except in the evaluation for causes or contributing factors to RLS (particularly ferritin and possibly magnesium level; in initial evaluation also consider renal function and B12 level).

Sleep testing is of limited utility in evaluating insomnia, with the following exceptions:

1. Nocturnal PSG should be obtained when sleep apnea (obstructive or central) or PLMS is suspected and can be useful in evaluating insomnia in which sleep is achieved but is described as restless or unsatisfying. PSG can also be useful in identifying sleep-state misperception but is not routinely performed solely for that purpose.
2. Actigraphy documents physical motion (of an arm) as a proxy for sleep and wakefulness. It is most commonly done when history suggests a circadian rhythm disorder or significant underreporting of sleep time (as in sleep-state misperception), but a proxy suggesting objective sleep time would be useful. For sleep-state misperception, PSG is more specific.

In studies using PSG to quantify sleep, people with chronic insomnia do tend to underestimate the amount of sleep they obtain, whereas people who routinely sleep 6 hours or less but are satisfied with their sleep tend overestimate their sleep duration.[25] When "sleep-state misperception" is severe, the term "paradoxical insomnia" is used.

Treatment

Sedating medication and sleep hygiene advice are often assumed to be the 2 approaches to treatment of insomnia. Instead, the first step is to evaluate for an underlying condition, as in identification of a specific condition crucial for identifying further diagnostic measures, specific medication approaches, and/or specific nonpharmacologic approaches. In addition, cognitive behavioral therapy for insomnia (CBT-I) has been shown to have better efficacy than medications at 6 weeks and in the long term for people with chronic insomnia due to primary insomnia (chronic unexplained insomnia), insomnia comorbid with psychiatric and medical disorders, and conditioned insomnia.

Acute insomnia should be treated pharmacologically if the patient desires that approach, with a medication quickly effective for insomnia (benzodiazepine receptor agonist—the "Z" drugs such as zolpidem—or benzodiazepine). The purposes of having a low threshold to treat acute insomnia include prevention of daytime impairment, reduction of acute suffering, and prevention of perpetuation with development of chronic insomnia.

Chronic insomnia warrants further evaluation as to type, to determine whether a specific approach or treatment may be effective, as above.

In either case, if an underlying cause can be identified, that cause should be addressed and treated.

Treatment of RLS and periodic limb movements of sleep

Symptomatic RLS and/or PLMS are treated with dopa agonists (pramipexole, ropinirole, or rotigotine; or, for intermittent use, levodopa) or $\alpha(2)\delta$ ligands (gabapentin enacarbil, gabapentin, or pregabalin). Clonazepam or opioids are sometimes used in refractory cases. The dopa agonists can cause impulse control behaviors including gambling and impulsive shopping, eating, and sex; patients on these medications should be warned about these possible side effects and should be queried regularly about any such problematic behavior arising during chronic use.[26] The dopa agonists in particular can cause "augmentation," in which RLS symptoms occur at other times of day and/or in other parts of the body, leading to progressive increase in medication use unless it is recognized, in which case stopping the medication and switching to another class is advised.[27]

A comprehensive approach to the evaluation and management of RLS is outlined in **Fig. 2**.

Obstructive and central sleep apnea

OSA is treated by reducing airway obstruction, either by introducing positive airway pressure to create a "pneumatic splint"[28] or by temporarily or permanently affecting the position of the tongue and other airway structures. The most standard treatment is CPAP (steady) or bilevel positive airway pressure, with that pressure conveyed from the machine to the person's airway via an interface to the nostrils (or to the nose and mouth). Low-tech single-use nasal valves that give higher resistance to outflow than inflow of air are also available. Supplemental oxygen without positive airway pressure improves oxygenation but does not address, and may even prolong, obstructive events during sleep.[29]

Avoiding the supine position for sleep can reduce apneas and improve sleep quality in more than half of people with OSA, particularly those who are younger and/or not as heavy.[30] Oral appliances worn at night advance the mandible and tongue to reduce obstruction; they are typically not covered by insurance in the United States. Where applicable, weight loss—and even exercise without loss of weight[31]—improves OSA, presumably by reducing adiposity affecting the upper airway. Bariatric surgery for morbid obesity improves OSA in 75% of patients and (after successful weight loss) serves as definitive OSA treatment for some.[32]

In some patients, surgery to remove obstructing tissue, such as large tonsils, can be curative. Multiple different surgeries or ablative approaches can be done to try to improve the anatomy of the airway, from nasal passages to hypopharynx, with reduction of tongue bulk or anterior advancement of the tongue base a common target.

People with OSA should avoid alcohol and other respiratory depressants before bedtime. If sleep medication is considered for a person with OSA, whether to better allow use of CPAP or for coexisting insomnia unrelated to CPAP, a medication that does not suppress respiration should be chosen. Typically, this would be a benzodiazepine receptor agonist such as zolpidem or eszopiclone.

CSA may be treated by treating the underlying cause, with respiratory stimulants if hypoventilation-type, and with CPAP, bilevel positive airway pressure, or adaptive servoventilation.

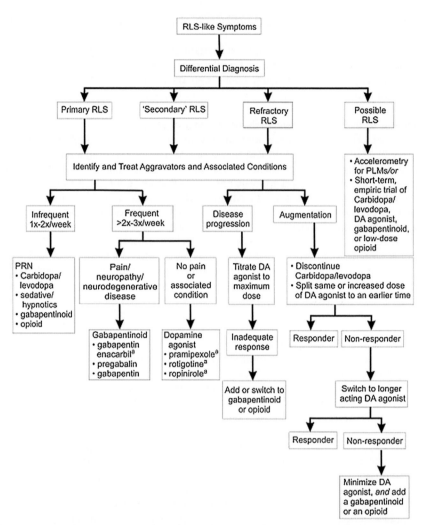

Fig. 2. A comprehensive approach to the evaluation and management of RLS. Accelerometry, also called actigraphy, monitors motor activity non-invasively. Its output showing timing of rest and activity may be used as a proxy for sleep/wake cycles or, when placed on a lower extremity, as a measure of limb movements during sleep. DA, dopamine agonist; PRN, pro re nata or as needed. (*From* Rye DB, Trotti LM. Restless legs syndrome and periodic leg movements of sleep. Neurol Clin 2012;30(4):1137–66.) [a] FDA-approved for RLS.

Circadian rhythm disorders

For the circadian sleep disorders presenting as insomnia, sleep medications are of quite limited benefit. The treatment approach is 4-fold:

a. Expectation management: If expectations can be changed to allow the person to sleep on his or her preferred schedule, this is likely to be the most effective long-term approach. However, responsibilities such as work or family may not allow this tactic.

b. Chronotherapy: The time at which sleep is attempted or allowed is gradually advanced or delayed toward a specific goal. The key is for the person to not only achieve *but also maintain* that "goal" sleep-wake schedule—including on days off and vacations—without letting it return to the problematic but more normal-feeling one. Long-term maintenance of a sleep-wake schedule that does not feel natural can be difficult.

c. Phototherapy: The person purposefully gets exposure to bright light at the time of day when he or she is sleepy but would like to be awake. For DSPS, that is light exposure right after awakening; for ASPS, it is light exposure in the evening. Sunlight (and artificial sources of the same range of wavelengths) is effective. Blue light with wavelengths around 450 to 470 nm is the most potent at suppressing melatonin.

d. Melatonin: Ingestion of melatonin 0.3 to 3 mg can be useful in shifting the sleep-wake time, whether due to jet lag or a chronic circadian disorder. A rule of thumb is that it is taken when it is dark out and other people are sleepy but the affected person is not, except that for DSPS it has been shown to be more effective when taken about 6 hours before the desired bed time rather than closer to bed time.[33] The melatonin serves as a signal that it is dark out and the brain and body should get ready for sleep. It helps keep the circadian clock on a desired schedule rather than reverting to the innate one.

Pharmacotherapy for insomnia

The pharmacotherapy of insomnia (**Table 2**) relies on 2 general approaches: stimulate a sleep-promoting system (via $GABA_A$ or melatonin receptors) or suppress one or more wake-promoting systems (particularly via histamine, acetylcholine, and/or serotonin receptors). All sedative-hypnotics have a mild to at-best moderate effect. All should be assumed to increase the risk of falls and to potentially impair functioning the next morning. The oldest of the US Food and Drug Administration (FDA)-approved, particularly the barbiturates, are global central nervous system depressants and therefore risky; they should not be used for the treatment of insomnia. Sedating medications (particularly antidepressants and antipsychotics) are commonly used off-label for the treatment of insomnia, but their use is most appropriate when warranted by another diagnosis. Otherwise, one of the newer nonbenzodiazepine sleep medications is preferred when pharmacologic treatment of insomnia is desired.

Melatonin receptor agonists

Melatonin, as a dietary supplement, is commonly taken for undifferentiated insomnia. It can have mildly beneficial effects in shortening the time to fall asleep and the total sleep time.[34] A melatonin-recepter agonist, ramelteon, is FDA-approved for the treatment of insomnia with difficulty falling asleep, for which it is modestly effective. No head-to-head trial has been published comparing it with melatonin. The manufacturer claims that ramelteon's preferential binding to MT1 and MT2 receptors over MT3 receptors may provide a safety benefit, but this claim has not been proven.

$GABA_A$ agonists

Benzodiazepines (BDZs) bind nonspecifically to GABA receptors, whereas the non-BDZ medications zaleplon, zolpidem, and eszopiclone (called "Z-drugs" or BDZ receptor agonists) bind specifically to $GABA_A$ and thus more specifically promote sleep without the anxiolytic, amnestic, and respiratory depressant effects of BDZs.

BDZs can provide a satisfying experience of sleep; however, the sleep achieved on them is objectively shallower (more time in stages 1 and 2, less in stages 3 and 4) than "normal" sleep and than sleep achieved on BDZ agonists.[35] BDZs may be used for acute insomnia in people without OSA and with normal respiratory function and are used chronically for some specific sleep disorders (eg, clonazepam used off-label for REM behavior disorder), but are not advised in the treatment of chronic insomnia.

Table 2
Medications used for nonspecific insomnia

	FDA-Approved as Sedative-Hypnotic	FDA Approved for Other Indications	Supplement (No FDA Oversight)
Benzodiazepine receptor agonist	Zolpidem Zaleplon Eszopiclone[a]	—	—
Benzodiazepine	Estazolam Flurazepam Quazepam Temazepam Triazolam	Clonazepam Lorazepam (All other approved BDZ not listed at left)	—
Melatonin receptor agonist	Ramelteon[a]	—	Melatonin
Histamine antagonist	Diphenhydramine[b] Doxylamine[b]	—	—
Histamine, adrenergic, and/or serotonin antagonist (as presumed mechanism for sedation)	Doxepin (one formulation)	Amitriptiline Doxepin (most formulations) Mirtazapine Quetiapine Trazodone	—
Global central nervous system depressant (use not advised)	Chloral hydrate (discontinued) Ethchlorvynol (discontinued) Butabarbital Pentobarbital/ carbromal Secobarbital	Sodium oxybate[c]	—

[a] Approved for chronic use for insomnia.
[b] Approved for over-the-counter use.
[c] Sodium oxybate (xyrem) is FDA-approved for treatment of cataplexy and excessive daytime sleepiness in narcolepsy but used off-label by some sleep specialists for severe insomnia. The medication can be dangerous and can be used for illicit purposes; its prescription and dispensing are tightly controlled.

For pharmacologic management of acute insomnia and chronic unexplained or co-morbid insomnia, the Z-drugs are preferred. These medications improve subjective and objective measures of sleep[36] and lead to minimal if any rebound insomnia on discontinuation.[37] Zolpidem in particular has been reported to cause complex sleep-related behaviors (including driving while asleep) in some cases; the plethora of reports regarding that medication may be due to its widespread use. This complex sleep-related behavior may be more likely to occur in situations of a higher blood level of zolpidem: in women, at higher doses, in hypoalbuminemia, and/or in conjunction with medications that increase zolpidem levels,[38] such as antifungals. Patients should be asked about a history of somnambulism (sleepwalking) before prescription, because the risk of these behaviors is higher in that situation.

Nonpharmacologic treatments
Improving satisfaction with the nighttime experience is the key in treating insomnia, and sometimes the person's attempts to achieve sleep are part of the problem. As with chronic pain, acceptance of some degree of symptoms can be helpful for sufferers.

Sleep hygiene advice encourages sleep-conducive behaviors and situations; some people with insomnia may benefit from this advice, but many people with insomnia are already following this advice—or not following some of it may make more sense to them. Sleep hygiene advice has been used for decades as the control intervention in studies on CBT-I and shown, at least for people enrolling in clinical trials on insomnia, not to be effective when used alone.[39,40]

Although little known to primary care physicians, CBT-I is effective in primary insomnia, conditioned insomnia, and insomnia comorbid with psychological and medical conditions; it should be considered first-line therapy for chronic insomnia.[41] CBT-I consists of several different approaches, among which sleep restriction therapy and stimulus control are the most effective components (**Box 1**).

CBT-I has been shown in double-blind randomized controlled trials to be more effective than relaxation therapy and to have persistent benefit for 6 months after a 6-week intervention.[42] CBT-I has been shown to be more effective than sleep medications beyond 6 weeks, although use of zolpidem during the initial CBT-I intervention improved the insomnia remission rate at 6 months more than CBT-I plus subsequent as-needed use of medication did, and more than CBT-I without initial use of medication did.[43]

Initial studies on CBT-I used 6 face-to-face individual or group sessions with a trained psychologist, but efficacy has been demonstrated when the intervention is shorter—2 sessions with a therapist followed by 2 phone calls[44]—or via other formats: by phone,[45] self-help booklet,[40,46] and Internet.[47]

CBT-I will likely become more accessible to patients in primary care practices in coming years.

REFERENCES

1. Edinger JD, Ulmer CS, Means MK. Sensitivity and specificity of polysomnographic criteria for defining insomnia. J Clin Sleep Med 2013;9(5):481–91.
2. Edinger JD, Bonnet MH, Bootzin RR, et al, American Academy of Sleep Medicine Work Group. Derivation of research diagnostic criteria for insomnia: report of an American Academy of Sleep Medicine Work Group. Sleep 2004;27(8): 1567–96.
3. American Psychiatric Association. Diagnostic and statistical manual of mental disorders. 5th edition. Arlington (VA): American Psychiatric Publishing; 2013.
4. Morin CM, Stone J, Trinkle D, et al. Dysfunctional beliefs and attitudes about sleep among older adults with and without insomnia complaints. Psychol Aging 1993;8(3):463–7.
5. Drake CL, Friedman NP, Wright KP, et al. Sleep reactivity and insomnia: genetic and environmental influences. Sleep 2011;34(9):1179–88.
6. Basta M, Chrousos GP, Vela-Bueno A, et al. Chronic insomnia and stress system. Sleep Med Clin 2007;2(2):279–91.
7. Arroll B, Fernando A 3rd, Falloon K, et al. Prevalence of causes of insomnia in primary care: a cross-sectional study. Br J Gen Pract 2012;62(595):e99–103.
8. Innes KE, Selfe TK, Agarwal P. Prevalence of restless legs syndrome in North American and Western European populations: a systematic review. Sleep Med 2011;12(7):623–34.
9. Phillips B, Young T, Finn L, et al. Epidemiology of restless legs symptoms in adults. Arch Intern Med 2000;160(14):2137–41.
10. Ohayon MM, O'Hara R, Vitiello MV. Epidemiology of restless legs syndrome: a synthesis of the literature. Sleep Med Rev 2012;16(4):283–95.

11. Allen RP, Walters AS, Montplaisir J, et al. Restless legs syndrome prevalence and impact: REST general population study. Arch Intern Med 2005;165(11):1286–92.

12. Hening W, Walters AS, Allen RP, et al. Impact, diagnosis and treatment of restless legs syndrome (RLS) in a primary care population: the REST (RLS epidemiology, symptoms, and treatment) primary care study. Sleep Med 2004;5(3):237–46.

13. Perez-Lloret S, Rey MV, Bondon-Guitton E, et al, French Association of Regional Pharmacovigilance Centers. Drugs associated with restless legs syndrome: a case/noncase study in the French Pharmacovigilance Database. J Clin Psychopharmacol 2012;32(6):824–7.

14. Bayard M, Bailey B, Acharya D, et al. Bupropion and restless legs syndrome: a randomized controlled trial. J Am Board Fam Med 2011;24(4):422–8.

15. Roenneberg T, Kuehnle T, Juda M, et al. Epidemiology of the human circadian clock. Sleep Med Rev 2007;11(6):429–38.

16. Wittmann M, Dinich J, Merrow M, et al. Social jetlag: misalignment of biological and social time. Chronobiol Int 2006;23(1–2):497–509.

17. Weitzman ED, Czeisler CA, Coleman RM, et al. Delayed sleep phase syndrome. A chronobiological disorder with sleep-onset insomnia. Arch Gen Psychiatry 1981;38(7):737–46.

18. Van Veen MM, Kooij JJ, Boonstra AM, et al. Delayed circadian rhythm in adults with attention-deficit/hyperactivity disorder and chronic sleep-onset insomnia. Biol Psychiatry 2010;67(11):1091–6.

19. Lichstein KL, Justin Thomas S, Woosley JA, et al. Co-occurring insomnia and obstructive sleep apnea. Sleep Med 2013;14(9):824–9.

20. Young T, Skatrud J, Peppard PE. Risk factors for obstructive sleep apnea in adults. JAMA 2004;291(16):2013–6.

21. Netzer NC, Hoegel JJ, Loube D, et al, Sleep in Primary Care International Study Group. Prevalence of symptoms and risk of sleep apnea in primary care. Chest 2003;124(4):1406–14.

22. Abrishami A, Khajehdehi A, Chung F. A systematic review of screening questionnaires for obstructive sleep apnea. Can J Anaesth 2010;57(5):423–38.

23. Myers KA, Mrkobrada M, Simel DL. Does this patient have obstructive sleep apnea?: The Rational Clinical Examination systematic review. JAMA 2013;310(7): 731–41.

24. Romero E, Krakow B, Haynes P, et al. Nocturia and snoring: predictive symptoms for obstructive sleep apnea. Sleep Breath 2010;14(4):337–43.

25. Fernandez-Mendoza J, Calhoun SL, Bixler EO, et al. Sleep misperception and chronic insomnia in the general population: role of objective sleep duration and psychological profiles. Psychosom Med 2011;73(1):88–97.

26. Voon V, Schoerling A, Wenzel S, et al. Frequency of impulse control behaviours associated with dopaminergic therapy in restless legs syndrome. BMC Neurol 2011;11:117.

27. Garcia-Borreguero D, Kohnen R, Silber MH, et al. The long-term treatment of restless legs syndrome/Willis-Ekbom disease: evidence-based guidelines and clinical consensus best practice guidance: a report from the International Restless Legs Syndrome Study Group. Sleep Med 2013;14(7):675–84.

28. Sullivan CE, Issa FG, Berthon-Jones M, et al. Reversal of obstructive sleep apnoea by continuous positive airway pressure applied through the nares. Lancet 1981;1(8225):862–5.

29. Mehta V, Vasu TS, Phillips B, et al. Obstructive sleep apnea and oxygen therapy: a systematic review of the literature and meta-analysis. J Clin Sleep Med 2013; 9(3):271–9.

30. Oksenberg A, Silverberg DS, Arons E, et al. Positional vs nonpositional obstructive sleep apnea patients: anthropomorphic, nocturnal polysomnographic, and multiple sleep latency test data. Chest 1997;112(3):629–39.

31. Kline CE, Crowley EP, Ewing GB, et al. The effect of exercise training on obstructive sleep apnea and sleep quality: a randomized controlled trial. Sleep 2011; 34(12):1631–40.

32. Sarkosh K, Switzer NJ, El-Hadi M, et al. The impact of bariatric surgery on obstructive sleep apnea: a systematic review. Obes Surg 2013;23(3):414–23.

33. Mundey K, Benloucif S, Harsanyi K, et al. Phase-dependent treatment of delayed sleep phase syndrome with melatonin. Sleep 2005;28(10):1271–8.

34. Ferracioli-Oda E, Qawasmi A, Block MH. Meta-analysis: melatonin for the treatment of primary sleep disorders. PLoS One 2013;8(5):e63773.

35. Dujardin K, Guieu JD, Leconte-Lambert C, et al. Comparison of the effects of zolpidem and flunitrazepam on sleep structure and daytime cognitive functions. A study of untreated unsomniacs. Pharmacopsychiatry 1998;31(1):14–8.

36. Huedo-Medina TB, Kirsch I, Middlemass J, et al. Effectiveness of non-benzodiazepine hypnotics in treatment of adult insomnia: meta-analysis of data submitted to the Food and Drug Administration. BMJ 2012;345:e8343.

37. Roehrs TA, Randall S, Harris E, et al. Twelve months of nightly zolpidem does not lead to rebound insomnia or withdrawal symptoms: a prospective placebo-controlled study. J Psychopharmacol 2012;26(8):1088–95.

38. Inagaki T, Miyaoka T, Tsuji S, et al. Adverse reactions to zolpidem: case reports and a review of the literature. Prim Care Companion J Clin Psychiatry 2010; 12(6). pii: PCC.09r00849.

39. Morin CM, Culbert JP, Schwartz SM. Nonpharmacological interventions for insomnia: a meta-analysis of treatment efficacy. Am J Psychiatry 1994;151(8): 1172–80.

40. Bjorvatn B, Fiske E, Pallesen S. A self-help book is better than sleep hygiene advice for insomnia: a randomized controlled comparative study. Scand J Psychol 2011;52(6):580–5.

41. Mitchell MD, Gehrman P, Perlis M, et al. Comparative effectiveness of cognitive behavioral therapy for insomnia: a systematic review. BMC Fam Pract 2012;13:40.

42. Edinger JD, Wohlgemuth WK, Radtke RA, et al. Cognitive behavioral therapy for treatment of chronic primary insomnia: a randomized controlled trial. JAMA 2001; 285(14):1856–64.

43. Morin CM, Vallières A, Guay B, et al. Cognitive behavioral therapy, singly and combined with medication, for persistent insomnia: a randomized controlled trial. JAMA 2009;301(19):2005–15.

44. Buysse DJ, Germain A, Moul DE, et al. Efficacy of brief behavioral treatment for chronic insomnia in older adults. Arch Intern Med 2011;171(10):887–95.

45. Arnedt JT, Cuddihy L, Swanson LM, et al. Randomized controlled trial of telephone-delivered cognitive behavioral therapy for chronic insomnia. Sleep 2013;36(3):353–62.

46. Jernelöv S, Lekander M, Blom K, et al. Efficacy of a behavioral self-help treatment with or without therapist guidance for co-morbid and primary insomnia—a randomized controlled trial. BMC Psychiatry 2012;12:5.

47. Cheng SK, Dizon J. Computerised cognitive behavioural therapy for insomnia: a systematic review and meta-analysis. Psychother Psychosom 2012;81(4): 206–16.

Diagnosing and Treating Dizziness

Alexandra Molnar, MD[a],*, Steven McGee, MD[b]

KEYWORDS

- Dizziness • Vertigo • Epley • Primary care

KEY POINTS

- Dizziness is a common presenting concern in primary care practice.
- History and physical examination usually suffice in making the diagnosis, without need for formal studies.
- Effective treatment can often be offered in the clinic, without need for medications.

INTRODUCTION

Dizziness that is severe enough to bring an individual into the clinic is remarkably common, affecting approximately 30%[1] of individuals aged 18 to 79 years during their lifetime. Prevalence of dizziness in the elderly and very elderly is even greater.[2]

Many primary care physicians find the care of the dizzy patient challenging, because of the vagueness and ambiguity of the patient's specific symptoms and the wide variety of possible diagnoses, ranging from benign to serious.[3] Even so, studies of many patients presenting with dizziness (**Table 1**)[4–6] have helped clarify the cause of dizziness. Whether the clinician works in the emergency department, the primary care clinic, or a specialized clinic for dizziness, the most common final diagnosis in dizzy patients is peripheral vestibular disease, usually benign paroxysmal positional vertigo (BPPV), less commonly Ménière disease or vestibular neuronitis.[5,7] The second most common diagnostic group in patients presenting acutely with dizziness to a primary care clinic or emergency room is orthostatic hypotension.

Many dizziness experts consider a condition called multiple sensory deficits to be particular common in elderly patients. This disorder describes the accumulation of multiple sensory insults (such as decreased vision, vestibular disease, peripheral

Disclosure: A. Molnar reports no financial conflicts of interest; S. McGee reports receiving royalties from Elsevier.
a Department of Medicine, Harborview Medical Center, University of Washington, Box 359895, 325–9th Avenue, Seattle, WA 98104, USA; b Department of Medicine, Veterans Affairs Puget Sound Healthcare System–Seattle Division, University of Washington, 1660 South Columbian Way, Seattle, WA 98108-1597, USA
* Corresponding author.
E-mail address: amolnar@uw.edu

Table 1 Cause of dizziness			
Cause	Emergency Room (n = 907[5]) (%)	Primary Care, Elderly (n = 1708[2]) (%)[a]	Specialized Dizziness Clinic (n = 125[6]) (%)
Peripheral vestibular disease (benign positional vertigo, vestibular neuronitis, Ménière disease)	32	40	38
Orthostasis/syncope	15	10	–
Multiple sensory deficits	–	8	13
Psychiatric	2	6	9
Infection	4	4	–
Central neurologic (serious)	5	4	5
Drug-related	5	3	–
Cardiac (serious)	4	2	4
Unknown	22	16	9

[a] Percentages rounded to the nearest integer.

neuropathy, poor perfusion of the brain, and orthopedic disorders), which, although by themselves are insufficient to be symptomatic, in combination deprive patients of enough sensory information about the environment to cause the presenting concern of dizziness.[8]

Serious cardiac or neurologic disorders (eg, arrhythmias, stroke) are uncommon causes of dizziness, affecting fewer than 1 in 10 patients. A diagnosis may be made in dizzy patients more than 80% of the time.

PATHOPHYSIOLOGY OF VESTIBULAR DISEASE

A basic understanding of the principal causes of peripheral vestibular disease helps clinicians recognize these disorders during their history and physical examination. For all of the causes discussed in this article, it can be helpful to recall that vertigo requires an imbalance between the 2 sides.

BPPV stems from detached otoliths that settle in the most dependent portion of the inner ear, most commonly the posterior semicircular canal[9] (otoliths are the tiny rocks that normally reside in the saccule and utricle and provide the body with information about our position in the gravitational field, ie, whether the body is upside down, upright, or tilting). Movements of the head in the plane of the affected posterior semicircular canal result in exaggerated movements of endolymph and cause vertigo.

The cause and pathophysiology of Ménière disease is poorly understood, thus, the alternative term of idiopathic endolymphatic hydrops.[10] The common histologic finding is dilated endolymph channels, although this abnormality has also been found in asymptomatic patients.[11] One theory is that obstruction causes increased endolymph pressure, leading to breaks in the intralabyrinthine membranes, and subsequent vertigo. The increased pressure also results in the tinnitus, aural fullness, and hearing loss,[12] which initially fluctuates but can progress to severe hearing loss in the affected ear.[9] Another theory redefines the problem as a dysfunction in 1 or more homeostatic systems that regulate the ionic composition of the endolymph. According to this theory, changes in endolymph composition result in dizziness and hearing fluctuation.[13,14]

Vestibular neuronitis is also called viral neuronitis, acute vestibulopathy, epidemic vertigo, and acute labyrinthitis. It stems from spontaneous mononeuropathy of the vestibular division of the eighth cranial nerve on 1 side. The mononeuropathy is usually believed to be virally mediated, in part because many patients report a viral prodrome and the illness may occur in epidemics. There is increasing evidence from animal studies and autopsy studies that many cases of vestibular neuronitis are caused by reactivation of latent herpes simplex virus type 1 infection.[15]

Central Vestibular Disease

Rarely, stroke may mimic vestibular neuronitis if it affects vestibular nuclei, as in cerebellar stroke and, less likely, lateral medullary stroke.

SYMPTOMS

Clinicians should attempt to categorize the patient's dizziness into 1 of 3 types: vertigo, light-headedness, or disequilibrium, an approach based on early investigations of chronic dizziness.[6] Vertigo is a sensation of movement (eg, twirling, tilting), perceived in the head, a symptom implying either peripheral or central vestibular disease. All vertigo is abrupt in onset, episodic, and aggravated by head movements; the various types are distinguished by duration, setting, and associated symptoms. Light-headedness is a feeling of faintness or graying of vision, implying hypotension and poor perfusion of the brain. Disequilibrium is a sensation of unsteadiness not in the head, implying proprioceptive or cerebellar disease. Nonetheless, this classification of dizziness fails in at least 10% of patients, despite the clinician's best efforts, because the patient's symptoms are too vague or ambiguous.[3,6]

Additional helpful questions to ask patients during the interview are given in **Table 2**.[16–20] A careful history may help to clarify nonspecific dizziness that does not easily fall into any 1 category. Some small percentage may be attributable to panic disorder or more rare causes, such as toxic exposure or infection (see **Tables 1** and **2**). Usually, a fairly certain diagnosis can be made by history alone, although physical examination helps confirm the diagnosis.[21]

PHYSICAL EXAMINATION

After the history, the most important step in evaluating dizziness is an attentive physical examination. Key components of examination are vital signs, gait, and special provocative tests. In patients with positional vertigo, the special provocational tests include the Dix-Hallpike test[22,23] (for posterior canal BPPV) and supine roll test (for lateral canal BPPV). In patients with acute, sustained vertigo (a symptom prompting consideration of vestibular neuronitis [common, benign] and posterior fossa stroke [uncommon but severe]), important additional tests are the head impulse test and a thorough neurologic examination.

If the physician is aware in advance that the patient's concern is dizziness, it is helpful to ask the nurse or medical assistant to perform orthostatic vital signs on the patient before the visit. Orthostatic hypotension, especially if it reproduces the patient's symptom of dizziness, helps confirm the diagnosis of presyncope. Nonetheless, presyncope or light-headedness itself is not a final diagnosis but merits further investigation, including careful review of recent medication changes and queries about fevers, bleeding, alteration in dietary habits, cardiac symptoms, and neurologic changes.

Observation of gait helps detect disequilibrium and other neurologic disorders, especially multiple sensory deficits among elderly patients who typically feel fine when resting but become conspicuously unsteady when walking. A useful diagnostic test in the office is to have the patient make several right-angle turns while walking

Table 2
Helpful questions to elicit the diagnosis of dizziness

Questions	Purpose	Answers: Suggested Diagnosis
What do you mean by "dizzy?"	Further elicit historical points without prejudicing a particular diagnosis	Vertigo, light-headedness, disequilibrium (see text)
What brings on the dizziness?	Ascertain the type	Turning my head: vertigo[16] Rolling over in bed: vertigo[16] Standing up: presyncope Stress: psychiatric Walking: disequilibrium or multiple sensory deficit[17] Darkness or uneven ground: disequilibrium or multiple sensory deficit[17]
How long does the dizziness last?	Helpful in subtyping vertigo	Less than 1 min: BPPV[16] Hours: Ménière[18] Days: vestibular neuronitis
What other symptoms have you had?	Helpful in evaluating for serious causes and subtyping vertigo	Other neurologic[a]: central vestibular disease[18] Hearing loss/tinnitus: Ménière, syphilis Palpitations: cardiac arrhythmia Fever: infection Viral prodrome: vestibular neuronitis
Any recent toxic exposures[17] or medication changes?[19]	Helpful in evaluating for precipitating causes	Gas heat in cold winter months: carbon monoxide poisoning[20] Recent medication change: untoward effect of medication

[a] Dysarthria, paresis, truncal instability, lethargy, ataxia, focal neurologic abnormality, imbalance, previous stroke.[5,8,26]

without assistance; if dizziness appears during this maneuver, the patient with multiple sensory deficit experiences immediate relief by touching the clinician's hand or the wall (a maneuver providing initial sensory information and thus relieving the unsteadiness).[17] Further support for the diagnosis of multiple sensory deficit includes documentation of a positive Romberg test (a test of proprioceptive loss), sensory loss in the legs (peripheral neuropathy), diminished visual acuity (eg, cataracts), or other abnormalities during musculoskeletal examination of the legs (eg, genu valgum). In all patients with dizziness, but especially those with disequilibrium, it is crucial to assess the patient's risk for fall-related or driving-related injury, issues that must be addressed in the treatment plan.[24]

SPECIAL PHYSICAL EXAMINATION MANEUVERS
Positional Vertigo

In patients with vertiginous symptoms related to change in position, the clinician should attempt to reproduce the symptom in the office using the Dix-Hallpike or supine roll maneuvers. The purpose of these maneuvers is not only to confirm the diagnosis but also to direct future therapy. Because most patients with positional vertigo have otoliths abnormally located in the posterior semicircular canal (reproduced by Dix-Hallpike maneuver) and only 10% to 15% have otoliths in the lateral semicircular canal (reproduced by the supine roll maneuver), the clinician usually begins testing with the Dix-Hallpike maneuver (**Fig. 1**).[22] During these tests, the clinician tests 1 ear at a time, beginning with the ear suspected to be abnormal, as suggested by the patient interview (eg, if the patient reports vertigo when rolling to the right, the clinician should suspect that the right ear is abnormal and begin testing with that ear).

A positive Dix-Hallpike maneuver has 3 key features: (1) it reproduces the patient's vertigo and nystagmus, (2) there is a latency period of several seconds to a minute before the vertigo and nystagmus are provoked, and (3) the vertigo and nystagmus resolve in less than 1 minute.[16]

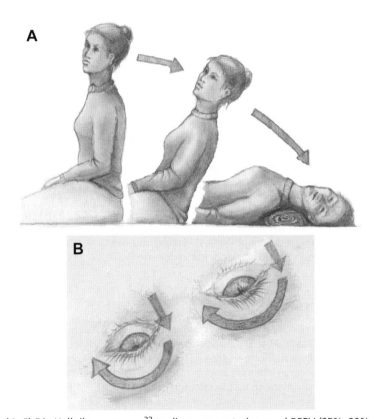

Fig. 1. (*A, B*) Dix-Hallpike maneuver[22] to diagnose posterior canal BPPV (85%–90% of cases of BPPV). Remember to test both sides. The undermost ear is the one being tested. To maximize the sensitivity of the test, the movement from upright to supine should take 1 to 2 seconds. It is important to warn the patient that this maneuver reproduces the vertigo and possibly even nausea, but the symptoms should resolve rapidly. Despite these symptoms, counsel the patient to keep their eyes wide open and focused on the examiner, so that the examiner may watch for nystagmus. The direction of the nystagmus (quick component) is upward and torsional, with the superior pole of the eyes rotating down toward the undermost ear. One often has to remind the patient throughout the maneuver about the importance of keeping the eyes open, because it is a natural reaction to close the eyes in response to the vertiginous symptoms. Usually, the examiner does not have the patient's head dangling off the end of the table as initially described,[23] because of the layout of many examination rooms and concerns about patient safety. Instead, the patient lies back with head fully supported by the table but the shoulders elevated on several rolled towels or a pillow, as shown in (*A*). (*Courtesy of* Jessica Stanton, MD.)

Some providers, when a history is strongly pointing toward BPPV but the Dix-Hallpike is negative bilaterally, go on to perform the supine roll maneuver (**Fig. 2**).[25]

Sustained Vertigo

Most patients with sustained vertigo suffer from vestibular neuronitis, although a few patients (especially elderly patients with cardiovascular risk factors) are having a stroke or other serious disease in the cerebellum or brainstem. One helpful bedside maneuver to help distinguish central and peripheral causes is the head impulse test (**Fig. 3**).[26–28]

Sustained vertigo implies an imbalance between the right and left vestibular systems, either peripheral or central. The head impulse test investigates the integrity of the peripheral vestibular system. Therefore, if the test is abnormal in patients with sustained vertigo, peripheral disease is suspected (ie, vestibular neuronitis); if the head impulse test is normal in patients with sustained vertigo, the peripheral system is normal and therefore central disease is suspected (ie, posterior fossa stroke). It is important to only do this test in someone with prolonged vertigo; if the vertiginous episodes are brief, then BPPV is the more likely diagnosis, and the Dix-Hallpike maneuver is more useful.

In addition to the finding of a normal head impulse test in patients with sustained vertigo, several other neurologic findings are compelling arguments that the patient is suffering from a posterior fossa stroke: truncal ataxia, skew deviation (**Fig. 4**),[26] saccadic pursuit, and direction-changing nystagmus (**Table 3**).[26,29] In clinical studies, these findings are sometimes more accurate than the initial diffusion-weighted magnetic resonance imaging (MRI) scans.[29,30]

Most patients with dizziness do not require additional laboratory testing. Important exceptions are patients with orthostatic hypotension (blood tests for anemia, electrolyte abnormalities, or renal insufficiency), suspected Ménière disease (audiometry, syphilis testing), or suspected posterior fossa disease (MRI). Vestibular testing is rarely indicated.[16]

TREATMENT

In patients with positional vertigo and a positive Dix-Hallpike test (posterior canalithiasis), the Epley maneuver (**Fig. 5**)[31] is indicated; if the supine roll test is positive (lateral or horizontal canalithiasis), no maneuver is indicated. The Epley maneuver addresses the anatomy of the canal affected and is specifically designed to move the patient through sequential positions to rid the affected canal of the abnormal otoliths, moving them back into the saccule. Canalith repositioning maneuvers may be performed immediately after the positive diagnostic maneuver and are easily and quickly achieved during the clinic visit. Other canalith repositioning maneuvers are available, but these other maneuvers have less robust data to support their successful application in the patient with vertigo.[16]

If a Dix-Hallpike is positive, the patient can maintain the position with the head down and be moved directly through the Epley maneuver (see **Fig. 5**). Even if the resolution does not occur in the clinic, 74% of patients report total resolution of symptoms within 1 week of undergoing an Epley maneuver,[16] although these data come from subspecialty clinics and the success rate for inexperienced practitioners may be less. The number of Epley attempts necessary to achieve success is unclear. Many experienced practitioners attempt the Epley more than once during a single clinic visit to maximize the chances of success, assuming the patient is willing and able.

For patients in whom the Dix-Hallpike is negative, but the supine roll is positive (ie, suspected horizontal canal BPPV), there is insufficient evidence to recommend

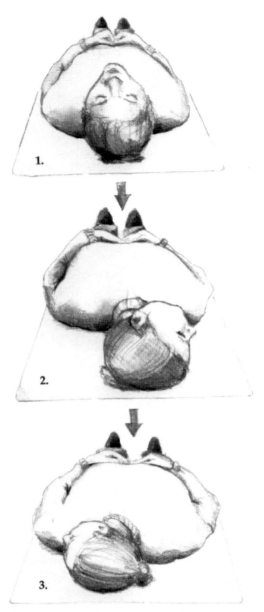

Fig. 2. The supine roll maneuver for diagnosis of lateral canal BPPV (10%–15% of cases of BPPV).[25] Remember to test both sides. The downward ear is the one being tested. (1) Lie supine facing the ceiling. (2) Quickly turn head to face right. If this provokes symptoms, the affected ear is the right ear. Return to facing the ceiling. (3) Quickly turn head to face left. If this provokes symptoms, the affected ear is the left ear. (*Courtesy of* Jessica Stanton, MD.)

PERIPHERAL VESTIBULAR DISEASE

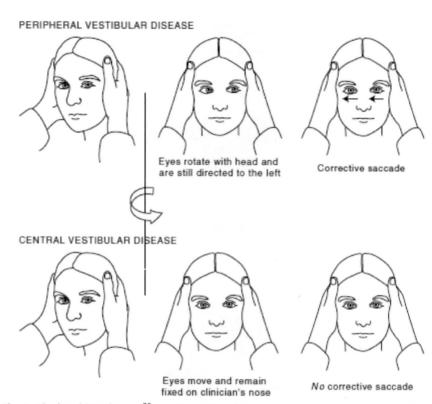

CENTRAL VESTIBULAR DISEASE

Fig. 3. The head impulse test[26] may be used to distinguish between a peripheral vestibular disease (such as vestibular neuronitis or Ménière disease[27]) and a central lesion (such as stroke or mass). The examiner sits in front of the patient and places a hand on each side of the patient's head. The patient is instructed to focus on the examiner's nose and the examiner focuses on the patient's eyes. The patient should keep their eyes open even if vertiginous symptoms worsen. An abnormal vestibulo-ocular reflex (peripheral disease) causes the eyes to move away with the head movement toward the abnormal side. At the end of rotation, the patient's eyes move quickly back to return the gaze to the clinician's nose. This is the corrective saccade. A normal vestibulo-ocular reflex (central disease) allows the patient to maintain gaze on the clinician's nose during rapid head movements to both sides without corrective saccades. There is improved sensitivity if the test is performed rapidly to aid in detection. The examiner should repeat the examination if initially normal or negative to make sure that saccades are not missed.[28] (*From* McGee SR. Evidence-based physical diagnosis. 3rd edition. Philadelphia: Elsevier/Saunders; 2012. p. 663; with permission.)

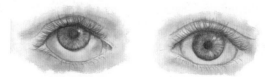

Fig. 4. Skew deviation.[26] One eye is aligned higher than the other, a sign of cerebellar or brainstem disease. (*Courtesy of* Jessica Stanton, MD.)

Table 3
Acute sustained vertigo and imbalance, detecting stroke: diagnostic accuracy of physical examination

Finding	Likelihood Ratio if Finding:	
	Present	Absent
Severe truncal ataxia	17.9	0.7
Skew deviation present	5.3	0.7
Saccadic pursuit	4.6	0.2
Direction-changing nystagmus	3.5	0.7
Normal head impulse test	9.6	0.2

Definition of findings: truncal ataxia: patient cannot sit unassisted; skew deviation: see **Fig. 4**; saccadic pursuit: when following the examiner's moving finger, the movements are not smooth but instead jerky or saccadic; direction-changing nystagmus: when patients with nystagmus look in the direction opposite the quick component of the initial nystagmus, the direction of the nystagmus changes.[29]
Data from McGee SR. Evidence-based physical diagnosis. 3rd edition. Philadelphia: Elsevier/ Saunders; 2012.

1 particular canalith repositioning maneuver.[16] Although the Lempert maneuver is 1 proposed remedy for this disorder, 1 study[32] found little advantage to this maneuver over watchful waiting; this same study found that horizontal canal BPPV tends to self-resolve more rapidly than posterior canal BPPV.

For individuals suffering from BPPV for whom the in-office canalith repositioning maneuvers are unsuccessful, home treatment can offer relief. Self-administered canalith repositioning procedures (CRPs), reviewed in the patient education handout in the supplementary appendix, are often effective for motivated patients with frequent attacks.[31] The self-administered Epley CRP is successful at least 64%[16] of the time. For patients who find this maneuver too complex to perform at home, the simpler Brandt-Daroff maneuver is recommended, although this maneuver completely relieves symptoms in only 23%[31] of patients. Like the Epley maneuver, the Brandt-Daroff maneuver reduces (fatigues) symptoms even if it does not bring about total resolution of symptoms.

For BPPV, there is a strong recommendation against medical treatments such as antihistamines and benzodiazepines. These treatments can increase risk of falls and urinary retention in older adults, and multiple studies have reported that they retard resolution of symptoms.[16] One study comparing CRP with medication showed CRP to be more successful at 2-week follow-up, with CRP giving 74% of individuals total relief and medication giving only 30% of individuals relief. Rarely, antiemetics are indicated for severe nausea or as prophylaxis for a planned maneuver that has provoked severe nausea during previous attempts.[16]

Treatment of Ménière disease is more challenging and usually requires further evaluation by audiologists or otolaryngologists. Traditional treatments include vestibular rehabilitation, sodium restriction, and thiazides.[14,33] In most patients, the episodes of vertigo become less common over time, although the patient's hearing loss progresses.

Vestibular neuronitis is also difficult to treat. Supportive care is important, and patients should be reassured that most cases resolve with time. Despite hopeful studies about the success of early steroid therapy,[34] further meta-analysis has found little difference between placebo and steroids[35] in patient symptoms and speed of recovery.

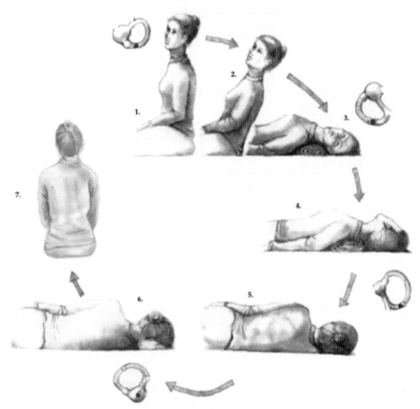

Fig. 5. Epley maneuver[31] shown for left ear (left ear downward initially). (1) Start by seating the patient on the table with the head turned 45° to the left. Place a pillow or rolled towel on the table so that on lying back it is under the shoulders. (2, 3) Lay the patient back quickly with shoulders on the pillow, neck extended, and head resting on the bed. In this position, the affected (left) ear is underneath. Wait for 30 seconds. (4) Turn the head 90° to the right (without raising it), and wait again for 30 seconds. (5, 6) Turn the body and head another 90° to the right, turning the head so that it is facing the ground, and wait for another 30 seconds. (7) Sit the patient up on the right side. Next to the patient positions are illustrations of the displaced otoliths moving through the semicircular canal with each position. Repeat maneuvers may be helpful. (*Courtesy of* Jessica Stanton, MD.)

Treatment of light-headedness depends on its cause, varying between simple counseling (arise slowly from a supine or seated position) and medication adjustments to specific treatments of serious underlying problems (eg, antiarrhythmic medications, pacemakers, mineralocorticoid medications).

Multiple sensory deficit can rarely be completely cured, but multidisciplinary efforts can improve functional status tremendously.[24] Interventions focus on providing the patient with more information about their environment through fall prevention efforts with a physical therapist, assistive devices, and home evaluation. Consideration of nightlights to improve nighttime sensory input and, for those with reduced visual acuity, updated spectacles prescription or cataract extraction might be necessary.

Psychiatric causes of dizziness can be challenging to treat.[6] Working closely with the patient and consideration of biofeedback, counseling, or medication may improve symptoms.

Serious conditions such as cerebellar stroke and unstable arrhythmia require emergent treatment, likely in an inpatient setting.

ADDITIONAL CONSIDERATIONS

Safety is a crucial consideration in managing patients with dizziness. Evaluating and mitigating fall risk with patients and their families reduces risk to the patient. Fall risk may be reduced with the assistance of physical therapists, home safety evaluations, and medication review. In addition, a careful discussion of risks related to driving or operating machinery reduces injury to the patient and the community. This discussion can be challenging for a variety of reasons, especially if loss of driving privileges isolates an elderly person. Enlisting the help of family or other social supports can reduce this isolation.

Recurrence is common, especially with BPPV. Counseling the patient that there may be recurrence but it is usually self-limited may help the patient be prepared if it does recur.

Follow-up is recommended at approximately 1 month for cases of BPPV. For most patients, symptoms of BPPV have resolved by this time. If it persists at 1 month, another Epley maneuver is indicated, with up to 98% success rates reported at follow-up attempts.[16]

SUMMARY

Dizziness is a common presenting concern in primary care practice. The history and physical examination distinguish almost all the different types of dizziness, and formal studies are rarely necessary. In most cases, effective treatments are available to administer in the clinic or at home, without need for medication.

Although providers may be tempted to order laboratory tests and prescribe medications for their patients with dizziness, a growing body of evidence indicates that the hands-on physical examination and therapeutic maneuvers are all that is necessary to care for patients with dizziness.[7] More than perhaps any other diagnosis, the presenting concern of dizziness allows providers to return to the healing touch that is the core of the doctor-patient relationship.

PATIENT EDUCATION MATERIAL

Your provider believes that your dizziness comes from a type of vertigo called benign paroxysmal positional vertigo (BPPV). This problem usually resolves without treatment within weeks. Some people with this type of dizziness experience more rapid relief by trying one of the maneuvers depicted below.

Epley maneuver[31]: start by determining which side is affected by turning your head to the left and right. The direction that gives you the most symptoms is the affected side. The maneuver will be most helpful if you practice it starting with the affected ear downward as you lean back. This maneuver will temporarily worsen symptoms, but can also help to make your vertigo go away entirely. The image below shows how to do the Epley maneuver with the left ear (affected ear) down (see **Fig. 5**).

The Epley maneuver has shown the most success when practiced at home, but can be complex. Some people find the Brandt-Daroff easier to do on their own at home. It also does not require that you know which ear is most affected (**Fig. 6**).

Keeping moving and active despite the dizziness does help to resolve symptoms more quickly, even though it may feel difficult. Please take extra caution while you are dizzy to avoid falls. Ask a friend or relative for help and sit down when possible.

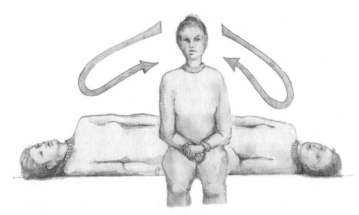

Fig. 6. The Brandt-Daroff maneuver: sitting upright on the side of a bed or couch, lie quickly down on 1 side, wait 30 seconds for dizziness to improve, and then sit up quickly. Repeat this maneuver on the other side. (*Courtesy of* Jessica Stanton, MD.)

If you are experiencing dizziness when you turn your head, *please do not drive a car* for your own safety and the safety of those around you.

If your symptoms get worse or new symptoms arise, contact your doctor immediately. If your symptoms do not improve after 2–3 weeks, please also contact your doctor's office.

ACKNOWLEDGMENTS

The authors would like to thank Jessica Stanton for donating her time, talent, and expertise in the creation of the figures for this article.

REFERENCES

1. Neuhauser HK, Radtke A, von Brevern M, et al. Burden of dizziness and vertigo in the community. Arch Intern Med 2008;168(19):2118–24.
2. Maarsingh OR, Dros J, Schellevis FG, et al. Dizziness reported by elderly patients in family practice: prevalence, incidence, and clinical characteristics. BMC Fam Pract 2010;11:2.
3. Herr RD, Zun L, Mathews JJ. A directed approach to the dizzy patient. Ann Emerg Med 1989;18(6):664–72.
4. Maarsingh OR, Dros J, Schellevis FG, et al. Causes of persistent dizziness in elderly patients in primary care. Ann Fam Med 2010;8(3):196–205.
5. Navi BB, Kamel H, Shah MP, et al. Rate and predictors of serious neurologic causes of dizziness in the emergency department. Mayo Clin Proc 2012; 87(11):1080–8.
6. Drachman DA, Hart CW. An approach to the dizzy patient. Neurology 1972;22(4): 323–34.
7. Kerber KA, Burke JF, Skolarus LE, et al. Use of BPPV processes in emergency department dizziness presentations: a population-based study. Otolaryngol Head Neck Surg 2013;148(3):425–30.
8. Sloane P, Blazer D, George LK. Dizziness in a community elderly population. J Am Geriatr Soc 1989;37(2):101–8.
9. Kutz JW. The dizzy patient. Med Clin North Am 2010;94(5):989–1002.

10. Marques PS, Perez-Fernandez N. Bedside vestibular examination in patients with unilateral definite Ménière's disease. Acta Otolaryngol 2012;132(5):498–504.
11. Rauch SD, Merchant SN, Thedinger BA. Meniere's syndrome and endolymphatic hydrops. Double-blind temporal bone study. Ann Otol Rhinol Laryngol 1989; 98(11):873–83.
12. Nelson JA, Viirre E. The clinical differentiation of cerebellar infarction from common vertigo syndromes. West J Emerg Med 2009;10(4):273–7.
13. Rauch SD. Clinical hints and precipitating factors in patients suffering from Meniere's disease. Otolaryngol Clin North Am 2010;43(5):1011–7.
14. Berlinger NT. Meniere's disease: new concepts, new treatments. Minn Med 2011; 94(11):33–6.
15. Strupp M, Brandt T. Peripheral vestibular disorders. Curr Opin Neurol 2013;26(1): 81–9.
16. Bhattacharyya N, Baugh RF, Orvidas L, et al. Clinical practice guideline: benign paroxysmal positional vertigo. Otolaryngol Head Neck Surg 2008;139(5 Suppl 4): S47–81.
17. McGee SR. Dizzy patients. Diagnosis and treatment. West J Med 1995;162(1): 37–42.
18. Chan Y. Differential diagnosis of dizziness. Curr Opin Otolaryngol Head Neck Surg 2009;17(3):200–3.
19. Renoir T. Selective serotonin reuptake inhibitor antidepressant treatment discontinuation syndrome: a review of the clinical evidence and the possible mechanisms involved. Front Pharmacol 2013;4:45.
20. Lakhani R, Bleach N. Carbon monoxide poisoning: an unusual cause of dizziness. J Laryngol Otol 2010;124(10):1103–5.
21. Kroenke K, Lucas CA, Rosenberg ML, et al. Causes of persistent dizziness. A prospective study of 100 patients in ambulatory care. Ann Intern Med 1992; 117(11):898–904.
22. Dix MR, Hallpike CS. The pathology, symptomatology and diagnosis of certain common disorders of the vestibular system. Proc R Soc Med 1952;45:341–54.
23. Citron L, Hallpike CS. Observations upon the mechanism of positional nystagmus of the so-called "benign paroxysmal type". J Laryngol Otol 1956;70(5):253–9.
24. Dros J, Maarsingh OR, Beem L, et al. Functional prognosis of dizziness in older adults in primary care: a prospective cohort study. J Am Geriatr Soc 2012;60(12): 2263–9.
25. Fife TD, Iverson DJ, Lempert T, et al. Practice parameter: therapies for benign paroxysmal positional vertigo (an evidence-based review): report of the Quality Standards Subcommittee of the American Academy of Neurology. Neurology 2008;70(22):2067–74.
26. McGee SR. Evidence-based physical diagnosis. 3rd edition. Philadelphia: Elsevier/ Saunders; 2012.
27. Seemungal BM, Bronstein AM. A practical approach to acute vertigo. Pract Neurol 2008;8(4):211–21.
28. Weber KP, Aw ST, Todd MJ, et al. Head impulse test in unilateral vestibular loss: vestibulo-ocular reflex and catch-up saccades. Neurology 2008;70(6):454–63.
29. Kattah JC, Talkad AV, Wang DZ, et al. HINTS to diagnose stroke in the acute vestibular syndrome: three-step bedside oculomotor examination more sensitive than early MRI diffusion-weighted imaging. Stroke 2009;40(11):3504–10.
30. Newman-Toker DE, Kattah JC, Alvernia JE, et al. Normal head impulse test differentiates acute cerebellar strokes from vestibular neuritis. Neurology 2008;70(24 Pt 2): 2378–85.

31. Radtke A, von Brevern M, Tiel-Wilck K, et al. Self-treatment of benign paroxysmal positional vertigo: Semont maneuver vs Epley procedure. Neurology 2004;63(1):150–2.
32. Sekine K, Imai T, Sato G, et al. Natural history of benign paroxysmal positional vertigo and efficacy of Epley and Lempert maneuvers. Otolaryngol Head Neck Surg 2006;135(4):529–33.
33. van Deelen GW, Huizing EH. Use of a diuretic (Dyazide) in the treatment of Menière's disease. A double-blind cross-over placebo-controlled study. ORL J Otorhinolaryngol Relat Spec 1986;48(5):287–92.
34. Karlberg ML, Magnusson M. Treatment of acute vestibular neuronitis with glucocorticoids. Otol Neurotol 2011;32(7):1140–3.
35. Fishman JM, Burgess C, Waddell A. Corticosteroids for the treatment of idiopathic acute vestibular dysfunction (vestibular neuritis). Cochrane Database Syst Rev 2011;(5):CD008607.

Fatigue

Jennifer Wright, MD*, Kim M. O'Connor, MD

KEYWORDS

- Fatigue • Obstructive sleep apnea • Depression • Ferritin

KEY POINTS

- Further defining a patient's complaint of "fatigue" as either sleepiness, dyspnea on exertion, weakness, generalized lack of energy, or feeling down or depressed can aid in evaluation and management.
- Laboratory evaluation rarely reveals a cause for fatigue but reasonable initial studies include complete blood count, basic metabolic panel, hepatic function testing, erythrocyte sedimentation rate, thyroid-stimulating hormone, ferritin, and screening for HIV and hepatitis C in at-risk populations.
- Even in the absence of anemia, in women of child-bearing age with a ferritin less than 50 ng/mL, iron replacement is associated with improvement of subjective fatigue.
- In situations where there is a low level of clinical concern for illness, additional diagnostic testing does not improve patient reassurance.

INTRODUCTION

Fatigue is a common symptom and the presenting concern for 5% to 10% of visits in primary care.[1] Time lost at work, medical visits, and evaluation result in significant costs to patients and society. Often the underlying cause of a patient's fatigue is not found, but rarely fatigue can be the initial symptom of a life-threatening disease, such as a yet undiagnosed malignancy or heart failure. For these reasons a guide to a rational, systematic approach to evaluation of fatigue is important.

HISTORY

History is the most important part of the evaluation of a patient presenting with fatigue and acts as a guide regarding the patient's subsequent work-up. The first key aspect is to define what the patient is describing; fatigue can be used by patients to describe

Conflict of Interest Disclosures: We have no conflicts of interest to report including no financial conflicts of interest.
Role in Authorship: All authors had access to the data and had a role in writing the article.
Division of General Internal Medicine, Department of Internal Medicine, General Internal Medicine Centre, University of Washington, Box 354760, 4245 Roosevelt Way Northeast, Seattle, WA 98105, USA
* Corresponding author.
E-mail address: sonic@u.washington.edu

Med Clin N Am 98 (2014) 597–608
http://dx.doi.org/10.1016/j.mcna.2014.01.010
0025-7125/14/$ – see front matter © 2014 Elsevier Inc. All rights reserved.

medical.theclinics.com

sleepiness, dyspnea on exertion, weakness, generalized lack of energy, or feeling down or depressed. However, to a medical professional the term fatigue is typically defined as a generalized lack of energy that does not improve with sleep and gets worse with activity.

A 56-year-old man with obesity, hypertension, and osteoarthritis presents to clinic with fatigue. He reports that he feels "run down." He continues to take part in moderate daily exercise without chest pain or increased shortness of breath but he reports that when he sits at his desk he finds himself nodding off, "too fatigued to make it through the day" without a nap.

"Fatigue" can describe sleepiness; ask the patient if the sensation improves with naps and activity, if they are describing a frequent desire to fall asleep primarily when at rest. If so these symptoms are consistent with sleepiness, typically caused by an underlying sleep disorder, such as obstructive sleep apnea. The patient in this case has risk factors and symptoms suggestive of obstructive sleep apnea. Work has been done regarding components of the patient history that may help tease out if the symptom they are describing is sleepiness or fatigue (**Table 1**).

A 36-year-old woman with history of migraines presents with fatigue. She reports the fatigue is "ruining my life," she is sleeping poorly, feels too fatigued to get out of bed in the morning, too fatigued to eat, too fatigued to play with her kids. She becomes tearful as she discusses her symptoms.

Fatigue can be a symptom of depression, can be caused by a medical condition that coexists with a patient's depression, or can be a way that a patient describes a depressed mood. The fatigue this patient describes is suggestive of fatigue associated with depression. Further questioning may be helpful. Consider using the Patient Health Questionnaire-9 (**Fig. 1**), a well-validated tool that asks patients to describe the frequency of many symptoms of depression, including lack of energy. If the patient also reports many other symptoms of depression (anhedonia; feeling down, depressed, or hopeless; sleep and appetite changes, a feeling of guilt or failure) it is reasonable to focus your initial management on depression. After treatment of the depression reassess their fatigue and evaluate further if this symptom persists.

As can be seen this initial clarification regarding what the patient is describing with the word fatigue can quickly focus the differential diagnosis. An additional example is patients using the term fatigue to describe shortness of breath limiting their ability to be active, what a medical professional would describe as dyspnea on exertion,

Table 1
Questions to assist is differentiating fatigue from sleepiness

Sleepiness	Fatigue
How likely are you to doze off or fall asleep in the following situations, in contrast to just feeling tired?	How strongly do you agree with the following statements?
Sitting and reading	Exercise brings on my fatigue
Watching television	I start things without difficulty but get weak as I go on
Sitting inactive in a public place (eg, theater, meeting)	I lack energy
As a passenger in a car for an hour when circumstances permit	
Sitting and talking to someone	
Sitting quietly after lunch without alcohol	

Adapted from Bailes S, Libman E, Baltzan M, et al. Brief and distinct empiric sleepiness and fatigue scales. J Psychosom Res 2006;60:605–13.

PATIENT HEALTH QUESTIONNAIRE (PHQ-9)—Depression Scale

Patient Name _____ Date _____

Read each item carefully, and circle your response.	Not at all	Several days	More than half the days	Nearly every day
1. Over the last 2 weeks, how often have you been bothered by any of the following problems?				
a. Little interest or pleasure in doing things				
b. Feeling down, depressed, or hopeless				
c. Trouble falling asleep or staying asleep, or sleeping too much				
d. Feeling tired or having little energy				
e. Poor appetite or overeating				
f. Feeling bad about yourself, feeling that you are a failure, or feeling that you have let yourself or your family down				
g. Trouble concentrating on things such as reading the newspaper or watching television				
h. Moving or speaking so slowly that other people could have noticed or being so fidgety or restless that you have been moving around a lot more than usual				
i. Thinking that you would be better off dead or that you want to hurt yourself in some way				
2. If you checked off any problem on this questionnaire so far, how difficult have these problems made it for you to do your work, take care of things at home, or get along with other people?	Not difficult at all	Somewhat difficult	Very difficult	Extremely difficult

How to score PHQ-9
Scoring Method for Diagnosis

Major Depressive Syndrome is suggested if:
• Of the nine items, five or more are circled as at least "More than half the days"
• Either item 1a or 1b is positive, that is, at least "More than half the days"
Minor Depressive Syndrome is suggested if:
• Of the nine items, b, c, or d is circled as at least "More than half the days"
• Either item 1a or 1b is positive, that is, at least "More than half the days"

Scoring Method for Planning and Monitoring Treatment

Question One:
• To score the first question, tally each response by the number value of each response:
Not at all = 0
Several days = 1
More than half the days = 2
Nearly every day = 3
• Add the numbers together to total the score
• Interpret the score by using the guide listed below:

Score	Action
≤4	The score suggests the patient may not need depression treatment.
≥5-14	Physician uses clinical judgment about treatment, based on patient's duration of symptoms and functional impairment
≥15	Warrants treatment for depression, using antidepressant, psychotherapy, and/or a combination of treatment

Question Two:
In question two the patient's responses can be one of four: Not difficult at all, Somewhat difficult, Very difficult, Extremely difficult. The last two responses suggest that the patient's functionality is impaired. After treatment begins, the functional status is again measured to see if the patient is improving.

Fig. 1. Patient Health Questionnaire (PHQ-9)—Depression Scale. (*Courtesy of* PHQ © 1999 Pfizer Inc. All rights reserved.)

concerning for cardiac or pulmonary causes of a patient's symptoms. See **Table 2** for differential diagnoses based on character of a patient's fatigue.

In patients who have fatigue manifesting in a lack of energy, without improvement with rest, additional questions are aimed at teasing out potential life-threatening and common diagnosis. Red flag symptoms include weight loss and/or night sweats

Table 2
Differential diagnosis based on further characterization of fatigue symptoms

Symptom	Sleepiness	Shortness of Breath	Weakness	Lack of Energy
Differential diagnosis	Sleep disorders: obstructive sleep apnea	Cardiac: congestive heart failure, arrhythmia, cardiac ischemia Pulmonary: chronic obstructive pulmonary disease, reactive airway disease, pulmonary embolism, pulmonary hypertension anemia	Neurologic disease: myopathies caused by endocrinopathy or autoimmune disease	Depression, fibromyalgia, infectious processes (hepatitis C, EBV, cytomegalovirus), medication side-effect, multiple sclerosis, malignancy

concerning for occult malignancy; a history of transient focal neurologic symptoms, such as focal weakness, vision loss, or urinary incontinence concerning of multiple sclerosis; and a history of melena concerning for gastrointestinal bleeding. Examples of symptoms that could lead one to make a diagnosis of a common cause of fatigue are constipation, weight gain, and menorrhagia associated with hypothyroidism; depressed mood and early morning awakenings associated with depression; or diffuse pain associated with fibromyalgia.

There are many other aspects of the history that are also important to consider. The chronicity can be telling; sudden onset of symptoms after a febrile illness with prominent pharyngitis is concerning of Epstein-Barr virus (EBV) or cytomegalovirus. In patients with a lifelong history of fatigue it is less likely that an underlying malignancy is the cause.

Medications are a common cause of secondary fatigue. Medications commonly associated with fatigue include β-blockers; antihistamines including the nonsedating second-generation agents; narcotics; muscle relaxants; sleep aids, such as zolpidem; benzodiazepines; and some antidepressants. Of the serotonin reuptake inhibitors, paroxetine is likely the most sedating. The serotonin-norepinephrine reuptake inhibitor venlafaxine is also more commonly associated with fatigue.

Substance use, including alcohol, can lead to fatigue and therefore needs to be explored. In addition, injection drug use greatly broadens the differential diagnosis. This is an important component of the history to obtain.

PHYSICAL EXAMINATION

As one collects the patient history considerable time is spent asking about concerning symptoms, typically ruling out possible causes of secondary fatigue. The physical examination has a similar focus. Does the patient have scleral icterus concerning for undiagnosed liver disease? Do they have a goiter concerning of undiagnosed thyroid dysfunction? Does the patient have crackles on pulmonary examination concerning for a cardiac or pulmonary cause of their fatigue?

It is estimated that physical examination aids in making clear diagnosis of the cause of a patient's fatigue only 2% of the time,[2] although it is still an important component of the initial evaluation. An additional value of a complete physical examination at the initial visit for the evaluation of fatigue is that it may help build trust in your patient that you are fully evaluating their concern.

LABORATORY EVALUATION

A 52-year-old woman with a history of menorrhagia, status post hysterectomy 1 year ago, depression, and generalized anxiety currently on duloxetine and clonazepam presents with fatigue of insidious onset, bothersome over the past 3 months. She brings in a list of laboratory work she would like performed, which includes urine testing for heavy metals, Lyme disease testing, and celiac disease testing.

Often one of the most challenging aspects of evaluating a patient with nonspecific fatigue characterized by a generalized lack of energy is deciding on the appropriate scope of laboratory evaluation. Although in general the data are sparse, it seems that laboratory studies only rarely reveal the cause of a patient's fatigue; diagnosis is made after laboratory evaluation in approximately 5% of cases.[2]

Standard recommendations regarding the initial, rational laboratory evaluation include complete blood count, a basic metabolic panel, hepatic function testing, an erythrocyte sedimentation rate, thyroid dysfunction screening with a thyroid-stimulating hormone, and pregnancy testing in women of childbearing age. HIV disease and hepatitis C screening should also be considered in those not screened previously or with ongoing risk factors. Hepatitis C screening is recommended in the "baby boomer" generation (those born between 1945 and 1965) and in patients with risk factors, such as a history of injection drug use. Fatigue is the most common symptom of hepatitis C. Routine HIV screening in all adult patients is also recommended by many organizations including the US Preventative Services Task Force, although the correlation of fatigue with otherwise undiagnosed HIV infection is unclear. Ferritin testing should be considered. In randomized controlled trials treatment of menstruating females with ferritin levels of less than 50 ng/mL, even in the absence of anemia, resulted in symptomatic improvement of fatigue (**Table 3**).[3,4]

Table 3
Recommended testing for patient presenting with fatigue

Test	Medical Conditions Potentially Identified	Notes
Complete blood count	Anemia, pancytopenia, hematologic malignancy, infection	
Erythrocyte sedimentation rate	May be elevated in occult rheumatologic disease or malignancy	
Basic metabolic panel including calcium levels	Electrolyte abnormalities, renal disease, diabetes	
Liver-function tests	Occult liver disease, low protein state	
Thyroid-stimulating hormone	Hypothyroidism or hyperthyroidism	In the elderly, hyperthyroidism may present with fatigue
HIV	Occult HIV disease	
Hepatitis C	Occult hepatitis C virus infection	Screening recommended in patients born between 1945 and 1965
Ferritin	Low iron stores	Studies support that even in the absence of anemia, treatment of ferritin <50 ng/mL with iron supplements may result in clinical improvements

There are many additional tests that are frequently ordered by providers, often at the request of their patients. Unless there are specific symptoms, risk factors, or abnormalities in the initial screening laboratory evaluation these are unlikely to be useful. As more tests are ordered the risk of false-positive results also increases (**Table 4**).

There are times when testing a vitamin D level is appropriate, but evidence that hypovitaminosis D causes isolated fatigue is lacking. For example, in patients presenting with low bone density and in those presenting with diffuse bony pain one should consider osteomalacia and check vitamin D levels.

It is common for patients to inquire regarding testing of their vitamin D level based on having read about associations between low vitamin D levels and a myriad of concerning conditions, such as cardiovascular disease and cancer. Reassure patients that although there is some controversy regarding when to test and when to supplement vitamin D, in the setting of fatigue there is little controversy: it is not recommended. A large Institute of Medicine review in 2011 did not identify good evidence that vitamin D was important in prevention of nonbone health conditions, such as cancer, heart disease, or fatigue.[5] The Endocrine Society recommends screening at-risk individuals, but the indication for treatment in these patients is limited to bone health and fall prevention, not improvement in pain, fatigue, or other health outcomes.[6] Studies support that vitamin D in combination with calcium supplementation can reduce the risk of fracture in community-dwelling adults, although there is controversy regarding what dose should be recommended and in which populations of patients.[7] In addition, the US Preventative Services Task force recommends vitamin D supplementation to prevent falls in community-dwelling adults 65 years of age and older.[8] Regardless, none of the recommendations for screening or testing are for evaluation or management of fatigue.

There are several potential presentations of vitamin B_{12} deficiency including macrocytic anemia, symmetric distal polyneuropathy, and cognitive deficits. However, to present with fatigue unaccompanied with these other findings is atypical. Fatigue in isolation is not an indication for vitamin B_{12} testing.

Heavy metal toxicity can present in a variety of ways, although it is very rare that heavy metal toxicity is the cause of a patient's fatigue. The following information may be of use in discussing a patient's concerns about potential heavy metal toxicity leading to their symptoms.

Chronic lead toxicity may present with vague symptoms including fatigue, but overall this is a very rare condition. Obtaining an occupational history may be helpful.

Table 4
Tests of low utility in evaluation of isolated fatigue

Test	Data to Support
Vitamin D	No evidence to support association of vitamin D deficiency and fatigue
Vitamin B_{12}	Consider if patient has other signs/symptoms of vitamin B_{12} deficiency (eg, macrocytic anemia, lower extremity paresthesias)
Heavy metal toxicity	Indicated if have history of exposure, obtain an occupational history
Lyme disease	Consider in patients with history consistent with potential exposure and symptoms consistent with Lyme disease, not isolated fatigue
EBV/cytomegalovirus	Consider in younger patients in the setting of viral symptoms before fatigue onset
Celiac disease	Recommended by the National Institute for Health and Clinical Excellence, United Kingdom; consider if other signs/symptoms of disease (diarrhea, iron deficiency)

Exposure in adults is typically related to a job, such as the manufacturing of batteries, lead smeltering, or steel welding or cutting.[9] Consuming home-distilled alcohol and Aryvedic medications have also been associated with cases of lead toxicity. However, without history of a potential exposure testing lead levels is not recommended for evaluation of fatigue. Should testing be perused, it should be serum (blood) testing.

Current exposures to mercury in the general population are from consumption of fish, amalgam dental fillings, and thimerosal-containing vaccines, none of which commonly result in toxicity.[10] Mercury toxicity symptoms may include fatigue, but the primary symptoms caused by ingestion of mercury, which would be the manifestation if the exposure were based on excessive fish consumption, are hand and feet paresthesias, ataxia, and visual field constriction. Inhalation of mercury vapor is characterized by tremor, changes in the gums, excessive salivation, and neuropsychiatric changes in severe cases, but more typically cases are mild and characterized by mild memory difficulties and kidney injury. Working with amalgam fillings in a dental office may be the setting for these inhalation exposures. The use of thimerosal, a preservative used in multidose vials of some vaccines, such as the seasonal flu vaccine, has been extensively studied and found to be safe.

In a study of patients with metal-on-metal hip implants, report of fatigue was common, as were elevated levels of cobalt and chromium presumed to be caused by the metal-on-metal hip implant.[11] But the fatigue did not correlate with the degree of elevation, arguing against a direct relationship between the elevated metal level and fatigue.

Lyme disease is another common concern in patients with nonspecific fatigue. Clearly fatigue is a common manifestation of infection in general, but there would be other characteristic symptoms of Lyme disease should this be the cause. In the case of early, localized disease 80% of patients have erythema migrans, a red rash at the site of the tick bite that slowly expands and may develop central clearing giving it a classic bull's-eye appearance.[12] In early disseminated disease more common symptoms include meningitis, cranial nerve palsies, and less commonly AV block. In late disease monoarthritis or oligoarthritis are the most common symptoms. Fatigue alone, without these other symptoms, is not an indication for Lyme disease testing.

A controversial condition termed chronic Lyme disease is also believed to exist by some practioners. This includes post–Lyme disease syndrome, a rare and poorly understood condition that involves fatigue, widespread musculoskeletal pain, and subjective cognitive difficulties after treatment of Lyme disease.[12] It is not an indication of persistent *Borrelia burgdorferi* infection and is not an indication for prolonged antibiotic therapy. Another group of patients who may be identified as having chronic Lyme disease includes patients without a clear or documented history of *B burgdorferi* infection but with nonspecific signs and symptoms, such as fatigue and arthralgias. In these cases, patients should not be treated with antibiotics either.

Testing for Lyme disease is in the form of serologic testing for antibodies. Not surprisingly in early, localized disease the antibodies are often not yet present leading to a low sensitivity of the test. Another difficulty in interpretation of the results of Lyme disease serology is that even after effective treatment the antibodies may remain positive for years. This would not be an indication of persistent infection or an indication for prolonged therapy.[12]

Fatigue is a common symptom in patients with infections, and there are many viral infections that can persist in the human body for prolonged to indefinite periods of time. Therefore, there has been significant interest in viral etiologies of fatigue, chronic fatigue syndrome (CFS) in particular. Associations between many viral infections and fatigue have been investigated with particular interest in EBV, cytomegalovirus, and human herpesvirus-6. Readers may recall a study released in 2009 that found an association between xenotropic murine leukemia virus–related virus and CFS, a study that was later retracted, the finding found to likely be caused by specimen contamination.[13] Chronic viral infection leading to fatigue remains an area of investigation, although at this point there is not sufficient evidence of a relationship to justify testing all patients with fatigue. EBV testing should primarily be reserved for patients younger than 40 years who present with fatigue that began after an episode of pharyngitis.[14]

Celiac disease, when undiagnosed and thus untreated, can result in many health problems, some of these associated with fatigue, such as iron deficiency. However, in the absence of symptoms and signs of celiac disease, such as diarrhea, unexplained iron deficiency, or profound vitamin D deficiency, testing for celiac disease as a standard screening test in patients with fatigue is not generally recommended. That said, there are some organizations that do recommend testing for this, such as the National Institute for Health and Clinical Excellence, out of the United Kingdom.[14] Classically, celiac disease has been thought to be a disease of people of Northern European descent; therefore, it is possible that the threshold for testing is lower in European nations. However, recent research has indicated that celiac disease is not isolated to patients of Northern European descent; it is a more globally distributed disease, and there is concern for increasing prevalence of the disease.[15] Screening recommendations could change in the future.

MANAGEMENT IN THE SETTING OF A NONDIAGNOSTIC EVALUATION

In a follow-up study of patients presenting to their primary care provider with fatigue, half were without a diagnosis to explain their symptoms in the year after their presentation.[16] There were a variety of diagnosis made in the other half of the patients that were possibly the cause of their fatigue. Of these, musculoskeletal problems were most common (19.4% of patients), most being lower extremity joint problems and back problems. Psychological problems were the second most common diagnosis category (16.5%), common diagnoses in this group being "strain," "burnout," depression, and anxiety. Only 8.2% of patients were given a diagnosis that the authors qualified as "clear somatic pathology" in the year after their presentation with fatigue, including anemia, thyroid dysfunction, diabetes, malignancy, rheumatoid arthritis, and heart failure.

In the 50% of patients without a diagnosis, what is to be done? Frequently the instinct is to order more tests. Even when providers suspect that a diagnosis may not be found, more tests are frequently ordered with the belief that this will offer the patient reassurance. In a systematic review assessing for evidence of patient reassurance after diagnostic testing in situations where there was a low level of clinician concern for serious illness (symptoms including dyspepsia, low back pain, and palpitations) there was no evidence of patient reassurance.[17] In this study 14 trials were identified comparing testing with nontesting for symptoms believed to be benign, meaning that based on clinical evaluation, the pretest probability of serious disease was low. There was no pattern of patient reassurance found, and patients did not have less concern about their illness, less health anxiety, or less symptoms based on having testing performed. The only possible benefit was a reduction in subsequent clinic visits, but the number of patients needed to test to avoid one clinic visit was on the order of 16 to 26 patients.

In the situation when the initial evaluation for fatigue is nondiagnostic there should be frank discussion with the patient regarding how to proceed. There are several key components: acknowledgment of the patient's symptoms, patient reassurance that there will be active on-going management in the form of symptom-focused treatments, and a plan for follow-up regarding their on-going symptoms and to assess for development of any new symptoms.

Acknowledgment of the patient's symptoms and in turn working to develop a collaborative, supportive relationship with the patient is recommended. It is often difficult for patients and providers to accept that there may not be a medical explanation for symptoms, but a shift of focus of your visits from diagnosis to symptom management is very important. This also needs to be something that the patient accepts in order for it to be successful. In a study regarding effective management of patients with medically unexplained symptoms, strategies to motivate patient involvement in their care and formulation of patient-centered treatment plans was successful in reducing symptom scores.[18] The provider should work with the patient to identify the most bothersome symptom they are experiencing, develop a treatment plan that is acceptable to the patient, and also develop a self-management plan. Schedule patients for frequent follow-up, slowly spacing out follow-up appointments over time. This too may foster a sense of support and encourage patient engagement in treatment recommendations.

Treatment of idiopathic fatigue is not highly evidence based, but there are several treatments that can be considered based on their benefit in similar conditions. A discussion of sleep quantity and quality should be part of treatment in all patients with fatigue. In the general population, high-quality sleep is associated with better overall sense of well-being and less fatigue.[19,20] The principles of good sleep hygiene should be reviewed with all patients with idiopathic fatigue (**Table 5**).

Physical activity is also something that should be recommended to all patients with idiopathic fatigue. Studies indicate that among patients with fatigue in the setting of otherwise good health, regular exercise decreases symptoms of fatigue.[21,22] When low-intensity versus moderate-intensity activity was compared, although both resulted in improved "vigor" or energy level, the benefit on fatigue was more impressive in patients taking part in low-intensity activity. An example of low-intensity activity is using an exercise bike for 30 minutes three times a week, benefits seen by week 6. The concept that low-intensity exercise may have more benefit on symptoms of fatigue than higher-intensity activity is consistent with the exercise interventions found to be of benefit in patients with two other conditions associated with significant

Table 5 Sleep hygiene measures	
Generally Agreed on Sleep Hygiene Measures	**Description**
Eliminate bedroom noise	Can use sound "screening," such as a white noise machine
Minimize napping	If napping necessary, limit to less than 20 min
Exercise	Exercise regularly but avoid exercising in the evening because this may result in difficulty initiating sleep
Avoid/limit caffeine	If drinking caffeinated beverage (eg, coffee) limit to one beverage in the morning
Avoid alcohol	Can result in awakenings after initially falling asleep
Eat light evening snack	Exception to this recommendation: patients with gastroesophageal reflux should not eat evening snack because this will likely cause reflux and in turn disturb sleep

Adapted from Hauri PJ. Sleep/wake lifestyle modifications: sleep hygiene. In: Barkoukis TJ, Matheson JK, Ferber R, et al, editors. Therapy in sleep medicine. Philadelphia: Elsevier; 2012. p. 151–60.

fatigue, fibromyalgia and CFS. In patients with CFS and fibromyalgia graded exercise therapy has been shown to be of benefit. This involves very slowly increasing a patient's level of physical activity over the course of weeks to months.[23,24]

Another therapy often recommended for treatment of fatigue in the setting of CFS and fibromyalgia is cognitive behavioral therapy. When available this therapy should also be extended to patients with idiopathic fatigue.

It is also critical to assess for comorbid conditions and treat those appropriately. Depression and anxiety can coexist with or be causative of fatigue. If an antidepressant medication is being considered take into account the patient's significant fatigue symptoms when choosing the agents to be prescribed. Of the serotonin reuptake inhibitors, paroxetine may be more sedating and therefore should be avoided in patients with significant fatigue. Bupropion is an antidepressant medication that tends to be activating and therefore should more strongly be considered. If the patient also has pain symptoms a serotonin-norepinephrine reuptake inhibitor may be a good choice, potentially treating mood symptoms and pain symptoms with a single agent.

Sleep disorders can also be causative or coexist with fatigue. Pharmacologic treatment may be challenging because medications to treat insomnia are by definition sedating, but cautious treatment should be considered because good sleep can in turn improve fatigue.

CHRONIC FATIGUE SYNDROME

A subset of patients with long-standing idiopathic fatigue may meet diagnostic criteria of CFS. In addition to fatigue lasting more than 6 months and unrevealing laboratory evaluation (overall consistent with the laboratory studies recommended previously) patients with CFS often have additional symptoms, such as sore throat, tender lymph nodes, and polyarthralgias (**Box 1**). Management of CFS is essentially the same as that

---

Box 1
Centers for Disease Control and Prevention diagnostic criteria for CFS

Consider a diagnosis of CFS if these three criteria are met:

1. The individual has severe chronic fatigue for 6 or more consecutive months that is not caused by ongoing exertion or other medical conditions associated with fatigue (these other conditions need to be ruled out by a doctor after diagnostic tests have been conducted)

2. The fatigue significantly interferes with daily activities and work

3. The individual concurrently has four or more of the following eight symptoms:

   - Postexertion malaise lasting more than 24 hours
   - Unrefreshing sleep
   - Significant impairment of short-term memory or concentration
   - Muscle pain
   - Multijoint pain without swelling or redness
   - Headaches of a new type, pattern, or severity
   - Tender cervical or axillary lymph nodes
   - A sore throat that is frequent or recurring

From Centers for Disease Control and Prevention. Chronic fatigue syndrome. Available at: http://www.cdc.gov/cfs/diagnosis/index.html.

suggested for long-standing idiopathic fatigue including graded exercise therapy; cognitive behavioral therapy; and treatment of comorbid conditions, such as depression and insomnia.[25]

In summary, although fatigue is a common symptom in primary care, frequently a clear biomedical cause is not identified and, in those cases, evaluation and management offers many challenges. On presentation, first work to discover what symptom the patient is describing with the word fatigue: perhaps sleepiness, depressed mood, or lack of energy. In the setting of fatigue that manifests as generalized lack of energy, made worse with activity and not improved with rest, then perform a thorough history followed by a limited initial laboratory screen. Should this be unrevealing, the management of patients' subjective symptoms and comorbid medical conditions should become the focus.

REFERENCES

1. Nijrolder I, van der Windt DA, van der Horst HE. Prognosis of fatigue and functioning in primary care: a 1-year follow-up study. Ann Fam Med 2008;6(6): 519–27.
2. Lane TJ, Matthews DA, Manu P. The low yield of physical examinations and laboratory investigations of patients with chronic fatigue. Am J Med Sci 1990;299(5): 313–8.
3. Verdon F, Burnand B, Stubi CL, et al. Iron supplementation for unexplained fatigue in non-anaemic women: double blind randomised placebo controlled trial. BMJ 2003;326(7399):1124.
4. Vaucher P, Druais PL, Waldvogel S, et al. Effect of iron supplementation on fatigue in nonanemic menstruating women with low ferritin: a randomized controlled trial. CMAJ 2012;184(11):1247–54.
5. Institute of Medicine (US). Committee to review dietary reference intakes for vitamin D and calcium. Institute of Medicine (US); 2011.
6. Holick MF, Binkley NC, Bischoff-Ferrari HA, et al. Evaluation, treatment, and prevention of vitamin D deficiency: an Endocrine Society clinical practice guideline. J Clin Endocrinol Metab 2011;96(7):1911–30.
7. Chung M, Lee J, Terasawa T, et al. Vitamin D with or without calcium supplementation for prevention of cancer and fractures: an updated meta-analysis for the U.S. Preventive Services Task Force. Ann Intern Med 2011;155(12): 827–38.
8. Moyer V. Prevention of falls in community-dwelling older adults: U.S. Preventive Services Task Force recommendation statement. Ann Intern Med 2012;157(3): 197–204.
9. Abadin H, Ashizawa A, Stevens YW, et al, ATSDR. Toxicologic profile for lead. US Department of Health & Human Services, Public Health Service Agency for Toxic Substances and Disease Registry; 2007.
10. Clarkson TW, Magos L, Myers GJ. The toxicology of mercury–current exposures and clinical manifestations. N Engl J Med 2003;349(18):1731–7.
11. Leikin JB, Karydes HC, Whiteley PM, et al. Outpatient toxicology clinic experience of patients with hip implants. Clin Toxicol (Phila) 2013;51(4):230–6.
12. Wright WF, Riedel DJ, Talwani R, et al. Diagnosis and management of Lyme disease. Am Fam Physician 2012;85(11):1086–93.
13. Lombardi VC, Ruscetti FW, Das Gupta J, et al. Detection of an infectious retrovirus, XMRV, in blood cells of patients with chronic fatigue syndrome. Science 2009;326(5952):585–9.

14. NICE: National Institute for Health and Care Excellence. Tiredness/fatigue in adults. NICE: National Institute for Health and Care Excellence guidelines; 2009.

15. Rubio-Tapia A, Murray JA. Celiac disease. Curr Opin Gastroenterol 2010;26(2): 116–22.

16. Nijrolder I, van der Windt D, de Vries H, et al. Diagnoses during follow-up of patients presenting with fatigue in primary care. CMAJ 2009;181(10):683–7.

17. Rolfe A, Burton C. Reassurance after diagnostic testing with a low pretest probability of serious disease: systematic review and meta-analysis. JAMA Intern Med 2013;173(6):407–16.

18. Smith RC, Lyles JS, Gardiner JC, et al. Primary care clinicians treat patients with medically unexplained symptoms: a randomized controlled trial. J Gen Intern Med 2006;21(7):671–7.

19. Alapin I, Fichten CS, Libman E, et al. How is good and poor sleep in older adults and college students related to daytime sleepiness, fatigue, and ability to concentrate? J Psychosom Res 2000;49(5):381–90.

20. Pilcher JJ, Ginter DR, Sadowsky B. Sleep quality versus sleep quantity: relationships between sleep and measures of health, well-being and sleepiness in college students. J Psychosom Res 1997;42(6):583–96.

21. Puetz TW, Flowers SS, O'Connor PJ. A randomized controlled trial of the effect of aerobic exercise training on feelings of energy and fatigue in sedentary young adults with persistent fatigue. Psychother Psychosom 2008;77(3):167–74.

22. O'Connor PJ, Puetz TW. Chronic physical activity and feelings of energy and fatigue. Med Sci Sports Exerc 2005;37(2):299–305.

23. White PD, Goldsmith KA, Johnson AL, et al. Comparison of adaptive pacing therapy, cognitive behaviour therapy, graded exercise therapy, and specialist medical care for chronic fatigue syndrome (PACE): a randomised trial. Lancet 2011; 377(9768):823–36.

24. Maquet D, Demoulin C, Croisier JL, et al. Benefits of physical training in fibromyalgia and related syndromes. Ann Readapt Med Phys 2007;50(6):363–8, 356–62.

25. Yancey JR, Thomas SM. Chronic fatigue syndrome: diagnosis and treatment. Am Fam Physician 2012;86(8):741–6.

Common Anal Problems

Jared Wilson Klein, MD, MPH

KEYWORDS

- Hemorrhoids • Perirectal abscess • Anal fistula • Anal fissure • Fecal incontinence

KEY POINTS

- Unusual presentations of common anal problems may herald underlying systemic disease.
- There are several medical therapies available for the treatment of anal fissures, including nitroglycerin, diltiazem, and botulinum toxin.
- Management of internal hemorrhoids depends on the severity of symptoms.
- Perirectal abscesses require drainage and commonly result in fistula formation.
- Fecal incontinence is common in elderly populations. In younger patients, it should prompt a thorough evaluation not only for sphincter dysfunction, but also neurologic and gastrointestinal disorders.
- Anal itching is most often related to poor anal hygiene.
- Rectal prolapse typically requires definitive surgical fixation.

INTRODUCTION

The anus has a critical, if thankless, function. It permits the retention and subsequent voluntary, timed evacuation of fecal matter.

Anatomic Pearls

The anus represents the terminus of the gastrointestinal tract and stretches from the pelvic floor (levator ani) to the skin surface (**Fig. 1**). The dentate line is the embryologic divide between endoderm and ectoderm; as such, tissue proximal to this point does not receive somatic innervation and is insensate. Distal from the dentate line, the anoderm is a transitional zone between columnar and squamous epithelium. The tripartite sphincter complex includes the internal sphincter (located more proximal and closer to the lumen of the anus), the external sphincter (slightly more distal and wrapping around the internal sphincter), and the puborectalis (a U-shaped, sling-like muscle at the anorectal junction).

Physiologic Refresher

The internal and external sphincters are the workhorses of the anus. The internal sphincter receives parasympathetic innervation and relaxes involuntarily with

Disclosures: None.
Division of General Internal Medicine, Department of Medicine, Harborview Medical Center, University of Washington, 325 Ninth Avenue, Box 359780, Seattle, WA 98104, USA
E-mail address: jaredwk@uw.edu

Med Clin N Am 98 (2014) 609–623
http://dx.doi.org/10.1016/j.mcna.2014.01.011
0025-7125/14/$ – see front matter © 2014 Elsevier Inc. All rights reserved.

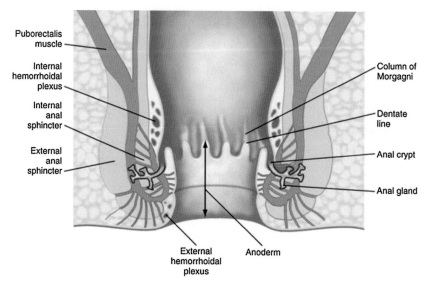

Fig. 1. Anal anatomy. (*From* Marcello PW. Diseases of the anorectum. In: Feldman M, Friedman LS, Brandt LJ, editors. Sleisenger and Fordtran's gastrointestinal and liver disease: pathophysiology, diagnosis and management. 9th edition. Philadelphia: Elsevier; 2010; with permission.)

distention of the rectal vault. This triggers the urge to defecate. The external sphincter, innervated by the pudendal nerve, is under voluntary control, and its integrity is crucial for maintaining fecal continence. The puborectalis plays an adjunctive role in maintaining continence. The anal glands (also called the crypts of Morgagni) and the venous hemorrhoidal plexuses facilitate lubrication during defecation.

ANAL FISSURES
Symptoms

The hallmark of an anal fissure is severe anal pain. This tends to be worse with bowel movements and with direct pressure on the site (eg, sitting). Some fissures are traumatic (eg, passage of hard stool, receptive anal intercourse, or insertion of a foreign body such as enema or endoscope), while others are idiopathic. Acute fissures, which have been present for days to weeks, tend to bleed slightly, and patients may report red blood on the tissue. Chronic fissures have been present for months or longer; they bleed less commonly and tend to have hyperkeratotic edges.

Diagnostic Test/Imaging Study

Anal fissures can be diagnosed with a classic history and simple external examination of the anus and perineum. By applying traction on the buttocks, the fissure can be visualized radiating out from the anus, typically in the midline and usually posterior in orientation. Acute fissures have the appearance of lacerations, while chronic lacerations are more fibrotic and may have a sentinel skin tag at the distal end (**Fig. 2**).[1]

Differential Diagnosis

Other causes of anal pain and bleeding can masquerade as fissures, including abscess, fistula, and hemorrhoids (**Box 1**). Additionally, anal fissures with any lateral orientation (not in the midline) should prompt investigation into secondary causes

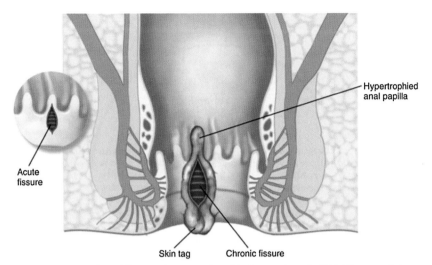

Fig. 2. Appearance of anal fissures (acute vs chronic). (*From* Marcello PW. Diseases of the ano-rectum. In: Feldman M, Friedman LS, Brandt LJ, editors. Sleisenger and Fordtran's gastrointestinal and liver disease: pathophysiology, diagnosis and management. 9th edition. Philadelphia: Elsevier; 2010; with permission.)

such as anal cancer, human immunodeficiency virus (HIV), inflammatory bowel disease, syphilis, or tuberculosis (**Fig. 3**).[2]

Management

Most acute anal fissures will resolve within a few weeks following institution of conservative measures such as sitz baths and stool softeners. There are several medical therapies available for chronic fissures aimed at reducing sphincter spasm (**Table 1**).[3,4] Both topical nitroglycerin and topical diltiazem have been shown to improve healing of chronic anal fissures, although a recent head-to-head trial suggested the superiority of diltiazem.[5] Botulinum toxin can be injected into the internal sphincter to alleviate spasm, although this may result in temporary incontinence of flatus and/or stool. Patients who fail these therapies are commonly referred for surgical sphincterotomy; however, this procedure comes with a risk of fecal incontinence.[6] For fissures associated with systemic disease, therapy should be directed at the underlying cause.

HEMORRHOIDS
Symptoms

Most often, patients with hemorrhoids report rectal bleeding. Although this is typically bright red in color, the quantity can range from scant blood on the tissue to more

---

Box 1
Anal fissure Differential diagnosis

- Anal fistula
- Perirectal abscess
- Thrombosed hemorrhoid
- If lateral orientation (not midline), consider underlying pathology (see **Fig. 3**)

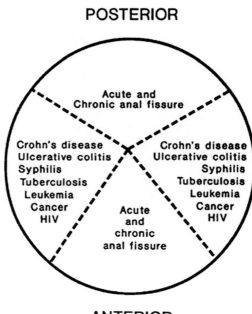

POSTERIOR

Acute and
Chronic anal fissure

Crohn's disease
Ulcerative colitis
Syphilis
Tuberculosis
Leukemia
Cancer
HIV

Crohn's disease
Ulcerative colitis
Syphilis
Tuberculosis
Leukemia
Cancer
HIV

Acute
and
chronic
anal fissure

ANTERIOR

Fig. 3. Etiology of anal fissures by location. (*From* Castillo E, Margolin DA. Anal fissures: diagnosis and management. Techniques in Gastrointestinal Endoscopy 2004;6(1):14; with permission.)

significant hemorrhage. This variation is caused by the vascularity of hemorrhoidal tissues, which act to cushion the anus during defecation (see **Fig. 1**). There may also be mucous-like discharge. Patients sometimes report discomfort, but usually this is dull in nature. Internal hemorrhoids are typically painless, as their innervation arises from above the dentate line, while external hemorrhoids can be acutely pruritic or painful, particularly when thrombosed (**Fig. 4**). Patients commonly note a mass protruding from or near the anus, usually worse with straining or Valsalva maneuver.

Diagnostic Test/Imaging Study

Like so many anal conditions, the diagnosis relies primarily upon history and physical examination. The buttocks should be spread to reveal the anus. Hemorrhoids are

Table 1
Medical therapies for chronic anal fissures

Regimen	Adverse Effects and Precautions
Topical nitroglycerin 0.2%–0.4% ointment, apply 1 in to anus every 12 h for up to 3 wk	Headache, should not be administered with PDE-5 inhibitors (eg, sildenafil)
Topical diltiazem 2% gel or ointment, apply small amount to anus 3 times daily[a,b]	Headache (less common than nitroglycerin)
Intrasphincteric botulinum toxin injection, 10–100 units once[a]	Temporary incontinence

Abbreviation: PDE, phosphodiesterase.
[a] Not approved by the US Food and Drug Administration.
[b] Not commercially available in the United States, must be compounded.

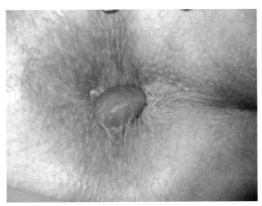

Fig. 4. Thrombosed external hemorrhoid. (*From* Madoff RD. Diseases of the rectum and anus. In: Goldman L, Schafer AI, editors. Goldman's Cecil medicine. 24th edition. Philadelphia: Elsevier; 2012; with permission.)

typically flesh-toned or slightly purple, mucous-covered nodules. If necessary, the examiner can ask the patient to bear down in order to expose nonexternal hemorrhoids. Anoscopy is an easy, in-office maneuver to better visualize the anus, particularly internal hemorrhoids. The device includes a cylinder and obturator component, typically disposable and made of clear plastic (**Fig. 5**). It is coated in water-soluble lubricant before being gently inserted into the anus. Leaving the external cylinder in place, the obturator can be removed, permitting the examiner to better visualize the entire anal mucosa for abnormalities.

Differential Diagnosis

Clinicians must be cautious not to misattribute rectal bleeding to hemorrhoids, thereby overlooking more proximal causes such as malignancy, inflammatory bowel disease, or arteriovenous malformations (**Box 2**). This is particularly important in older adults and patients with risk factors for these diseases. It is also necessary to differentiate the presence of protruding hemorrhoids (containing only mucosa) from rectal prolapse (including full thickness of the bowel wall; more details in subsequent section).

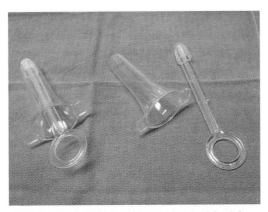

Fig. 5. Anoscope with obturator inserted (*left*) and removed (*right*).

Box 2
Hemorrhoid Differential diagnosis (DDx)

- Proximal GI bleeding
  - Malignancy
  - Arteriovenous malformation
  - Inflammatory bowel disease
  - Diverticuli
- Rectal prolapse
- Anal fissure
- Anal fistula

Management

The foundation of therapy for all hemorrhoids is treatment of constipation in order to reduce straining. Adequate hydration and increased fiber intake, either in the form of foods rich in fiber or fiber supplements (eg, psyllium), should be recommended to all patients.[7] Sitz baths can also ameliorate acute symptoms. There are several topical remedies used for relief of acute symptoms, many of which are available over the counter and include topical corticosteroids (hydrocortisone 1% cream/ointment), astringents (witch hazel), and topical anesthetics (dibucaine and pramoxine). Evidence is lacking that these preparations speed resolution of the hemorrhoids. Nevertheless, these treatments are often recommended, particularly in the acute phase. Although analgesia is sometimes required, opioids should be avoided because of their adverse effects on gastrointestinal (GI) motility. Treatment of internal hemorrhoids is guided by the stage, which is based on the patient's symptoms (**Table 2**).[8] Patients with significant symptoms and grade 3 and especially grade 4 symptoms may be offered more invasive treatments, including ligation banding and surgical hemorrhoidectomy.[9] Although these procedures can be performed in the office, patients are often referred to a specialist, particularly for hemorrhoidectomy. The presence of a thrombosed external hemorrhoid often requires surgical management with thrombectomy, particularly within 72 hours of symptom onset. Adverse effects of invasive treatments include local pain, abscess formation (or other infection), and bleeding.

Table 2
Grading and treatment of internal hemorrhoids

Stage	Diagnostic Features	Treatment
1	Bleeding, often painless	• Avoid constipation, increase fiber intake
2	Protrusion with spontaneous reduction	• Avoid constipation, increase fiber intake • Rubber band ligation • Sclerotherapy
3	Protrusion requiring manual reduction	• Avoid constipation, increase fiber intake • Rubber band ligation • Sclerotherapy • Elective referral for hemorrhoidectomy
4	Protrusion with inability to manually reduce	• Avoid constipation, increase fiber intake • Elective referral for hemorrhoidectomy
Thrombosed	Severe pain, purple color change	• Urgent surgical thrombectomy

PERIRECTAL ABSCESSES
Symptoms

Abscesses of the perirectal and perianal areas typically occur when the anal glands or crypts (see **Fig. 1**) become occluded, permitting retention of bacteria and inflammatory cells.[10] These lesions commonly present with dull, aching pain in the perineum as well as fevers. Patients with perirectal abscess can occasionally present with sepsis and critical illness, as is the case with Fournier gangrene. For this reason, rectal examination is mandatory in the evaluation of febrile patients without an obvious source, although caution is urged in patients with neutropenia.

Diagnostic Test/Imaging Study

Most perirectal abscesses can be diagnosed based on a typical history as well as rectal examination. Anoscopy is uncomfortable and often unnecessary. Abscesses are categorized based on location, with perianal and ischiorectal abscesses being the most common (**Fig. 6**).[11] Supralevator abscesses are much less common. Advanced imaging techniques, such as computed tomography (CT) or ultrasound, are occasionally necessary to identify the location and extent of infections, particularly for deeper abscesses (eg, supralevator and ischiorectal sites). These tests may also be helpful in excluding the presence of other entities.

Differential Diagnosis

Anal fistulas are part of the same disease continuum as perirectal abscesses and can also present with pain and swelling, although there is often also drainage (**Box 3**). It may be important to exclude the presence of prostatitis or a prostatic abscess in men without an obviously visible perirectal abscess. This can be done via physical

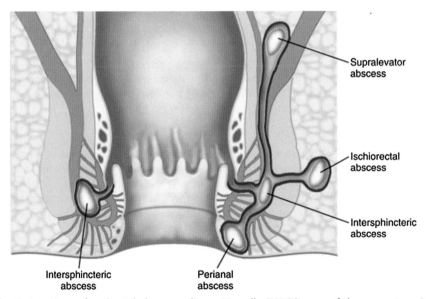

Fig. 6. Locations of perirectal abscesses. (*From* Marcello PW. Diseases of the anorectum. In: Feldman M, Friedman LS, Brandt LJ, editors. Sleisenger and Fordtran's gastrointestinal and liver disease: pathophysiology, diagnosis and management. 9th edition. Philadelphia: Elsevier; 2010; with permission.)

Box 3
Perirectal abscess DDx

- Anal fistula
- Prostatitis/prostatic abscess (men only)
- Infected pilonidal cyst
- Thrombosed hemorrhoid (rare)

---

examination, sometimes in concert with advanced imaging techniques. Pilonidal cysts can occasionally become infected, but will typically be located in the midline and posterior from the anal verge. Thrombosed hemorrhoids, although similarly painful, are much less common and have a typical purpuric appearance. It is always important to consider the possibility of underlying bowel pathology (particularly inflammatory bowel disease, malignancy or sexually transmitted disease) in patients with recurrent, severe, or deep abscesses.

Management

As antibiotics will not penetrate the abscess cavity, it is crucial to drain these pockets. For perianal abscesses, bedside incision and drainage can be performed after appropriate preparation of the site. Postdrainage care should involve sitz baths, stool bulking, and wound care. Deeper abscesses and those involving the anal sphincter require surgical consultation in order to ensure complete drainage and to maintain sphincter integrity. The use of antibiotics after drainage is controversial, although they are often prescribed for patients with immunocompromising conditions, underlying bowel pathology, or diabetes.[12] If prescribed, antibiotics should cover common enteric pathogens (**Box 4**).[13] Despite treatment, upwards of 50% of perirectal abscesses will result in the formation of an anal fistula.[14]

ANAL FISTULAS
Symptoms

Anal fistulas, most often the sequelae of perirectal abscesses, typically present with drainage. This is a result of the persistent tract between the abscess cavity and the anus. There may also be pain, bleeding, or swelling in the area.

Diagnostic Test/Imaging Study

Given the discomfort that occurs with probing these lesions, anal fistulas may need to be examined after administration of sedation or anesthesia. Fistulas will often appear as an opening in the skin beyond the anal verge. Occasionally a fibrous cord or tract may be palpable. Anoscopy can aid in the identification of an internal opening, although the patient may not tolerate this examination. Fistula severity is based on the degree of sphincter involvement (**Fig. 7**).

Box 4
Oral antibiotics covering common enteric pathogens

- Trimethoprim-sulfamethoxazole and metronidazole
- Amoxicillin with clavulanic acid
- Moxifloxacin

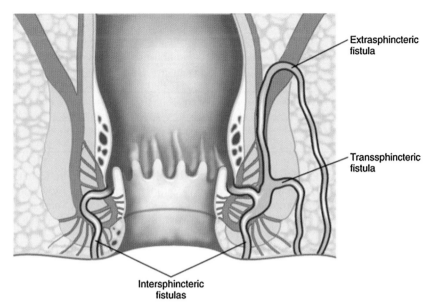

Extrasphincteric
fistula

Transsphincteric
fistula

Intersphincteric
fistulas

Fig. 7. Locations of anal fistulas. (*From* Marcello PW. Diseases of the anorectum. In: Feldman M, Friedman LS, Brandt LJ, editors. Sleisenger and Fordtran's gastrointestinal and liver disease: pathophysiology, diagnosis and management. 9th edition. Philadelphia: Elsevier; 2010; with permission.)

Differential Diagnosis

Rarely, anal fistulas may be caused by underlying systemic diseases, including inflammatory bowel disease, malignancy, sexually transmitted infections, or pelvic radiation (**Box 5**). This is particularly true in the case of extrasphincteric fistulas, which connect from the exterior directly to the rectum, as well as with multiple or chronic fistulas. It is also important to exclude the possibility of an inadequately drained abscess cavity.

Management

Anal fistulas require referral for surgical treatment, typically by opening the fistulous tract and allowing it to heal via secondary intent (**Table 3**).[12,15] This can be challenging, depending on the degree of involvement of the sphincter, and may lead to postoperative incontinence. High-grade fistulas require advanced surgical techniques in an attempt to reconstruct the sphincter musculature and maintain continence.

FECAL INCONTINENCE
Symptoms

Incontinence of stool is defined as involuntary loss of external sphincter control resulting in inadvertent passage of fecal matter. Passing small amounts of stool with flatus

---

Box 5
Anal fistula DDx

- Incompletely drained perirectal abscess
- Extrasphincteric or extensive fistulas, consider underlying pathology

Table 3
Categorization of anal fistulas

Location	Sphincter Involvement	Risk of Incontinence	Treatment
Intersphincteric	Internal	Uncommon (0%–15%)	Fistulotomy, fibrin glue injection, fistula plug
Trans-sphincteric	Internal and external	Intermediate	Fistulotomy, fibrin glue injection, fistula plug
Extrasphincteric	Internal and external	Significant (25%–50%)	Fistulotomy, endorectal flap, seton drain

or immediately following bowel movements can be physiologic, but more significant incontinence requires additional investigation. Often episodes are provoked by increased intra-abdominal pressure (eg, straining, coughing, bending). Fecal incontinence may represent a late-effect of vaginal delivery; therefore it is more prevalent in women with pelvic floor weakness and comorbid urinary incontinence. The incidence of fecal incontinence also increases with advancing age as well as comorbid GI symptoms, particularly diarrhea or constipation. It is a common symptom in patients over the age of 80, with a prevalence of 10.4% in older women.[16] In is more common in elderly patients with dementia, and in institutionalized patients. It is important to remember that patients may be reluctant to discuss their symptoms due to social stigma and embarrassment.

Diagnostic Test/Imaging Study

Although history is the primary diagnostic tool for eliciting the presence and underlying etiology of fecal incontinence, there are several other diagnostic tools available.[17] Simple rectal examination provides the examiner a general sense of sphincter tone as well as pointing to underlying diseases. Patients may require endoscopic examination of the colon to identify underlying malignancy or inflammation. More advanced methods include anal manometry (to quantify sphincter tone), pudendal nerve testing (to assess for delayed conduction, suggesting nerve damage), and anal ultrasound (to look for anatomic muscle damage or other structural abnormalities).[18] These tests are best performed in a specialized laboratory and require referral to a gastroenterologist or colorectal surgeon. In elderly patients, in whom the prevalence of fecal incontinence is so common, work up should be focused on history and examination, and testing reserved only for those patients whose history and examination point to a secondary cause.

Differential Diagnosis

There is a broad differential for the symptom of fecal incontinence (**Box 6**). The primary task is to differentiate primary fecal incontinence (eg, as a result of pelvic floor weakness and/or sphincter dysfunction) from secondary incontinence (eg, related to an underlying neurologic or GI disorder) (**Table 4**).

Box 6
Primary fecal incontinence DDx

- Obstetric sphincter damage
- Surgical sphincter damage (fistulectomy, hemorrhoidectomy)
- Pelvic floor weakness

Table 4
Selected secondary causes of fecal incontinence

	Etiology	Typical Symptoms
Neurologic	Dementia	Memory impairment, comorbid urinary incontinence
	Stroke	Acute, focal neurologic impairment
	Brain mass	Subacute, focal neurologic impairment
	Caudaequina syndrome	Back pain, leg weakness, groin or leg numbness
	Diabetic neuropathy	Comorbid peripheral neuropathy, retinopathy
	Multiple sclerosis	Gait abnormalities, sensory disturbances
Neuromuscular	Myasthenia gravis	Diplopia, bulbar symptoms (dysphagia, dysarthria)
	Muscular dystrophy	Proximal weakness, gait abnormalities
	Toxin (organophosphate, snake venom)	Acute onset, appropriate exposure history
Gastrointestinal	Inflammatory bowel disease	Diarrhea (may be bloody), abdominal pain
	Severe diarrhea	Usually apparent on history
	Fecal impaction	Rectal pain, mixed constipation/diarrhea
	Proctitis	Rectal pain, history of pelvic radiation or ulcerative colitis

Management

Once secondary causes have been identified and treated, the management of primary fecal incontinence involves supportive and surgical options.[19] Supportive measures include protective undergarments and scheduled voiding. Some patients have found significant improvement in symptoms via biofeedback techniques.[20] In patients with significant diarrhea, bulking agents (eg, psyllium) and antidiarrheal medications (eg, loperamide) may provide some relief. Various injectable materials, including silicone and polymer gels, can be injected into the mucosa to narrow the anal canal.[21] These may be considered for patients who have failed other conservative approaches or have focal internal sphincter dysfunction. Sphincteroplasty is the gold standard therapy, but it is reserved for patients who have failed conservative measures or who have significant incontinence.

PRURITIS ANI
Symptoms

Anal itching (also termed pruritis ani or anusitis) is a common symptom.[22] The itching is usually centered around the sphincter, but may also involve the perineum and gluteal cleft. Pain and irritation are commonly associated complaints. Scant bleeding may be present, and some patients report a rash, although this is often difficult to self-identify.

Diagnostic Test/Imaging Study

The primary diagnostic tool is a careful physical examination of the perianal region for signs of poor hygiene and/or primary anal disorders. A specimen can be collected, if indicated. Options include skin scraping, punch biopsy, and transparent tape testing (**Table 5**).

Table 5
Diagnostic testing options for pruritis ani

Test Name	Used to Diagnose...	How to Obtain Sample
Skin scraping	*Candida* or tinea infection	Gently scrape the leading edge of a rash with a scalpel, collect skin flakes onto slide, treat with potassium hydroxide, visualize fungal or yeast elements with light microscopy
Punch biopsy	Malignancy or primary dermatologic condition	Infiltrate local anesthetic, stabilize the skin, apply firm pressure with 3 or 6 mm punch tool, squeeze the site and snip the peduncle with scissors, ensure hemostasis, send the specimen in buffered formalin (or other solution, depending on laboratory specifications and requested testing)
Transparent tape test	Pinworm infection	Drape clear tape around the end of a glass microscope slide with adhesive surface outwards, spread buttocks and gently dap slide on anus, flip tape so adhesive surface adheres to slide, visualize nematodes with light microscopy

Differential Diagnosis

The most common cause of pruritis ani is poor perianal hygiene with a cycle of itching and scratching (**Box 7**). This symptom is thus more common in the setting of fecal incontinence and various other primary anal disorders. There are numerous other

Box 7
Pruritis ani DDx

- Poor perianal hygiene
- Anal disorder
  - Prolapsing hemorrhoids
  - Fissure
  - Fistula
- Dermatologic disorder
  - Contact dermatitis
  - Psoriasis
  - Lichen sclerosus
- Infection
  - Fungus/yeast (tinea cruris or *Candida*)
  - Sexually transmitted infection (condyloma, herpes)
  - *Enterobias vermicularis* (pinworm)
- Malignancy/neoplasia
  - Squamous cell neoplasia or carcinoma
  - Adenocarcinoma

diagnoses associated with anal itching, including dermatologic, infectious, and malignant etiologies.

Management

The foundation of managing pruritis ani involves ensuring adequate perianal hygiene, including regular bathing with warm, soapy water. The area should be kept dry, and talcum powder can be applied if necessary. In the setting of significant skin breakdown or excoriations, a barrier ointment (eg, zinc oxide) can be applied. Topical steroids (eg, hydrocortisone 1% cream or ointment) can be used briefly for symptomatic relief. If present, an underlying cause should be confronted.

RECTAL PROLAPSE
Symptoms

Also called procidentia, rectal prolapse classically presents with a large rectal mass. There is typically pain, bleeding, and fecal incontinence with difficulty maintaining anal hygiene. Most patients report difficulty with constipation and straining during bowel movements, but also suffer from incontinence.[23] Occasionally patients have complete outlet obstruction, and rarely they may have associated mucosal ulceration. Patients tend to be women, and the condition occurs more commonly with advancing age.

Diagnostic Test/Imaging Study

Rectal prolapse can be diagnosed purely on rectal examination and is characterized by circumferential mucosal folds, as opposed to radial folds seen in hemorrhoidal disease (**Fig. 8**). If necessary, the patient can be instructed to strain to elicit the prolapse. More advanced imaging techniques are rarely necessary.

Differential Diagnosis

The primary diagnosis to differentiate from rectal prolapse is large, protruding internal hemorrhoids, which can be differentiated based on the orientation of the mucosal folds.

Management

Initial management for rectal prolapse involves manual reduction, which is particularly important if there is any concern for strangulation of the blood supply. Patients

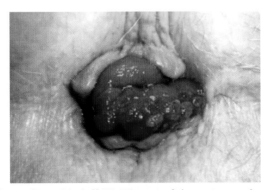

Fig. 8. Rectal prolapse. (*From* Madoff RD. Diseases of the rectum and anus. In: Goldman L, Schafer AI, editors. Goldman's Cecil medicine. 24th edition. Philadelphia: Elsevier; 2012; with permission.)

should be advised to avoid constipation by maintaining adequate hydration and fiber intake. Pelvic floor exercises (Kegels) may be suggested, although rigorous evidence of their benefit is lacking. Definitive management relies heavily upon surgical fixation, which can be accomplished through transabdominal (preferred) or transperineal approaches.[24,25]

SUMMARY

Anal problems are pervasive, embarrassing and vexing to patients. Primary care providers should be well versed in addressing these concerns, which uncommonly require referral for specialty care. Additionally, anal symptoms and findings may herald previously undiagnosed underlying illness.

REFERENCES

1. Castillo E, Margolin DA. Anal fissures: diagnosis and management. Tech Gastrointest Endosc 2004;6(1):12–6.
2. Oh C, Divino CM, Steinhagen RM. Anal fissure: 20-year experience. Dis Colon Rectum 1995;38(4):378–82.
3. Clinical Practice Committee. American Gastroenterological Association medical position statement: diagnosis and care of patients with anal fissure. Gastroenterology 2003;124:233–4.
4. Perry WB, Dykes SL, Buie WD, et al, The Standards Practice Task Force of The American Society of Colon and Rectal Surgeons. Practice parameters for the management of anal fissures. Dis Colon Rectum 2010;53:1110–5.
5. Ala S, Saeedi M, Hadianamrei R, et al. Topical diltiazem vs. topical glyceril trinitrate in the treatment of chronic anal fissure: a prospective, randomized, double-blind trial. Acta Gastroenterol Belg 2012;75(4):438–42.
6. Garcia-Acuilar J, Belmonte C, Wong WD, et al. Open vs. closed sphincterotomy for anal fissures. Dis Colon Rectum 1996;39(4):440–3.
7. Alonso-Coello P, Guyatt GH, Heels-Ansdell D, et al. Laxatives for the treatment of hemorrhoids. Cochrane Database Syst Rev 2005;(4):CD004649.
8. Clinical Practice Committee. American Gastroenterological Association medical position statement: diagnosis and treatment of hemorrhoids. Gastroenterology 2004;126:1461–2.
9. The Standards Practice Task Force of The American Society of Colon and Rectal Surgeons. Practice parameters for the management of hemorrhoids (revised 2010). Dis Colon Rectum 2011;54:1059–64.
10. Whiteford MH. Perianal abscess/fistula disease. Clin Colon Rectal Surg 2007; 20(2):102–9.
11. Boe JM. Anorectal disorders. In: Adams JG, editor. Emergency medicine: clinical essentials. 2nd edition. Philadelphia: Saunders; 2013. p. 336–46.
12. The Standards Practice Task Force of The American Society of Colon and Rectal Surgeons. Practice parameters for the treatmentof perianal abscess and fistula-in-ano (revised). Dis Colon Rectum 2005;47(7):1337–42.
13. Gilbert DN, Moellering RC, Eliopoulos GM, et al, editors. The Sanford guide to antimicrobial therapy. 39th edition. Sperryville (VA): Antimicrobial Therapy Inc; 2009. p. 20.
14. Sainio P. Fistula-in-ano in a defined population. Incidence and epidemiological aspects. Ann Chir Gynaecol 1984;73(4):219.
15. Stremnitzer S, Strobl S, Kure V, et al. Treatment of perianal sepsis and long-term outcome of recurrence and continence. Colorectal Dis 2011;13:703–7.

16. Halland M, Koloski NA, Jones M, et al. Prevalence correlates and impact of fecal incontinence among older women. Dis Colon Rectum 2013;56(9):1080–6.

17. Shah BJ, Chokhavatia S, Rose S. Fecal Incontinence in the Elderly: FAQ. Am J Gastroenterol 2012;107:1635–46.

18. Clinical Practice and Practice Economics Committee. American Gastroenterological Association medical position statement on anorectal testing techniques. Gastroenterology 1999;116:732–60.

19. The Standards Practice Task Force of The American Society of Colon and Rectal Surgeons. Practice parameters for the treatment of fecal incontinence. Dis Colon Rectum 2007;50:1497–507.

20. Heymen S, Jones KR, Ringel Y, et al. Biofeedback treatment of fecal incontinence: a critical review. Dis Colon Rectum 2001;44:728–36.

21. Maeda Y, Laurberg S, Norton C. Perianal injectable bulking agents as treatment for faecal incontinence in adults. Cochrane Database Syst Rev 2013;(2):CD007959.

22. Nelson RL, Abcarian H, Davis FG, et al. Prevalence of benign anorectal disease in a randomly selected population. Dis Colon Rectum 1995;38(4):341–4.

23. Kairaluoma MV, Kellokumpu IH. Epidemiologic aspects of complete rectal prolapse. Scand J Surg 2005;94:207–10.

24. The Standards Practice Task Force of The American Society of Colon and Rectal Surgeons. Practice parameters for the management of rectal prolapse. Dis Colon Rectum 2011;54:1339–46.

25. Fargo MV, Latimer KM. Evaluation and management of common anorectal conditions. Am Fam Physician 2012;85(6):624–30.

Involuntary Weight Loss

Christopher J. Wong, MD

KEYWORDS

- Involuntary weight loss • Unintentional weight loss • Unintended weight loss
- Unexplained weight loss • Malignancy • Diagnosis • Prognosis • Etiology

KEY POINTS

- Involuntary weight loss is a common clinical problem that frequently is a sign of underlying illness.
- The most common identified causes of involuntary weight loss are malignancy, gastrointestinal disorders, and psychiatric conditions; unknown etiologies represent a significant portion.
- Patients with normal history, physical examination, laboratory tests, and basic imaging studies are less likely to have a malignancy as the cause of involuntary weight loss; however, malignancy cannot be completely excluded.
- Treatment of involuntary weight loss is directed at the underlying causes.

INTRODUCTION

Involuntary weight loss is truly a generalist's syndrome. There is no specialty for it, and the differential diagnosis is as broad as any. It may be present as a patient's chief complaint but also may be found by astute observation by a clinician or family member. It requires a comprehensive evaluation to determine its cause. Involuntary weight loss poses a clinical problem of opposing tensions: on one hand, the specter of malignancy urges the clinician to undertake extensive workup so as not to miss it; on the other, most patients who present with involuntary weight loss do not have a malignancy, and these patients may incur the cost of the diagnostic workup, including the risk of invasive tests and procedures that may follow incidental findings. Frequently patients with involuntary weight loss are elderly and already have comorbid medical conditions, and the prognostic implications may be serious.

IS INVOLUNTARY WEIGHT LOSS A CONCERN? INSIGHTS FROM EPIDEMIOLOGY

It is often now presumed that intentional weight loss is desirable, whereas unintentional weight loss is a marker for serious illness. However, the relationship between

Division of General Internal Medicine, Department of Medicine, University of Washington, 4245 Roosevelt Way Northeast, Box 354760, Seattle, WA 98105, USA
E-mail address: cjwong@uw.edu

Med Clin N Am 98 (2014) 625–643
http://dx.doi.org/10.1016/j.mcna.2014.01.012
0025-7125/14/$ – see front matter © 2014 Elsevier Inc. All rights reserved.

medical.theclinics.com

weight and health has had a storied epidemiologic history. The Metropolitan Life Insurance Company was one of the early pioneers in identifying obesity as a risk factor for mortality in its actuarial life tables from the 1950s. Although there remain concerns regarding measurement standardization and smoking status in that data set,[1] the concept of obesity as a risk factor for mortality eventually became consensus. The range of body mass index at which mortality is increased is still a subject of research and controversy.[2]

The next epidemiologic question was whether *changes* in weight were associated with positive or negative health outcomes. In the 1980s and 1990s debate took place with the concern that weight loss may be harmful.[3,4] Other approaches sought to associate health risk with weight fluctuation or "weight cycling" in general.[5–7] However, studies that attempted to control for preexisting illnesses have not shown a definite risk from weight fluctuation alone.[8,9] Several studies sought to demonstrate that intentional weight loss was favorable for health outcomes, and in doing so were able to show an association between unintentional weight loss and mortality in select populations.[10,11] By contrast, a study of men in Israel beginning in the 1960s reported increased mortality with weight loss regardless of dieting status.[12] An analysis of data of the more modern era from the Iowa Women's Health Study showed that unintentional weight loss, but not intentional weight loss, of more than 20 lb (9 kg) was associated with increased mortality.[13] After adjusting for comorbid conditions, this association appeared to be present in the 55-year and older age group. Wannamethee and colleagues[14] sought to further explore intentional versus unintentional weight loss in a study of more than 4000 British men, and found that unintentional weight loss (over 4 years, mean −3.91 kg, as reported by participants) was associated with increased risk of total mortality, even after adjustment for preexisting disease. Of note, intentional weight loss was only associated with mortality if the weight loss was undertaken on the advice of a physician or if the patient was in ill health.

Finally, studies examining shorter-term weight loss are likely more relevant to the clinical problem of involuntary weight loss. In the United States, Gregg and colleagues[15] found that intentional weight loss over the preceding year was associated with a decreased mortality rate over the ensuing 9 years, whereas unintentional weight loss was associated with an approximately 30% increase in mortality. Sahyoun and colleagues[16] found an association between weight loss of 5% or more within the preceding 6 months and increased total mortality.

Thus despite the limitations in epidemiology-based methods to differentiate between voluntary and involuntary weight loss, there are at least moderate data suggesting that unintentional weight loss is harmful.

WHAT DEFINES INVOLUNTARY WEIGHT LOSS?

These epidemiology studies suggest that unintentional weight loss may be harmful. When approaching a patient, however, there is need to have a clinical definition for use in practice. Although there is as yet no consensus definition of involuntary weight loss, certain terms may still be reasonably defined (**Table 1**).

First, the term involuntary: in the literature, "involuntary" is used interchangeably with "unintended" or "unintentional." These terms may be defined as the condition whereby the patient does not purposefully set out to lose weight for any reason, and excluding weight loss as an expected consequence of treatment of a known illness, such as diuretic therapy for heart failure. In addition, there are several terms used in the literature to describe weight loss of unknown etiology. For this review, the terms "unexplained" or "isolated" or "unknown" refer to weight loss without an

Table 1
Terms used to describe involuntary weight loss and associated conditions

Term	Description
Involuntary weight loss	Synonyms: unintended weight loss, unintentional weight loss
	Weight loss that is not intended by the patient, and is not a consequence of the expected treatment of a known condition
	≥5% weight loss within 6–12 mo (no consensus definition for degree or duration)
	Weight loss measured or by clinical criteria (see text)
Unexplained weight loss	Synonyms: Isolated involuntary weight loss
	Weight loss that is not intended, and of which the cause is not found after a workup
	The exact amount of workup and time is not precisely defined: see **Fig. 2**
Sarcopenia	Geriatric syndrome consisting of low muscle mass (2 standard deviations below reference) and poor physical performance[29]
Cachexia	Metabolic syndrome: loss of muscle mass caused by an underlying illness
	Weight loss of 5% or greater over 12 mo or less and 3 of 5[28]:
	Decreased muscle strength
	Fatigue
	Anorexia
	Low fat-free mass index
	Abnormal laboratory tests (increased inflammatory markers, anemia, low serum albumin)

apparent cause after a workup has been performed. There is no consensus as to the amount of workup required to label the weight loss as unexplained, but one could reasonably consider such a workup to include history, physical examination, laboratory and imaging studies, and the passage of time without a diagnosis.

Second, one must consider the extent of weight loss to consider involuntary weight loss as a clinical entity or syndrome. There are 3 characteristics to consider: the degree of weight loss, how weight loss is assessed, and the time frame in which the weight loss occurs.

Degree of Weight Loss

What is a normal and what is an abnormal amount of weight loss? Although it is widely believed that day-to-day fluctuations of up to 5 lb (2.2 kg) may be normal based on changes in intake and output and time of measurement, there are few data available to gauge what is normal fluctuation in weight in healthy people. In addition, weight may fluctuate throughout the day, as much as 1% to 2% in one small study of hospitalized patients.[17] The normal amount of weight loss in the elderly population (ie, weight loss that is physiologic and not associated with increased morbidity or mortality) may be in the range of 0.1 to 0.2 kg/y[18] to 0.5% per year.[19] Involuntary weight loss, then, should merit a diagnostic workup when exceeding these thresholds. Most of the published case series of involuntary weight loss used an inclusion criteria of 5% or greater weight loss compared with usual body weight,[20–26] with some studies using criteria up to 7.5% to 10%.[20,23,27] Wallace and colleagues[19] assessed the degree of weight loss that is significant in a prospective cohort study of elderly veterans. Using a receiver-operator characteristic curve, they assessed the optimal weight-loss percentage to be 4% over the preceding year with regard to the balance of sensitivity (75%) and specificity (61%) associated with subsequent mortality. In another epidemiology study, involuntary weight loss of 5% or more (but not <5%) over the preceding 6 months was associated with subsequent mortality.[16] However, the optimal cutoff for weight-loss percentage described as pathologic that would apply broadly to all populations remains uncertain.

Assessment of Weight Loss

How weight loss is measured is also a matter of some discretion. Excessively stringent criteria such as requiring weights measured at the same time of day on a standardized office scale would miss patients who have not been previously followed regularly and frequently; these patients may nevertheless on presentation have a serious illness and would be harmed by a delay in diagnostic workup. Conversely, criteria that are too vague may result in unnecessary testing of patients without underlying illness. Published case series often replicated the measurement method of Marton and colleagues[21]: either documented weight loss, or at least 2 of the following 3 criteria: change in clothing size, a friend or relative corroborating the weight loss, or the patient's estimate of amount of weight lost. These criteria remain useful, although this method has not been validated as a prognostic tool.

In addition to the magnitude of weight loss, the duration is worth considering. Too short a time frame may select for only the most acute illnesses; too long a time frame may reflect other long-term physiologic changes rather than an underlying serious illness. From a clinical perspective, an intermediate time frame on the order of months to a year is likely to be most relevant. Published case series used criteria for weight loss occurring in the preceding 3 to 12 months (**Table 2**).[20–25] One study had no duration requirement.[26] Requiring a longer duration before a workup may miss a serious diagnosis that may progress. Involuntary weight loss that occurred many years prior with subsequent stabilization or reversal is not likely to reflect a progressive illness, although it may be the sign of a relapsing-remitting condition.

It is reasonable, therefore, to define the degree of weight loss as 5% or more of usual body weight within the preceding 6 to 12 months, to use weights measured in the clinic when available, and to use the criteria of Marton and colleagues if standardized measurements are unavailable (see **Table 1**).

OTHER SYNDROMES

Cachexia is not synonymous with involuntary weight loss; it is a clinical syndrome characterized by loss of muscle mass, and is caused by inflammatory metabolic derangements attributable to an underlying illness. The consensus definition as of 2008 is as follows: weight loss of at least 5% in 12 months or less, the presence of an underlying illness, and 3 of 5 of the following: decreased muscle strength, fatigue, anorexia, low fat-free mass index, and abnormal laboratory testing consisting of increased inflammatory markers, anemia, or low serum albumin (see **Table 1**).[28] Patients presenting with involuntary weight loss may have or may develop cachexia, depending on the cause of the weight loss.

Sarcopenia is a term used to describe a geriatric syndrome characterized by the loss of muscle mass and muscle function; although weight loss is not a criterion for sarcopenia, patients may have common underlying mechanisms causing both sarcopenia and cachexia.[29]

PATHOPHYSIOLOGY

Weight homeostasis is a complex system affected by gastrointestinal hormones, hormones from adipose tissue, and the hypothalamus, as well as reward centers and social factors. Involuntary weight loss is a striking problem in many nations when juxtaposed with epidemics of obesity. Much of the focus with regard to weight homeostasis has been either the pathophysiology of obesity or the mechanisms underpinning weight-losing syndromes such as cancer cachexia (**Fig. 1**).

In obesity, the long-term increase in weight is governed by numerous factors, including availability of high-calorie food and decrease in physical activity, with possible contributions from exposures to toxins, viruses, and medications.[30] At the gastrointestinal level, satiety is sensed by gastric distension sending signals to the brain via the nervous system, and by release of peptides such as cholecystokinin, peptide YY, glucagon-like peptide 1 (GLP-1), and amylin, while feeding is stimulated by ghrelin.[31] Leptin is responsible for decreased food intake, and is secreted by adipocytes in response to body fat mass, affecting receptors in the hypothalamus. Evolutionarily, it is thought that low leptin levels in response to low fat mass stimulate hunger and energy efficiency in an effort to return to the fat mass set point.[31] Over time, the set point for the body's fat mass may increase under the influence of multiple factors, leading to obesity.[31]

Involuntary weight loss, however, is not merely the opposite aspect of pathologic weight gain in obesity. What happens to patients who lose weight involuntarily, when it is so difficult for others to lose weight intentionally or even to maintain weight without gaining? One such model is the weight loss associated with cancer, or cancer cachexia. Cancer cachexia is thought to be mediated by the production of cytokines such as tumor necrosis factor (TNF)-α and interleukin-6, and other factors including myostatin and activin, to a susceptible host.[32] These factors suppress the appetite and promote muscle and fat breakdown. In addition, they may promote inefficient energy expenditure. The normal response to decreased energy intake is to reduce energy expenditure; in cancer cachexia, in the face of decreased energy intake resulting from multiple factors, instead of decreasing energy consumption, continued gluconeogenesis, lactate recycling, and protein turnover occur, driven in some models by TNF.[33] The expected physiologic decrease in leptin in response to decreased fat mass does not occur in cancer cachexia.[33] Weight loss in acute illnesses such as sepsis is also likely mediated by cytokines. The cachexia in other states is not just about losing total weight; rather, it is a transformation of body mass, as exemplified by cachexia resulting from chronic obstructive pulmonary disease (COPD).[34] By contrast, the weight loss attributable to inadequate food intake alone has normal leptin signaling and is reversible with nutritional repletion.

INCIDENCE AND PREVALENCE

Estimates of the incidence of involuntary weight loss vary. The yearly incidence in case series from referral centers varies between 0.6% and 7.3% per year.[20,22,24,35,36]

These estimates depend on the particular patient populations and referral patterns, as well as the definition of involuntary weight loss used. A series of elderly veterans reported a higher incidence of 13% per year using a cutoff of 4% weight loss.[19] In a general population, the incidence would be expected to be much lower than that in referral centers or in subsets of higher-risk patients. However, an epidemiology study of 5% or more weight loss over the preceding 6 months reported a 7% prevalence.[16] Nursing home and home care populations may have increased prevalence of involuntary weight loss.[37–39] Other epidemiology studies spanned a longer period of time. These prevalences vary, from a 4-year 11% prevalence in men in Great Britain[8] to a 6-year 19% prevalence in women in the United States.[13]

Table 2
Involuntary weight loss case series

Study,[Ref.] Year	Type of Study, No. of Patients	Setting	Patients	Follow-Up	Median Age (y)	Malignancy (%)	Gastrointestinal (%)	Infection (%)	Psychiatric (%)	Unknown (%)
Marton et al,[21] 1981	Prospective N = 91	Veterans Administration, California, United States	≥5% weight loss over 6 mo 70% inpatient, 30% outpatient	6–12 mo	59	19	14	3	9	26
Rabinovitz et al,[24] 1986	Retrospective N = 154	Internal medicine department, Israel	≥5% weight loss Inpatient	24–36 mo	64	36	17	4	10	23
Thompson & Morris,[27] 1991	Prospective N = 45	Family practice clinics, southeastern United States	Age ≥63 y ≥7.5% weight loss over 6 mo Outpatient	24 mo	72	16	11	2	18	24
Lankisch et al,[22] 2001	Prospective N = 158	Referral center, single site, Germany	≥5% weight loss within 6 mo Inpatient	12–36 mo	68	24	19	a	11	16

Study	Design	Setting	Definition	Time frame						
Bilbao-Garay et al,[20] 2002	Prospective N = 78	Internal medicine referral clinic, Spain	≥5% weight loss over 3 mo, or ≥10% over 6 mo Outpatient Used diagnostic protocol	6 mo	59	23	6	5	33	11
Metalidis et al,[23] 2008	Prospective N = 101	University general internal medicine clinic, Belgium	≥5% weight loss over 6–12 mo Inpatient and outpatient	6 mo	64	22	15	8	16	28
Wu et al,[25] 2011	Retrospective N = 136	Veterans hospital, Taiwan	≥5% weight loss over 6–12 mo Elderly, inpatient	1 admission	80	17	b	b	b	26
Chen et al,[26] 2010	Retrospective N = 50	Veterans hospital, Taiwan	≥5% weight loss, no time frame Elderly, inpatient.	12 mo	79	6	22	6	13	16

a Etiology listed by organ system; infectious causes not reportedly separately.
b Not reported separately.
Data from Refs.[20–27]

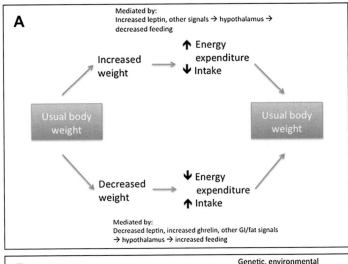

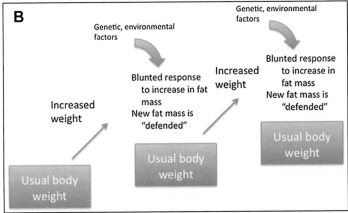

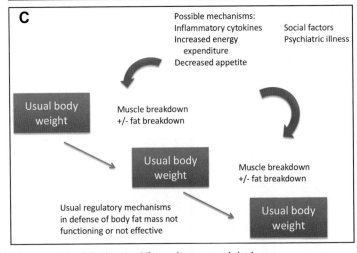

Fig. 1. (*A*) Homeostasis. (*B*) Obesity. (*C*) Involuntary weight loss.

DIFFERENTIAL DIAGNOSIS

The causes of involuntary weight loss are many (**Table 3**). In the literature, weight loss associated with clinical diseases may be reported as a symptom, a quantified amount of weight loss, or, in the case of certain diseases such as heart failure, COPD, and cancer, it may be characterized by extensive research into the phenomenon of cachexia (see **Table 1**).

Cardiovascular Disease

The most well-described condition is cardiac cachexia associated with advanced heart failure. This wasting process is likely mediated via inflammatory and hormonal mechanisms[40] and is associated with increased mortality independent of New York Heart Association (NYHA) class, with a prevalence as high as 16%.[41] Involuntary weight loss caused by cardiac cachexia presents as loss of muscle mass and fat, and is distinct from intentional weight loss such as produced by diuretic therapy. In most cases, one would expect the diagnosis of heart failure to be already known or evident on presentation.

Respiratory Disease

Advanced COPD can cause involuntary weight loss. Low body weight and, more specifically, low muscle mass (fat-free mass) is associated with mortality.[42] Studies of COPD have generally used static measurements of weight or fat-free mass rather than measuring loss of weight per se; the prevalence of cachexia using these measurements is estimated at between 20% and 40%.[34] Cachexia caused by advanced COPD is likely due to a combination of increased energy expenditure from work of breathing as well as neurohormonal changes. In most cases, the presence of severe COPD should be evident on history and physical examination, and readily confirmed

Table 3	
Causes of involuntary weight loss: examples	
Cardiovascular	**Heart Failure/Cardiac Cachexia**
Respiratory	COPD, interstitial lung disease, vasculitides, lung cancer
Gastrointestinal	Malabsorption, diarrhea, autoimmune/inflammatory, mesenteric ischemia
Renal	Uremic cachexia
Malignancy	Solid tumors, eg, lung, prostate, colorectal, pancreatic > hematologic malignancies
Neurologic	Dementia, stroke, Parkinson disease, neuromuscular diseases, multiple sclerosis
Endocrine	Diabetes, adrenal insufficiency, hyperthyroidism
Rheumatologic	Rheumatoid arthritis, sarcoidosis
Infectious disease	HIV, tuberculosis, other chronic infections
Psychiatric	Depression, anxiety, anorexia nervosa
Medications	Antiepileptics, antidepressants, antianxiety drugs, stimulants, diuretics, laxatives
Substance abuse and dependence	Alcohol, opiates; smoking as risk factor for malignancy
Social	Poverty, abuse, neglect; oral health

Abbreviations: COPD, chronic obstructive pulmonary disease; HIV, human immunodeficiency virus.

by imaging and pulmonary function testing. Other respiratory diseases that may present with involuntary weight loss include malignancy, rheumatologic disease such as antineutrophil cytoplasmic antibody (ANCA)-associated vasculitides, interstitial lung disease, and infections such as tuberculosis. Because smoking is a common risk factor for both COPD and lung cancer, the patient with known COPD who presents with involuntary weight loss should not be assumed to have COPD cachexia; rather, workup of lung cancer should be considered.

Gastrointestinal

Gastrointestinal causes of weight loss include malabsorptive syndromes such as pancreatic insufficiency and celiac disease, diarrheal illnesses, inflammatory bowel disease, peptic ulcer disease, mesenteric ischemia, and protein-losing enteropathies. An important cause, especially in the elderly, is dental disease, with difficulty chewing leading to decreased caloric intake.[43]

Renal

Renal failure may result in weight gain caused by inadequate renal excretion; advanced renal failure may lead to protein energy malnutrition.[44] Inflammatory cytokines and neuropeptide signaling to the hypothalamus have been implicated in the uremia cachexia syndrome.[45] As with advanced heart failure, involuntary weight loss in advanced chronic kidney disease must be distinguished from weight loss resulting from medical treatments, including diuretic therapy and dialysis.

Cancer

Cancer is estimated to cause involuntary weight loss of at least 5% in approximately one-third of patients,[44] and becomes nearly universal when terminal. Weight loss appears to be greater in patients with solid tumors, especially gastrointestinal, pancreatic, and lung cancers, and is associated with increased mortality.[44,46] Unlike advanced heart failure or COPD, cancer as the cause of weight loss may not be readily apparent on initial history and physical, and may require additional laboratory testing and imaging studies. Weight loss may be rapid in gastrointestinal and head and neck cancers.

Neurologic

Neurologic conditions may cause weight loss from decreased functional status owing to cognitive impairment such as dementia, reduced swallowing and gastrointestinal function such as in Parkinson disease, multiple sclerosis, and neuromuscular disorders.

Endocrinopathies

Weight loss is a common presenting feature of hyperthyroidism, occurring in 40% to 60% of those affected, even in elderly patients who may not have as many other classic features of hyperthyroidism.[47–49] Other endocrinopathies that may present with weight loss include diabetes, adrenal insufficiency (25%–60%),[50,51] hypopituitarism, and carcinoid syndrome, among others.

Inflammatory and Rheumatologic Conditions

Conditions such as rheumatoid arthritis,[52] sarcoidosis, and ANCA-associated vasculitides may present with weight loss.

Infectious Diseases

Human immunodeficiency virus (HIV) may lead to weight loss and cachexia, from the virus itself as well as from the medications used to treat it. Other chronic infections such as tuberculosis may lead to chronic inflammatory states and consequent weight loss.

Psychiatric

Psychiatric conditions such as depression and anxiety may be associated with both weight gain and weight loss. These disorders must also be distinguished from adverse effects of medications used to treat these conditions.

Medications

Medications used to treat other conditions may inadvertently cause weight loss. The antiepileptic drugs topiramate and zonisamide have been shown to cause weight loss,[53–55] and are often used for conditions other than epilepsy. Psychiatric medications commonly associated with weight loss include selective serotonin reuptake inhibitors, which can have variable effects on weight; bupropion; and stimulants such as those used for attention-deficit hyperactivity disorder. Many medications may have gastrointestinal side effects that may secondarily cause weight loss resulting from diarrhea. Metformin and GLP-1 agonists used to treat diabetes, and diuretics and laxatives through appropriate use or misuse all may cause weight loss. Antibiotics may cause weight loss through diarrhea or direct effects.

Substance Abuse and Dependence

Likely through multifactorial mechanisms, substance abuse can cause involuntary weight loss. Abuse of cocaine may lead to fat dysregulation in addition to appetite suppression.[56] Other substance dependence frequently leads to malnutrition,[57] including alcoholism, heroin dependence, and methamphetamine dependence.

Social

Just as ready access to high-calorie foods can be one factor in the development of obesity, inadequate access to food through poverty or neglect and abuse may be a factor in causing weight loss. Weight loss caused by inadequate intake produces appropriate downregulation of leptin and a decrease in energy expenditure, and, unlike the weight loss from cancer cachexia, is reversible by reinstituting proper nourishment.

ETIOLOGY OF INVOLUNTARY WEIGHT LOSS: INSIGHTS FROM CASE SERIES

Given such a wide differential diagnosis, it is useful to explore what is found in published case series of patients with involuntary weight loss.

What Causes are Found?

With the caveat that the different case series included different populations, countries, age groups, and inclusion criteria, the following overall representation is seen (see **Table 2**).[20–27] Malignancy represented 6% to 36% of cases, with all but one series being greater than 15%; nonmalignant gastrointestinal illnesses 6% to 19%; and psychiatric illnesses 9% to 33%. Infection was a relatively small percentage of cases (2%–8%) and in a significant portion of cases, no cause was found (11%–28%).

What Percentage of Patients are Unknown After an Initial Workup?

How often a diagnosis is found after the initial workup depends on the content of the initial workup and on the final percentage of unknown causes in the cohort. The aforementioned case series were heterogeneous in population, and only 2 of the studies[20,23] used a protocol for the initial workup. Few series reported the percentage of patients able to be diagnosed after the initial workup (the extent of which varied by series), and this value was between 33% and 60%.[21,24,27]

Hernandez and colleagues[35] studied the characteristics and outcomes specifically of patients who had a negative initial workup. These patients initially received a complete blood count (CBC), basic metabolic panel (glucose, blood urea nitrogen, creatinine, potassium, sodium), chest radiograph, and abdominal radiograph, in addition to history and examination. After 6 months, no diagnosis was found in 25% of patients; these patients were considered to have "isolated involuntary weight loss." Excluding those lost to follow-up, approximately 94% of these patients with a negative initial workup were eventually found to have a diagnosis. Malignancy represented 38%, followed by psychiatric (23%) and gastrointestinal diseases (10%). A smaller study in France, by contrast, had very few malignancies in a population who had already undergone workup.[58]

Based on these limited data, one could expect to find a diagnosis after initial workup in most cases, with another 10% to 20% yield after additional workup, and subsequently leaving 10% to 25% of patients still without a diagnosis after extended follow-up.

What About Unintended Weight Loss in the Elderly?

Increasingly old age, loss of a spouse, disability, and previous hospital admission are being reported as risk factors for weight loss in the elderly.[59] Unintentional weight loss in the elderly is very common, occurring in 15% to 20% of elderly patients.[59]

Older patients are at greater risk than younger patients for decreased caloric intake. Olfactory function declines with age, and increasing dental problems and dry mouth can cause decreased interest in food intake because of pain, difficulty chewing, and decreased enjoyment in the taste of food. Eating is usually a very social behavior, and elderly persons who are alone are less likely to eat adequate calories.

What Factors Portend a More Serious Diagnostic Etiology?

Various prediction rules have been described (**Table 4**), but are mainly based on small case series. Marton and colleagues[21] developed a discriminant function score for weight loss being due to a physical cause, but did not specifically assess prediction of malignancy. The variables that were associated with less likelihood of a physical cause of weight loss were a smoking history of less than 20 pack-years and a lack of decrease in activity. Factors that were more predictive were nausea/vomiting, recent increase in appetite, recently changed cough, or positive physical examination findings.

Hernandez and colleagues[60] found that age greater than 80 years, white blood cell count greater than 12,000, alkaline phosphatase greater than 300 IU/L, and lactate dehydrogenase (LDH) greater than 500 IU/L were predictive of malignancy in a multivariate analysis, with albumin greater than 3.5 g/dL being negatively associated. The amount of weight loss was associated with a diagnosis of malignancy in the univariate analysis, but not in the multivariate analysis. A clinical predictive rule was developed and validated using point scores for these variables: likelihood ratios were 0.07, 1.2, and 28 for scores of less than 0, 0 to 1, and greater than 1, respectively. Therefore,

Table 4
Diagnostic models for patients presenting with involuntary weight loss

Marton	Physical cause of involuntary weight loss less likely: <20 pack-year smoking history Lack of decrease in activity Physical cause of involuntary weight loss more likely: Nausea/vomiting Recent increase in appetite Recently changed cough Positive physical examination findings	Developed a discriminant function model using these factors Smoking +3, no decrease in activities +5, nausea −3, increased appetite −2, changed cough −1, examination findings −1; +8 correction factor Physical cause by score: 1–6, 100%; 7–8, 78%; 9–11, 14%, 12–16, 0% Not validated in separate sample or population
Hernandez	Malignancy more likely: Age >80 y WBC >12,000 Alkaline phosphatase >300 IU/L LDH >500 IU/L Malignancy less likely: Albumin >3.5 g/dL	Prediction rule developed, +1 for age and WBC, +2 for alkaline phosphatase, +3 for LDH, −2 for albumin Score <0, LR 0.07; score >1, LR 28
Baicus	Malignancy more likely: Age >62 y Hemoglobin <10 g/dL ESR >29 mm/h	All 3 present: 9% risk All 3 absent: 64% risk

Abbreviations: ESR, erythrocyte sedimentation rate; LDH, lactate dehydrogenase; LR, likelihood ratio; WBC, white blood cells.
  Data from Refs.[21,36,59]

a score less than 0 or greater than 1 is clinically useful. However, the overall negative predictive value of this prediction model was 85%, not necessarily enough to exclude malignancy in a clinical situation.

Baicus and colleagues[36] assessed inpatients with involuntary weight loss and derived a formula for the risk of cancer based on age older than 62 years, hemoglobin less than 10 g/dL, and erythrocyte sedimentation rate (ESR) greater than 29 mm/h. The risk for all 3 factors not being present was 9%, compared with 64% if all 3 were positive.

From the other case series, there are some associative data regarding malignancy risk. In the case series of Metalidis and colleagues,[23] no patients with malignancy had a completely normal baseline evaluation, which consisted of history, examination, chest radiograph, abdominal ultrasonogram, and laboratory tests that included CBC, C-reactive protein (CRP), aspartate aminotransferase, alanine aminotransferase, LDH, alkaline phosphatase, albumin, ferritin, thyroid function tests, fasting glucose, and a urinalysis. However, the number of patients with malignancy was relatively small (n = 22). Rabinovitz and colleagues[24] showed that patients with malignancy were more likely to have a low albumin level or elevated alkaline phosphatase.

What is the Prognosis for Patients Who Present with Involuntary Weight Loss?

In the published case series, overall mortality was high, at 16% to 38%.[19–24] Mortality tended to be higher in patients diagnosed with malignancy. The amount of weight loss may be predictive: Chen and colleagues[26] reported that of elderly patients with unexplained, unintentional weight loss, those with cancer had the most rapid weight loss, of approximately 6.5% per month. However, this study had fewer patients with malignancy in comparison with other studies. Conversely, Rabinovitz and colleagues[24] did not find a difference in degree of weight loss with respect to etiology.

SUGGESTED ALGORITHM

A suggested algorithm is shown in **Fig. 2**. Patients who present with involuntary weight loss have serious illness, including malignancy, a significant percentage of the time. All

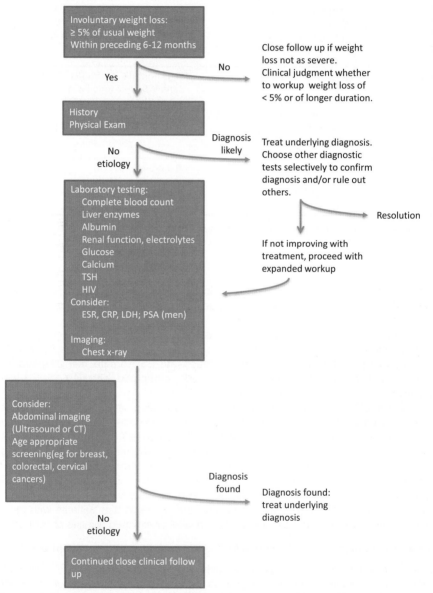

Fig. 2. Suggested algorithm. CRP, C-reactive protein; CT, computed tomography; ESR, erythrocyte sedimentation rate; HIV, human immunodeficiency virus; LDH, lactate dehydrogenase; PSA, prostate-specific antigen; TSH, thyroid-stimulating hormone.

patients who present with involuntary weight loss should be evaluated, whether it is the patient's chief complaint or is incidentally found. A working definition of 5% or greater loss of usual weight within the preceding 6 to 12 months is a reasonable starting point for evaluation. Failing to precisely meet this criterion should not preclude a workup if the clinical suspicion is high; as noted earlier, Wallace and colleagues[19] found a 4% cutoff to be optimal in a sample of elderly veterans. In addition, weight loss over a period longer than 12 months may still be of importance to merit a workup. If weight measurements are not known, the methodology of Marton and colleagues[21] remains reasonable (see earlier discussion). Note should be made of the obese patient for whom intended weight loss changes unexpectedly from difficult to easy; although there are few data to support it, it is reasonable to investigate whether this presentation represents involuntary weight loss.

Workup should include a discussion of the risks of the testing in the context of the patient's overall goals of care.

A thorough history should include assessment of cardiac, respiratory, and gastrointestinal symptoms, as well as systemic signs of infection or malignancy. Assessment of depression, anxiety, or other psychiatric causes of weight loss should be undertaken, as well as screening for substance abuse and dependence. Risk factors for infection should be identified. Identification of social factors and a comprehensive medication/supplement history should be compiled.

Examination should be complete, to include the major cardiovascular, respiratory, gastrointestinal, genitourinary, dermatologic, and musculoskeletal organ systems, as well as a neurologic examination, mental status examination, and assessment for lymphadenopathy. Breast and prostate examinations should be considered.

The workup should be conducted according to a patient-centered approach. Many patients who present with involuntary weight loss are elderly with significant comorbid conditions. Elderly patients are more likely to have complex causes including social isolation, depression, and underlying frailty. Appropriate history should be taken (focusing on sense of smell, food intake, swallowing, dental pain, social support systems, and symptoms of depression) and physical examination carried out, focusing on oral-cavity examination in elderly patients with unintended weight loss.

If a leading diagnosis is suggested at the initial presentation, patients should receive confirmatory testing, if needed, and treatment begun. If treatment does not result in weight gain the workup should be reassessed, with consideration for additional testing. It is important not to provide premature diagnostic closure; though some patients with progressive chronic disease may develop weight loss as a result, there may be a separate illness that precipitates the involuntary weight loss.

If the cause is not evident after the initial history and examination, a reasonable laboratory testing strategy includes a CBC, liver function panel, renal function, blood sugar, electrolytes, calcium, thyroid-stimulating hormone, ESR, CRP, and LDH; although not specific, these are reasonable screening tests. An HIV test is now recommended as universal screening and should be ordered if a patient's status is not known. A prostate-specific antigen test in male patients should be considered, although other tumor markers should not be routinely ordered. Appropriate imaging studies start with a chest radiograph.

Although some clinicians, in light of the case series results discussed here, would favor only performing imaging interventions if there are directed abnormalities in the initial workup, one must recognize that the case series are varied and have small sample sizes. In a patient with ongoing weight loss, it is reasonable to add abdominal imaging even if the initial laboratory tests are not revealing—either with ultrasonography, as was used in some case series, or an abdomen/pelvis computed tomography (CT) scan. The increased sensitivity of the CT must be weighed against the risks of radiation and contrast exposure. In addition, one should consider age-appropriate cancer screening if it has not already been done, to include colorectal cancer screening, breast cancer screening, and cervical cancer screening. One must balance whether screening has already been discontinued in the elderly or medically frail patient, and whether the advent of involuntary weight loss would alter the decision making regarding the potential findings of these screening tests.

If no cause is found initially, during the course of follow-up it might be expected that a diagnosis will be found in another 10% to 20% of patients. Patients should be followed closely for ongoing weight loss, and for localizing symptoms or signs that may suggest a diagnosis.

TREATMENT

Treatment of involuntary weight loss is generally directed toward identifying and treating the underlying illness, with the presumption that treating this illness will reverse the weight loss. A systematic review of megestrol treatment for patients with cachexia caused by HIV, cancer, COPD, cystic fibrosis, and in the elderly found an increase in weight but no effect on quality of life.[61] Another review found that there may be a small increase in weight in patients with advanced HIV treated with anabolic steroids and resistance exercise.[62] The question is whether there is an effective treatment for involuntary weight loss of unknown etiology or while the workup is proceeding. Performing a nutritional assessment is a reasonable step, but there is as yet no conclusive data pertaining to interventions such as megestrol, cannabinoids, nutritional supplements, or enteral or parenteral feeding, in the setting of involuntary weight loss without an etiologic diagnosis.

SUMMARY

Involuntary weight loss remains an important and challenging clinical problem, with a high degree of morbidity and mortality. Because of the frequency of finding a serious underlying diagnosis, clinicians must be thorough in assessment, keeping in mind a broad range of possible causes. Although prediction scores exist, they have not been broadly validated; therefore, clinical judgment remains ever essential.

REFERENCES

1. Willet WC, Dietz WH, Colditz GA. Guidelines for healthy weight. N Engl J Med 1999;341:427–34.
2. Flegal KM, Kit BK, Orpana H, et al. Association of all-cause mortality with overweight and obesity using standard body mass index categories. JAMA 2013; 309:71–82.
3. Pamuk ER, Williamson DF, Serdula MK, et al. Weight loss and subsequent death in a cohort of U.S. adults. Ann Intern Med 1993;119:744–8.
4. Reynolds MW, Fredman L, Langenberg P, et al. Weight, weight change, and mortality in a random sample of older community-dwelling women. J Am Geriatr Soc 1999;47:1409–14.
5. Lissner L, Odell PM, D'Agostino RB, et al. Variability of body weight and health outcomes in the Framingham population. N Engl J Med 1991;324:1839–44.
6. Blair SN, Shaten J, Brownell K, et al. Body weight change, all-cause mortality, and cause-specific mortality in the multiple risk factor intervention trial. Ann Intern Med 1993;119:749–57.

7. Folsom AR, French SA, Zheng W, et al. Weight variability and mortality: the Iowa Women's Health Study. Int J Obes Relat Metab Disord 1996;20:704–9.
8. Wannamethee SG, Shaper AG, Walker M. Weight change, weight fluctuation, and mortality. Arch Intern Med 2002;162:2575–80.
9. Iribarren C, Sharp DS, Burchfiel CM, et al. Association of weight loss and weight fluctuation with mortality among Japanese American men. N Engl J Med 1995; 333:686–92.
10. Williamson DF, Pamuk E, Thun M, et al. Prospective study of intentional weight loss and mortality in overweight white men aged 40-64 years. Am J Epidemiol 1999;149:491–503.
11. Williamson DF, Pamuk E, Thun M. Prospective study of intentional weight loss and mortality in never-smoking overweight US white women aged 40-64 years. Am J Epidemiol 1995;141:1128–41.
12. Yaari S, Goldbourt U. Voluntary and involuntary weight loss: associations with long term mortality in 9,228 middle-aged and elderly men. Am J Epidemiol 1998;148:546–55.
13. French SA, Folsom AR, Jeffery RW, et al. Prospective study of intentionality of weight loss and mortality in older women: the iowa women's health study. Am J Epidemiol 1999;149:504–14.
14. Wannamethee SG, Shaper AG, Lennon L. Reasons for intentional weight loss, unintentional weight loss, and mortality in older men. Arch Intern Med 2005; 165:1035–40.
15. Gregg EW, Gerzoff RB, Thompson TJ, et al. Intentional weight loss and death in overweight and obese U.S. adults 35 years of age and older. Ann Intern Med 2003;138:383–9.
16. Sahyoun NR, Serdula MK, Galuska DA. The epidemiology of recent involuntary weight loss in the United States population. J Nutr Health Aging 2004; 8:510–7.
17. Vivanti A, Yu L, Palmer M, et al. Short-term body weight fluctuations in older well-hydrated hospitalised patients. J Hum Nutr Diet 2013;26:429–35.
18. Wallace JI, Schwartz RS. Epidemiology of weight loss in humans with special reference to wasting in the elderly. Int J Cardiol 2002;85:15–21.
19. Wallace JI, Schwartz RS, LaCroix AZ, et al. Involuntary weight loss in older outpatients: incidence and clinical significance. J Am Geriatr Soc 1995;43: 329–37.
20. Bilbao-Garay J, Barba R, Losa-Garcia JE, et al. Assessing clinical probability of organic disease in patients with involuntary weight loss: a simple score. Eur J Intern Med 2002;13:240–5.
21. Marton KI, Sox HC, Krupp JR. Involuntary weight loss: diagnostic and prognostic significance. Ann Intern Med 1981;95:568–74.
22. Lankisch PG, Gerzmann M, Gerzmann JF, et al. Unintentional weight loss: diagnosis and prognosis. The first prospective follow-up study from a secondary referral centre. J Intern Med 2001;249:41–6.
23. Metalidis C, Knockaert DC, Bobbaers H, et al. Involuntary weight loss. Does a negative baseline evaluation provide adequate reassurance? Eur J Intern Med 2008;19(5):345–9.
24. Rabinovitz M, Pitlik SD, Leifer M, et al. Unintentional weight loss: a retrospective analysis of 154 cases. Arch Intern Med 1986;146:186–7.
25. Wu JM, Lin MH, Peng LN, et al. Evaluating diagnostic strategy of older patients with unexplained unintentional body weight loss: a hospital-based study. Arch Gerontol Geriatr 2011;53:e51–4.

26. Chen SP, Peng LN, Lin MH, et al. Evaluating probability of cancer among older people with unexplained, unintentional weight loss. Arch Gerontol Geriatr 2010; 50(Suppl 1):S27–9.
27. Thompson MP, Morris LK. Unexplained weight loss in the ambulatory elderly. J Am Geriatr Soc 1991;39:497–500.
28. Evans WJ, Morley JE, Argiles J, et al. Cachexia: a new definition. Clin Nutr 2008; 27:793–9.
29. Rolland Y, Abellan van Kan G, Gillete-Guyonnet S, et al. Cachexia versus sarcopenia. Curr Opin Clin Nutr Metab Care 2011;14:15–21.
30. Bray GA, Champagne CM. Beyond energy balance: there is more to obesity than kilocalories. J Am Diet Assoc 2005;105:S17–23.
31. Guyenet SJ, Schwartz MW. Regulation of food intake, energy balance, and body fat mass: implications for the pathogenesis and treatment of obesity. J Clin Endocrinol Metab 2012;97:745–55.
32. Fearon KC, Glass DJ, Guttridge DC. Cancer cachexia: mediators, signaling, and metabolic pathways. Cell Metab 2012;16:153–66.
33. Argiles JM, Busquets S, Felipe A, et al. Molecular mechanisms involved in muscle wasting in cancer and ageing: cachexia versus sarcopenia. Int J Biochem Cell Biol 2005;37:1084–104.
34. Wagner PD. Possible mechanisms underlying the development of cachexia in COPD. Eur Respir J 2008;31:492–501.
35. Hernandez JL, Riancho JA, Matorras P, et al. Clinical evaluation for cancer in patients with involuntary weight loss without specific symptoms. Am J Med 2003; 114:631–7.
36. Baicus C, Ionescu R, Tanasescu C. Does this patient have cancer? The assessment of age, anemia, and erythrocyte sedimentation rate in cancer as a cause of weight loss. A retrospective study based on a secondary care university hospital in Romania. Eur J Intern Med 2006;17(1):28–31.
37. Sorbye LW, Schroll M, Finne-Soveri H, et al. Unintended weight loss in the elderly living at home: the aged in Home Care Project (AdHOC). J Nutr Health Aging 2008;12:10–6.
38. Wright BA. Weight loss and weight gain in a nursing home: a prospective study. Geriatr Nurs 1993;14:156–9.
39. Knoops KT, Slump E, de Groot LC, et al. Body weight changes in elderly psychogeriatric nursing home residents. J Gerontol A Biol Sci Med Sci 2005;60: 536–9.
40. von Haehling S, Lainscak M, Springer J, et al. Cardiac cachexia: a systematic overview. Pharmacol Ther 2009;121:227–52.
41. Anker SD, Ponikowski P, Varney S, et al. Wasting as independent risk factor for mortality in chronic heart failure. Lancet 1997;349:1050–3.
42. Schols AM, Broekhuizen R, Weling-Scheepers CA, et al. Body composition and mortality in chronic obstructive pulmonary disease. Am J Clin Nutr 2005;82:53–9.
43. Sullivan DH, Martin W, Flaxman N, et al. Oral Health Problems and Involuntary Weight Loss in a Population of Frail Elderly. J Am Geriatr Soc. 1993;41:725–31.
44. Tan BH, Fearon KC. Cachexia: prevalence and impact in medicine. Curr Opin Clin Nutr Metab Care 2008;11:400–7.
45. Mak RH, Cheung W. Cachexia in chronic kidney disease: role of inflammation and neuropeptide signaling. Curr Opin Nephrol Hypertens 2007;16:27–31.
46. Utech AE, Tadros EM, Hayes TG. Predicting survival in cancer patients: the role of cachexia and hormonal, nutritional and inflammatory markers. J Cachexia Sarcopenia Muscle 2012;3:245–51.

47. Rotman-Pikielny P, Borodin O, Zissin R, et al. Newly diagnosed thyrotoxicosis in hospitalized patients: clinical characteristics. QJM 2008;101:871–4.
48. Boelaert K, Torlinska B, Holder RL, et al. Older subjects with hyperthyroidism present with a paucity of symptoms and signs: a large cross-sectional study. J Clin Endocrinol Metab 2010;95:2715–26.
49. Trivalle C, Doucet J, Chassagne P, et al. Differences in the signs and symptoms of hyperthyroidism in older and younger patients. J Am Geriatr Soc 1996;44: 50–3.
50. Burke CW. Adrenocortical insufficiency. Clin Endocrinol Metab 1985;14:947–76.
51. Ross IL, Levitt NS. Addison's disease symptoms—a cross sectional study in Urban South Africa. PLoS One 2013;8:e53526.
52. von Haehling S, Anker SD. Cachexia as a major underestimated and unmet medical need: facts and numbers. J Cachexia Sarcopenia Muscle 2010;1:1–5.
53. Lim J, Ko YH, Joe SH. Zonisamide produces weight loss in psychotropic drug-treated psychiatric outpatients. Prog Neuropsychopharmacol Biol Psychiatry 2011;35:1918–21.
54. Stephen LJ, Kelly K, Wilson EA. A prospective audit of adjunctive zonisamide in an everyday clinical setting. Epilepsy Behav 2010;17:455–60.
55. Li Z, Maglione M, Tu W, et al. Meta-analysis: pharmacologic treatment of obesity. Ann Intern Med 2005;142:532–46.
56. Ersche KD, Stochl J, Woodward JM, et al. The skinny on cocaine: insights into eating behavior and body weight in cocaine-dependent men. Appetite 2013;71: 75–80.
57. Santolaria-Fernández FJ, Gómez-Sirvent JL, González-Reimers CE, et al. Nutritional assessment of drug addicts. Drug Alcohol Depend 1995;38:11–8.
58. Leduc D, Rouge PE, Rousset H, et al. Etude clinique de 105 cas d'amaigrissements isolees en medecine interne. Rev Med Interne 1988;9:480–6.
59. Newman AB, Yanez D, Harris T. Weight change in old age and its association with mortality. J Am Geriat Soc 2001;49:1309–18.
60. Hernandez JL, Matorras P, Riancho JA, et al. Involuntary weight loss without specific symptoms: a clinical prediction score for malignant neoplasm. QJM 2003;96:649–55.
61. Ruiz Garcia V, López-Briz E, Carbonell Sanchis R, et al. Megestrol acetate for treatment of anorexia-cachexia syndrome. Cochrane Database Syst Rev 2013;(3):CD004310. http://dx.doi.org/10.1002/14651858.CD004310.pub3.
62. Payne C, Wiffen PJ, Martin S. Interventions for fatigue and weight loss in adults with advanced progressive illness. Cochrane Database Syst Rev 2012;(1):CD008427. http://dx.doi.org/10.1002/14651858.CD008427.pub2.

Identifying and Treating the Causes of Neck Pain

Ginger Evans, MD

KEYWORDS

- Neck pain • Cervical spondylosis • Radiculopathy • Myelopathy • Chronic pain

KEY POINTS

- The first step in evaluating neck pain is to look for red flags to suggest serious underlying disease, analogous to the evaluation of low back pain.
- It is important to distinguish mechanical neck pain from radiculopathy or myelopathy based on history and physical examination; techniques are reviewed herein.
- The role of magnetic resonance imaging in mechanical neck pain is dubious.
- Many conservative treatment options are available. Those options with the best support in the literature include educational videos, select exercise interventions, mobilization accompanied by exercise, some medications, and possibly, acupuncture.
- There is no role for surgery in mechanical neck pain.
- Patients with severe or progressive radiculopathy or myelopathy are appropriately referred for surgery; those with mild to moderate radiculomyelopathy have short-term benefits from surgery, but long-term outcomes may be similar to conservative treatment.

INTRODUCTION

Neck pain is a common condition, with approximately 15% to 20% of people reporting neck pain each year and 1.5% to 1.8% of adults seeking ambulatory health care for this complaint annually.[1] Despite the frequency of this presenting complaint, a clear understanding of the cause and the best treatment course is often elusive. This review is aimed at primary care providers evaluating patients in clinic with the complaint of neck pain. Workup of neck pain in trauma victims is outside the scope of this review.

Anatomy

A brief review of the anatomy of the neck sets the stage for a better appreciation of potential causes of pain in the region. There are 7 cervical vertebrae. C1 and C2, atlas and axis, have no intervertebral disk between them. The remaining C3-7 vertebrae are

The author has no conflicts of interest to disclose.
Department of Medicine, VA Puget Sound Health Care System, University of Washington, 1660 South Columbia Way, S-123-PCC, Seattle, WA 98108, USA
E-mail address: gingere@u.washington.edu

Med Clin N Am 98 (2014) 645–661
http://dx.doi.org/10.1016/j.mcna.2014.01.015
0025-7125/14/$ – see front matter Published by Elsevier Inc.

connected superiorly and inferiorly to intervertebral disks, and articulate with adjacent vertebrae through 2 important joints:

- Uncovertebral joints (also called the joints of Luschka)
- Zygapophyseal joints (also called z-joints or facet joints)

To help envision the important structures in the vertebrae, we can begin at C4 and imagine moving posterolaterally from the vertebral body as it arches around toward the spinous process. First, a protuberance called the uncinate process is encountered (which abuts the C3-4 intervertebral disk and C3 vertebral body, forming the uncovertebral joints and comprising the anterior wall of the intervertebral foramen for the exiting C4 spinal nerve). Second, the uncinate process is followed by a depression (which forms the inferior wall of the intervertebral foramen). Third, there is another protuberance, called the articular facet (which connects, through a true synovial joint, to the C3 vertebra to form the zygapophyseal joint and the posterior wall of the intervertebral foramen). Therefore, (1) the anteromedial wall of the intervertebral foramen is the uncovertebral joint, which is not a true synovial joint and is a frequent site of bony overgrowth, and (2) the posterolateral wall of the intervertebral foramen is composed of the zygapophyseal joint, which is a true synovial joint and provides stability to the spine.[2–4]

There are 8 cervical spinal nerves; C1-7 exit superiorly to their named vertebra. C8 exits between C7 and T1.

- Motor efferent fibers have cell bodies in the anterior horn of the ventral spinal cord, exiting the cord to the ventral root, and then merging with sensory afferents to become the spinal nerve (a short nerve located inside the intervertebral foramen).
- Sensory afferents ascend from the periphery. The cell bodies form the dorsal root ganglion, which is located within the intervertebral foramen, just before merging with the spinal nerve (also inside the foramen). Sensory afferents enter the spinal cord through the dorsal root.[2,4,5]

Other surrounding structures to highlight include:

- The vertebral artery, which ascends adjacent laterally to the intervertebral foramina
- The intervertebral disks, comprising a gelatinous nucleus pulposis surrounded by an annulus fibrosis, and protected in the midline from herniating into the spinal cord by the posterior longitudinal ligament
- Cervical muscles and soft tissue

Diagnostic Uncertainty

Significant uncertainty still surrounds the pathophysiology of chronic neck pain, and in many cases, the chance of a clinician accurately identifying a specific cause is low.[1,6] A more critical task is to evaluate patients with neck pain for the following: cervical radiculopathy, cervical myelopathy, and dangerous underlying causes of pain (eg, cancer, fractures, osteomyelitis).[6,7]

Categorization of Neck Pain and Associated Cervical Spine Disorders

Radiculopathy

Radiculopathy is the constellation of symptoms caused by dysfunction of 1 or more cervical spinal nerve roots. It is less common than mechanical neck pain, with 1 population-based study[8] showing an average annual age-adjusted incidence of 83.2 per 100,000 people. Although noncompressive causes should be considered (eg, diabetes, herpes zoster, root avulsion), most (approximately 90%) radiculopathies result from compressive causes. In a large retrospective review at Mayo Clinic,[8] 21.9% of all radiculopathy cases were believed to have a probable cause of disk herniation (based on radiologic or surgical findings). Spondylosis is the major contributor to the remaining cases. Spondylosis usually refers to progressive, age-associated, degenerative changes of the vertebrae and intervertebral disks. These changes can lead to radiculopathy through bony hypertrophy of the uncovertebral joints and, less commonly, the zygapophyseal joints, both of which may cause narrowing of the intervertebral foramen and consequent compression of the spinal nerve.

Myelopathy

Myelopathy is related to narrowing of the spinal canal, most often from spondylosis (including osteophytes of the uncovertebral or zygapophyseal joints, or degenerative hypertrophy of the ligamentum flavum or posterior longitudinal ligaments). Pathophysiology may involve direct spinal cord or nerve root compression or ischemia from compression of arterial or venous supplies to the cord.[9]

Neck pain

Neck pain in the absence of radiculopathy, myelopathy, or clear serious underlying disease is also called mechanical neck pain, and has less well-understood pathophysiology. Among other things, this type of pain may be labeled as cervical muscle strain, myofascial pain, cervical spondylosis, cervical facet joint pain, and diskogenic pain. Because these structures are innervated, all of the muscles, synovial joints, intervertebral disks, dura mater, and vertebral arteries may theoretically generate pain.[2,7] Some studies attempting to more specifically delineate which of these features to implicate have focused on zygapophyseal joints and intervertebral disks. Examples of methods used include delivery of noxious stimuli (eg, saline or contrast injection) to specified structures in asymptomatic volunteers,[10,11] delivery of noxious stimuli to symptomatic volunteers (eg, provocation diskography),[12] and delivery of localized anesthesia in symptomatic volunteers (eg, anesthetic block to zygapophyseal joint either directly or through medial branch blocks).[13]

Some general conclusions from this research include[7,14,15]:

1. Zygapophyseal joints may be a source of pain in some subsets of patients with chronic neck pain caused by minor trauma or degenerative changes. The zygapophyseal joints may also produce referred pain to the head and upper extremities (referred pain is believed to stem from nociceptive afferents from facet joints that converge in the spinal cord with nociceptive afferents from other distal sites).[7,14,15] Attempts to map typical locations of pain derived from each zygapophyseal joint have been created and revised.[14] The prevalence of zygapophyseal pain in a primary care clinic population has not been determined. One estimate from a small population of specialty clinic patients (based on serial positive local anesthetic blocks) was reported at 36%.[16]

2. Although possible, there is no strong evidence that intervertebral disks (through degenerative or other changes) are a source of pain (diskogenic pain). This area remains controversial.[17–19]

3. Other potential sources of pain (eg, soft tissue, muscles, arteries) have not been rigorously studied.

These diagnostic techniques and the conclusions drawn from their use remain controversial.[20,21] Some systematic reviews find adequate evidence to support them,[15,22] but a recent systematic review and guidelines from the Bone and Joint 2000–2010 Task Force on Neck Pain do not endorse these injection techniques as a diagnostic maneuver.[1,19] Furthermore, per the literature review of this task force, there is no "evidence [that was deemed scientifically admissible] demonstrating that disk degeneration is a risk factor for neck pain."[23] Coauthors of related guidelines concur that there is "no evidence that common degenerative changes on cervical magnetic resonance imaging (MRI) are strongly correlated with neck pain symptoms."[19]

Summary

Recent guidelines state, "in most settings a simple descriptive clinical diagnosis might be preferable to a speculative tissue diagnosis as the origin of pain."[1] These guidelines propose a clinically practical grading system to guide workup and therapy by categorizing patients as follows:

Grade I: neck pain with no signs of major disease and no or little interference with daily activities

Grade II: neck pain with no signs of major disease, but interference with daily activities

Grade III: neck pain with neurologic signs of nerve compression

Grade IV: neck pain with signs of major disease

SYMPTOMS
Radiculopathy

The hallmark of radicular pain is some combination of diminished motor strength (described by about 15% of patients at presentation), reflexes, or sensation (paresthesias described by about 90% of patients at presentation) in a nerve root distribution. Lower cervical nerve roots (C5-8) are the most commonly involved in compressive radiculopathies. C7 is involved more than half the time; C6 is involved about 35% of the time.[8] Only a few patients describe trauma or physical exertion preceding their pain.[8] **Table 1** gives a description of history and examination findings for each nerve root. This table represents a compilation of several sources of information; the most distinguishing and consistently reported findings are in bold type.[2,3,6,7]

Pain is not a universal symptom of radiculopathy. Pain associated with radiculopathy may occur directly if the dorsal root ganglion is compressed.[24] Herniated disks, themselves, may also release inflammatory mediators, which may incite pain.[4] Although sensory symptoms like tingling may be felt in a dermatomal distribution, pain does not readily follow this same distribution. Instead, it is often deep feeling and is described as extending through the shoulder, arm, forearm, and hand (the hand being more common in C6-8 involvement).[4,7,8,25]

Myelopathy

Onset of symptoms of cervical myelopathy is often subtle and gradual; years may go by before the patient presents for medical care.[9,26] However, patients can present with sudden or episodic worsening, especially associated with trauma such as sudden hyperextension. If symptoms are mild at onset, the most common clinical course is to remain stable. Less frequently, a steady progression in symptoms is seen.[27,28]

Symptoms are variable and may include[9,29]:

1. Significant pain in the neck, shoulders, or arms (although not present in most patients)[30]
2. Gait spasticity
3. Upper extremity numbness, which is often in a nonspecific distribution but can be dermatomal, especially with a coexisting radiculopathy

Table 1
Signs and symptoms of cervical radiculopathy by involved nerve root

	C5	C6	C7	C8
Pain	Neck Scapula Shoulder	Neck Scapula Shoulder Radial forearm	Neck Scapula Chest Hand	Neck Medial forearm Hand
Sensation	**Clavicle, lateral shoulder** (Anterior forearm)	(Lateral arm, forearm) **Thumb** (Index finger)	(Thumb) **Index finger** **Middle finger** (Ring finger) (Palm)	(Medial forearm, arm) **Ring finger** **Little finger** (Medial hand)
Muscles innervated	Deltoid Biceps brachii Brachialis	Biceps brachii Brachialis Extensor carpi radialis longus and brevus	Extensor carpi radialis longus, brevus Triceps brachii Flexor digitorum superficialis, profundus	Triceps brachii
Motor	**Shoulder abduction** **Elbow flexion** **Wrist extension**	(Shoulder abduction) **Elbow flexion** (Forearm supination) (Forearm pronation) **Wrist extension** Finger extension	Elbow extension Forearm pronation **Wrist extension** **Finger, thumb extension**	Elbow extension Wrist flexion **Finger, thumb extension** Finger, thumb flexion Finger, thumb abduction Finger, thumb adduction
Reflexes	(Biceps) (Brachioradialis)	Biceps Brachioradialis	Triceps	

This table represents a compilation of several sources of information[2,3,6,7]; the most distinguishing and consistently reported findings are in bold type.

4. Loss of fine motor control in the hands
5. Lower extremity weakness
6. Bowel or bladder dysfunction, including urgency, frequency, retention

Mechanical Neck Pain

As discussed earlier, in the absence of these nerve dysfunction syndromes, the cause of neck pain is not well understood. The prevalence of neck pain increases with age, declining again in late life, and it frequently coexists with other comorbidities such as low back pain, headache, and poor self-rated health.[23] These same comorbidities also portend a worse prognosis. Workers' compensation payments and work-related stress are also reported predictors of persistent pain.[6] Most people who present to primary care clinic with neck pain experience recurrent or persistent problems.[31] In one population-based study of primary care patients with neck pain,[32] only one-third of patients reported resolution of symptoms at 1-year follow-up. Other studies suggest that between 15% and 50% of people in the general population report resolution at one year.[1]

DIAGNOSTIC TESTS/IMAGING STUDIES

Ordering imaging studies for neck pain is tricky. Although neck pain may be causing significant disability, imaging studies are often unhelpful and potentially misleading. A strong correlation between physical examination and imaging studies is paramount.

As most investigators on this subject have advocated, the clinician's first task is to ascertain any symptoms that might suggest serious underlying disease (such as trauma/fracture, osteomyelitis, cancer, inflammatory arthritides, or spinal cord compromise). These red flags,[6,19] as outlined in **Box 1**, should be similar to those

---

Box 1
Red flags for serious underlying disease

Cancer or infection

    Fever, chills, weight loss

    History of cancer

    Age >50 years or <20 years

    Intravenous drug use

    Immunosuppression (steroids, human immunodeficiency virus, transplant)

    Recent infection, especially with bacteremia

    Pain that is worse when supine

    Severe night time pain

    Fail to improve >6 weeks

    Tenderness over vertebral body

Fracture

    Significant trauma

    Osteoporosis

Systemic disease

    History of ankylosing spondylitis or inflammatory arthritis

Myelopathy

    Lower extremity spasticity

    Bowel or bladder changes

    Upper motor neuron signs (eg, Babinski, Hoffman)

reported in patients with low back pain.[33] Such symptoms warrant appropriate, expedited evaluation.

The second and related task is to discern any potential for spinal cord or nerve root compression. This task may be accomplished via the history and physical examination, as described in the next section (see section on symptoms also).

Radiculopathy, History, and Physical Examination

Findings of radiculopathy on examination might include decreased sensation as well as lower motor neuron signs (weakness, hyporeflexia, and less commonly, atrophy or hypotonia). Classically, sensory findings follow a dermatomal distribution, but in clinical practice, sensory findings on examination only follow this distribution in a few patients,[3,8] probably because of significant overlap in dermatomes. Pain into the arm rarely follows a dermatomal pattern, but may run more similar to a myotomal pattern.[4,7,8,25] **Table 1** compiles commonly reported associated findings depending on spinal nerve involved.[2,3,6,8,34] In practice, the experience of pain is variable, and dermatomal/myotomal boundaries overlap significantly. Lower cervical nerve roots are more commonly affected; C7 is the most frequent.[8]

Several provocative maneuvers have been reported for cervical radiculopathy.[19,35,36]

The upper limb tension test (ULTT), also called the brachial plexus tension test or test of Elvey, has been reported as the straight leg raise of the upper extremities; Rubinstein and colleagues[35] reviewed the literature and concurred that it has high sensitivity (97%), with a reasonable negative likelihood ratio (reported at 0.12, but with a large confidence interval). However, it has low specificity (22%–90%).[19,36,37] The ULTT is performed with the patient in a supine position. Provide (1) scapular depression with one hand, while (2) abducting the shoulder to 90°, with the elbow in 90° of flexion. (3) Supinate the forearms and wrist. Extend the wrist and fingers. (4) Push forward on the hand to laterally rotate the shoulder. (5) Extend the elbow. (6) Provocation of pain into the arm can also be further elicited in the final position by having the patient bend their head contralaterally (which should elicit or exacerbate pain)[36,38]; an ipsilateral head bend should diminish pain (**Fig. 1**).[36]

Neck distraction is performed by grasping under the patient's chin while they are supine and applying a modest upward distracting force, which should relieve symptoms. Wainner and colleagues[36] reported low sensitivity (44%) but reasonably high specificity (90%), with a reasonable positive likelihood ratio of 4.4 (although again with a large confidence interval).

Likewise, a positive Spurling sign (**Fig. 2**), Valsalva (pain with 3 seconds of breath holding/bearing down), or abduction relief sign (resolution of pain with placing hand on the patient's head) also have reasonably high specificity (86%–93%, 94%, and 75%–92%, respectively). Their sensitivity is low. They could support a diagnosis of radiculopathy in the context of corroborating history and other examination findings, but their absence does not rule out the disease.[35,36,39–41]

Myelopathy, History, and Physical Examination

In contrast to radiculopathy, the physical examination hallmarks of myelopathy are primarily upper motor neuron findings in a distribution below the level of compression. These findings may include upper or lower extremity weakness, spastic gait, and hyperreflexia. The plantar reflex (Babinski sign) and Hoffman reflex are important to perform, and their presence should alert the clinician to possible myelopathy.[6] The Hoffman reflex is performed by applying a quick pressure (flicking) to the middle finger and then looking for reflexive flexion of the thumb. Please note, this response can be

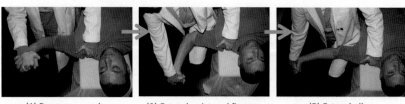

| (1) Depress scapula,
(2) Abduct shoulder | (3) Extend wrist and fingers,
(4) Laterally rotate shoulder | (5) Extend elbow |

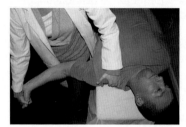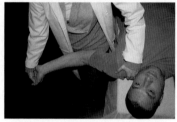

| Contralateral head bend worsens symptoms | Ipsilateral head bend improves symptoms |

Fig. 1. ULTT. (*Data from* Wainner RS, Fritz JM, Irrgang JJ, et al. Reliability and diagnostic accuracy of the clinical examination and patient self-report measures for cervical radiculopathy. Spine (Phila Pa 1976) 2003;28(1):52–62.)

nonpathologic in naturally hyperreflexic patients. There can be coexisting lower motor neuron findings in myelopathy because of simultaneous nerve root compression; these are classically at the level of involvement, not lower.

Laboratory Tests and Imaging

Blood work is rarely useful in the evaluation of neck pain, except perhaps in the evaluation of someone with red flag symptoms that suggest infection, cancer, and so forth (see **Box 1**).

Plain radiographs for the evaluation of nontraumatic neck pain in primary care clinic, are rarely, if ever, useful. They should be considered only in cases in which the history and examination have yielded red flags for serious disease (in which case the need for more advanced imaging might supersede radiographs, depending on the situation).

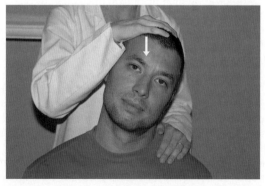

Fig. 2. Spurling maneuver: pain with axial pressure while head is bent ipsilaterally.

Abnormal curvature does not predict muscle spasm as sometimes believed.[42] In one series of 85 patients referred for radiographs based on neck pain,[43] there were no unexpected findings of malignancy or infection. In another series of 848 patients referred for radiographs,[44] there were no unexpected serious diagnoses.

MRI is clearly the test of choice if serious underlying disease, such as infection or cancer, is being considered. However, MRI findings of spinal cord or nerve root compression must be interpreted with caution and always correlated with the patient's history and examination. Degenerative changes, herniated disks, and compression of neural structures on MRI are common, age-related findings.[19] Review of cervical spine MRI scans performed in 100 asymptomatic patients showed herniated disks in 57% of patients older than 64 years, with spinal cord impingement in 26%. Asymptomatic spinal cord compression was observed in 7% of all the patients.[45] MRI can reliably show compression of neural structures, but these findings should then be correlated with any myelopathic or radicular symptoms.[19] Showing degenerative changes in the absence of nerve or cord compression usually does not change management.

Electromyography should be used in conjunction with the physical examination and MRI to evaluate a suspected radiculopathy. It has little role in evaluation of suspected myelopathy, except to rule out alternative explanations of symptoms/findings.[46]

Diskography and diagnostic (anesthetic) injections are controversial, and, although advocated by some investigators, they are generally not recommended based on current evidence for mechanical neck pain.[1,19]

DIFFERENTIAL DIAGNOSIS

A specific cause for neck pain is frequently not found. Rare causes should be considered, especially if red flags are present in the history or physical examination to suggest these. **Table 2** gives a list of common and rare causes.[6,7,19,47–49]

TREATMENT

Because neck pain is a common and sometimes disabling problem, it is not surprising that numerous methods of treatment are routinely used to mitigate symptoms. The scientific literature on treatment is often sparse, conflicting or mired in methodological flaws, making it difficult for the practicing clinician to feel confident about what course of action to recommend. It is not even clear what the benefits and harms of giving a diagnostic label (such as degenerative joint disease) may be for a patient.

Multiple challenges exist in both treating and studying the treatment of patients with neck pain. Lack of clarity on the basic understanding of the cause of neck pain without radiculopathy or myelopathy makes targeted interventions challenging. Gold standards for diagnosis of purported causes are murky. Patients with neck pain are probably a heterogeneous group of patients who respond differently to various interventions. For example, response to treatment may vary depending on (1) presence of radiculopathy, myelopathy or neither, (2) comorbid psychiatric disease or personality,[50] or (3) other premorbid musculoskeletal pains,[23] to name a few. With the inherently subjective nature of pain reporting, it can be hypothesized that a patient's preference for certain treatments (eg, if a friend had a good experience with one type of treatment) may influence a patient's perception or reporting of pain after treatment.

As mentioned earlier, distinctions should be drawn between mechanical neck pain, neck pain with radiculopathy or myelopathy, and neck pain with serious underlying disease (eg, fracture, cancer, infection). Treatment of patients in this final category (serious underlying disease) is often appropriately more aggressive, with excellent

Table 2
Common and rare causes of neck pain, radiculomyelopathy or both

	Neck Pain Alone	Neck Pain with Radiculopathy/ Myelopathy	Radiculopathy/ Myelopathy Symptoms Alone	
Common				
Disk herniation	x	x	x	
Neuroforaminal stenosis (from spondylosis, disk herniation, or both)		x	x	
Spinal canal stenosis (from spondylosis, large central disk herniation, ligament calcification, or combination)		x	x	
Nonspecific pain (also known as mechanical pain) from unknown cause; sometimes, this is labeled as cervical muscle strain, facet joint pain, and so forth	x			
Rare				
Tumor	x	x	x	
Benign tumors (hemangioma, osteoid osteoma, osteoblastoma, osteochondroma, giant cell tumor)		x	x	
Serious infections (diskitis, osteomyelitis, epidural abscess, septic arthritis, meningitis)	x	x	x	
Vascular causes (eg, vertebral artery, internal carotid or aortic dissection)	x	x	x	
Nerve root infarction (vasculitis)		x	x	
Trauma: fracture, root avulsion, spinal cord injuries	x	x	x	
Polymyalgia rheumatica/ temporal arteritis	x			Stiffness should be primary
Inflammatory arthropathies (rheumatoid arthritis, crystal arthropathy, ankylosing spondylitis)	x			Typically multiple joint involvement and systemic inflammatory symptoms
				(*continued on next page*)

Table 2
(continued)

	Neck Pain Alone	Neck Pain with Radiculopathy/ Myelopathy	Radiculopathy/ Myelopathy Symptoms Alone	
Fibromyalgia	x			Should not be isolated neck pain
Synovial cyst			x	
Torticollis	x			Not necessarily painful
Diffuse idiopathic skeletal hyperostosis			x	Classically painless, except at risk for cervical fractures from minimal trauma. Stiffness and dysphagia more common symptoms
Paget disease			x	Cervical spine lesions only seen in 11% of patients. In a series of 180 patients, none reported neck pain and only 2 patients had spinal cord compression[48]
Thoracic outlet syndrome		x	x	
Shoulder diseases	x			
Multiple sclerosis			x	
Amyotrophic lateral sclerosis, Guillain-Barré syndrome, normal pressure hydrocephalus			x	
Noncompressive radiculopathies (rare)				
Diabetic monoradiculopathy			x	
Herpes zoster			x	
Lyme disease			x	
Tuberculosis	x		x	
Syphilis			x	
Brucellosis			x	
Cytomegalovirus			x	
Lyme disease			x	
Histiocytosis X			x	
Sarcoidosis			x	
Human immunodeficiency virus–related neuropathy			x	

support in the literature. This subject is outside the scope of this discussion and we focus instead on the first two categories.[1]

Multiple helpful systematic reviews have been published for individual treatment methods, combinations of treatment methods, and overall surgical versus conservative treatment courses.[51–65]

Conservative Treatments

A panoply of conservative treatments are available. Typically, in the absence of severe myelopathic or radicular motor weakness, these treatments are the first attempted courses of action. Of the available options, those believed to have the weight of evidence in support include educational videos after whiplash injury; select exercise interventions; mobilization when used with exercise; some medications; and possibly, acupuncture.

Although reassurance and education are often given at initial consultations, there is no evidence that such counseling is superior to any other noninvasive treatments for mechanical neck pain.[53] Specifically, after whiplash injury, an educational video was shown to predict lower pain ratings at 24 weeks.[66] There is low-quality to moderate-quality evidence for the use of specific cervical and scapular stretching and strengthening exercises for chronic neck pain,[55,67,68] but not upper extremity stretching and strengthening or a general exercise program. The improvement from these stretching and strengthening exercises is often limited to immediately after treatment and decreases after the intermediate-term.

Manual therapies encompass a range of hands-on interventions, which might typically be used by a physical therapist, occupational therapist, chiropractor, or doctor of osteopathic medicine. One type of manual therapy is joint mobilization. Joint mobilizations are a type of passive movement of a skeletal joint, graded and distinguished by positioning of the joint and velocity and amplitude of the movement. Within the spectrum of mobilizations, a high-velocity, low-amplitude thrust has several synonymous terms: manipulation, a grade V mobilization, or an adjustment. Multiple systematic reviews have looked at the evidence for joint mobilization, manipulation, or other manual therapies as a treatment of mechanical neck pain and come to slightly different conclusions. Mior[69] concluded that evidence is limited and that these therapies may or may not be effective. Gross and colleagues[56] in their Cochrane review concluded that mobilization or manipulation when used with exercise is beneficial, but when performed alone is not. The Bone and Joint Task Force[53] concluded that mobilization or exercise sessions alone or in combination with medications are beneficial in the short-term (6–13 weeks).

Several classes of oral medications are frequently used for chronic, mechanical neck pain, including nonsteroidal antiinflammatory drugs, muscle relaxants, opiates, antidepressants, and other analgesics. They all have limited evidence and unclear benefits.[57]

Two systematic reviews of acupuncture[53,58] reported moderate-quality or inconsistent evidence of benefit compared with sham controls.

Because of limited evidence, conclusions cannot be drawn about the effectiveness of massage,[59] and multiple investigators have concluded that passive modalities (transcutaneous electrical nerve stimulation, ultrasonography, diathermy, electrotherapy) are not associated with short-term or long-term pain or functional improvements.[53,60]

Specifically for radiculopathy, traction has been advocated; it is intuitively believed to decrease pressure on the exiting spinal nerve. It is contraindicated in patients with significant or severe spondylosis, who have myelopathy, a positive Lhermitte sign, or rheumatoid arthritis with atlantoaxial subluxation.[70] A recent Cochrane review[61] found only one study deemed to have a low risk of bias and concluded that there was no evidence of benefit. Graham and colleagues[62] also found few high-quality trials and concluded that there was no evidence of benefit to continuous traction and low-quality evidence for intermittent traction. Others have determined that poor methodological quality precludes any conclusions.[4,63]

In a practice environment with a dearth of high-quality evidence, perhaps patient preference should strongly influence choice of therapy. Future research is critical.

Invasive Treatments

Steroid injections may be considered for radiculopathy, with evidence supporting short-term symptom improvement.[54,71] For more significant manifestations of radiculopathy, steroid injections do not seem to decrease the rate of open surgery.[54] Zygapophyseal injections are a controversial therapy for mechanical neck pain (without radiculopathy) and are not endorsed by the Bone and Joint Task Force.[54]

Surgery

For a detailed discussion of surgical outcomes, the reader is referred to the surgical literature. There is not convincing evidence to support the role of surgery in mechanical neck pain,[54] and there is wide variation in current practice with regards to who is referred for surgery.[72]

For patients with severe or progressive radiculomyelopathy, surgery is appropriately considered.[9]

In the presence of mild to moderate radiculopathy, short-term outcomes of pain relief, decreased numbness, and weakness are better with surgery compared with conservative management, but that difference disappears with longer-term (1–2 year) follow-up.[64] In the presence of mild to moderate myelopathy, short-term benefits have been reported, but long-term follow-up (3 years) does not delineate benefits over conservative treatment.[28,54,64]

MANAGEMENT

Mechanical neck pain is frequently a chronic or recurrent problem for individual patients. Regular follow-up with a provider should focus on vigilance for clues to underlying serious disease and monitoring for the onset or progression of radiculopathy or myelopathy. Conservative management is usually the recommended course, and various options were discussed earlier. Given the lack of evidence that one conservative management tool is superior to another,[73] patient preference and availability can figure prominently in the decision. Other pillars of chronic pain management also apply here, such as validating the patient's experience of pain, managing expectations of treatments, refocusing goals of treatment toward functionality, and treating comorbidities such as depression. Although it has not yet been validated in the literature,[65] considering a multidisciplinary approach seems reasonable.

SUMMARY/FUTURE CONSIDERATIONS

Future studies are needed to further understand the pathophysiology of mechanical neck pain. Robust scientific evidence is sparse on which noninvasive treatments are the most beneficial and how to better select patients for particular noninvasive or invasive treatments.

REFERENCES

1. Guzman J, Haldeman S, Carroll L, et al. Clinical practice implications of the Bone and Joint Decade 2000-2010 Task Force on Neck Pain and its associated disorders: from concepts and findings to recommendations. Spine 2008;33(4S): S199–213.
2. Netter FH. Atlas of human anatomy. 3rd edition. Teterboro (NJ): Icon Learning Systems; 2003.
3. Robinson J, Kothari M. Clinical features and diagnosis of cervical radiculopathy. Available at: http://www.uptodate.com/. Accessed September 28, 2013.
4. Carette S, Fehlings MG. Cervical radiculopathy. N Engl J Med 2005;353: 392–9.
5. Zhang J, Tsuzuki N, Hirabayashi S, et al. Surgical anatomy of the nerves and muscles in the posterior cervical spine: a guide for avoiding inadvertent nerve injuries during the posterior approach. Spine 2003;28(13):1379–84.
6. Honet JC, Ellenberg MR. What you always wanted to know about the history and physical exam of neck pain but were afraid to ask. Phys Med Rehabil Clin N Am 2003;14:473–91.
7. Bogduk N. The anatomy and pathophysiology of neck pain. Phys Med Rehabil Clin N Am 2011;22:367–82.
8. Radhakrishnan K, Litchy WJ, O'Fallon WM, et al. Epidemiology of cervical radiculopathy. A population based study from Rochester, Minnesota 1876 through 1990. Brain 1994;117:325–35.
9. McCormick WE, Steinmetz MP, Benzel EC. Cervical spondylotic myelopathy: make a difficult diagnosis, then refer for surgery. Cleve Clin J Med 2003; 70(10):899–904.
10. Dreyfuss P, Michaelsen M, Fletcher D. Atlanto-occipital and lateral atlanto-axial joint pain patterns. Spine 1994;19(10):1125–31.
11. Dwyer A, Aprill C, Bogduk N. Cervical zygapophyseal joint pain patterns. I: a study in normal volunteers. Spine 1990;15(6):453–7.
12. Fukui S, Ohetso K, Shiotani M, et al. Referred pain distribution of the cervical zygapophyseal joints and cervical dorsal rami. Pain 1996;68:79–83.
13. Aprill C, Dwyer A, Bogduk N. Cervical zygapophyseal joint pain patterns. II: a clinical evaluation. Spine 1990;15(6):458–61.
14. Cooper G, Bailey B, Bogduk N. Cervical zygapophysial joint pain maps. Pain Med 2007;8(4):344–53.
15. Sehgal N, Dunbar EE, Shah RV, et al. Systematic review of diagnostic utility of facet (zygapophysial) joint injections in chronic spinal pain: an update. Pain Physician 2007;10:213–8.
16. Speldewinde GC, Bashford GM, Davidson IR. Diagnostic cervical zygapophyseal joint blocks for chronic cervical pain. Med J Aust 2001;174(4): 174–6.
17. Schellhas KP, Smith MD, Gundry CR, et al. Cervical discogenic pain. Prospective correlation of magnetic resonance imaging and discography in asymptomatic subjects and pain sufferers. Spine 1996;21(3):311–2.
18. Slipman CW, Plastaras C, Patel R, et al. Provocative cervical discography symptom mapping. Spine 2005;5(4):381–8.
19. Nordin M, Carragee EJ, Hogg-Johnson S, et al. Assessment of neck pain and its associated disorders. Results of the Bone And Joint Decade 2000– 2010 Task Force on Neck Pain and its Associated Disorders. Spine 2008;33(Suppl): S101–22.

20. Hogan QH, Abram SE. Neural blockade for diagnosis and prognosis. Anesthesiology 1997;86(1):216–41.
21. Ackerman WE, Munir MA, Zhang JM, et al. Are diagnostic lumbar facet injections influenced by pain of muscular origin? Pain Pract 2004;4(4):286–91.
22. Falco FJ, Erhart S, Wargo BW, et al. Systematic review of diagnostic utility and therapeutic effectiveness of cervical facet joint interventions. Pain Physician 2009;12(2):323–44.
23. Hogg-Johnson S, van der Velde G, Carroll LJ, et al. The burden and determinants of neck pain in the general population: results of the Bone and Joint Decade 2000-2010 Task Force on Neck Pain and its Associated Disorders. Spine 2008;33(4S):S39–51.
24. Song XJ, Hu SJ, Greenquist KW, et al. Mechanical and thermal hyperalgesia and ectopic neuronal discharge after chronic compression of dorsal root ganglia. J Neurophysiol 1999;82(6):3347–58.
25. Slipman CW, Plastaras CT, Palmitier RA, et al. Symptom provocation of fluoroscopically guided cervical nerve root stimulation: are dynatomal maps identical to dermatomal maps? Spine 1998;23(20):2235–42.
26. Brain WR, Northfield D, Wilkinson M. Neurological manifestations of cervical spondylosis. Brain 1952;75(2):187–225.
27. Kadanka Z, Mares M, Bednaríka J, et al. Predictive factors for mild forms of spondylotic cervical myelopathy treated conservatively or surgically. Eur J Neurol 2005;12(1):16–24.
28. Kadanka Z, Mares M, Bednaník J, et al. Approaches to spondylotic cervical myelopathy: conservative versus surgical results in a 3-year follow-up study. Spine 2002;27(20):2205–10.
29. Tracy JA, Bartleson JD. Cervical spondylotic myelopathy. Neurologist 2010; 16(3):176–87.
30. Lunsford LD, Bissonette DJ, Zorub DS. Anterior surgery for cervical disc disease. Part 2: treatment of cervical spondylotic myelopathy in 32 cases. J Neurosurg 1980;53(1):12–9.
31. Carroll L, Hogg-Johnson S, van der Velde G, et al. Course and prognostic factors for neck pain in the general population. Results of the Bone and Joint Decade 2000-2010 Task Force on Neck Pain and its Associated Disorders. Spine 2008;33(4S):S75–82.
32. Cote P, Cassidy JD, Carroll LJ, et al. The annual incidence and course of neck pain in the general population: a population-based cohort study. Pain 2004; 112(3):267–73.
33. Chou R, Qaseem A, Snow V, et al. Diagnosis and Treatment of Low Back Pain: A Joint Clinical Practice Guideline from the American College of Physicians and the American Pain Society. Ann Intern Med 2007;147(7):478–91.
34. Yoss RE, Corbin KB, MacCarlty CS, et al. Significance of symptoms and signs in localization of involved root in cervical disk protrusion. Neurology 1957;7(10): 673–83.
35. Rubinstein S, Pool JJ, van Tulder MW. A systematic review of the diagnostic accuracy of provocative tests of the neck for diagnosing cervical radiculopathy. Eur Spine J 2007;16(3):307–19.
36. Wainner RS, Fritz JM, Irrgang JJ, et al. Reliability and diagnostic accuracy of the clinical examination and patient self-report measures for cervical radiculopathy. Spine 2003;28(1):52–62.
37. Sandmark H, Nisell R. Validity of five common manual neck pain provoking tests. Scand J Rehabil Med 1995;27(3):131–6.

38. Elvey RL. The investigation of arm pain: signs of adverse responses to the physical examination of the brachial plexus and related tissues. In: Boyling JD, Palastanga N, editors. Grieve's modern manual therapy. 2nd edition. New York: Churchill Livingstone; 1994. p. 577–85.

39. Tong HC, Haig AJ, Yamakawa K. The Spurling test and cervical radiculopathy. Spine 2002;27(2):156–9.

40. Davidson RI, Dunn EJ, Metzmaker JN. The shoulder abduction test in the diagnosis of radicular pain in cervical extradural compressive monoradiculopathies. Spine 1981;6(5):441–6.

41. Viikari-Juntura E, Porras M, Laasonen EM. Validity of clinical tests in the diagnosis of root compression in cervical disc disease. Spine 1989;14(3):253–7.

42. Matsumoto M, Fujimura Y, Suzuki N, et al. Cervical curvature in acute whiplash injuries: prospective comparative study with asymptomatic subjects. Injury 1998;29(10):775–8.

43. Heller CA, Stanley P, Lewis-Jones B, et al. Value of x ray examinations of the cervical spine. Br Med J (Clin Res Ed) 1983;287(6401):1276–8.

44. Johnson MJ, Lucas GL. Value of cervical spine radiographs as a screening tool. Clin Orthop Relat Res 1997;340:102–8.

45. Teresi LM, Lufkin RB, Reicher MA, et al. Asymptomatic degenerative disk disease and spondylosis of the cervical spine: MR imaging. Radiology 1987; 164(1):83–8.

46. So YT, Weber CF, Campbell WW. Practice parameter for needle electromyographic evaluation of patients with suspected cervical radiculopathy: summary statement. American Association of Electrodiagnostic Medicine. American Academy of Physical Medicine and Rehabilitation. Muscle Nerve 1999;22(S8): S209–11.

47. Shelerud RA, Paynter KS. Rarer causes of radiculopathy: spinal tumors, infections, and other unusual causes. Phys Med Rehabil Clin N Am 2002;13:645–96.

48. Harinck HI, Bijvoet OL, Vellenga CJ, et al. Relation between signs and symptoms in Paget's disease of bone. Q J Med 1986;58(226):133–51.

49. Mazières B. Diffuse idiopathic skeletal hyperostosis (Forestier-Rotes-Querol disease): what's new? Joint Bone Spine 2013;80(5):466–70. http://dx.doi.org/10.1016/j.jbspin.2013.02.011.

50. Van der Donk J, Shouten J, Passchier J, et al. The associations of neck pain with radiological abnormalities of the cervical spine and personality traits in a general population. J Rheumatol 1991;18(12):1884–9.

51. Nikolaidis I, Fouyas IP, Sandercock PA, et al. Surgery for cervical radiculopathy or myelopathy. Cochrane Database Syst Rev 2010;(1):CD001466. http://dx.doi.org/10.1002/14651858.CD001466.pub3.

52. Vernon H, McDermaid CS, Hagino C. Systematic review of randomized clinical trials of complementary/alternative therapies in the treatment of tension-type and cervicogenic headache. Complement Ther Med 1999;7(3):142–55.

53. Hurwitz EL, Carragee EJ, van der Velde G, et al. Treatment of neck pain. Noninvasive interventions: results of the bone and Joint Decade 2000-2010 Task Force on Neck Pain and its Associated Disorders. Spine 2008;33(4S):S123–52.

54. Carragee EJ, Hurwitz EL, Cheng I, et al. Treatment of neck pain. Injections and surgical interventions: results of the Bone and Joint Decade 2000-2010 Task Force on Neck Pain and its Associated Disorders. Spine 2008;33(4S):S153–69.

55. Kay TM, Gross A, Goldsmith CH, et al. Exercises for mechanical neck disorders. Cochrane Database Syst Rev 2012;(8):CD004250. http://dx.doi.org/10.1002/14651858.CD004250.pub4.

56. Gross A, Hoving JL, Haines TA, et al. A Cochrane review of manipulation and mobilization for mechanical neck disorders. Spine 2004;29(14):1541–8.
57. Peloso PM, Gross A, Haines T, et al, Cervical Overview Group. Medicinal and injection therapies for mechanical neck disorders. Cochrane Database Syst Rev 2007;(3):CD000319. http://dx.doi.org/10.1002/14651858.CD000319.pub4.
58. Trinh K, Graham N, Gross A, et al. Acupuncture for neck disorders. Spine 2007; 32(2):236–43.
59. Patel KC, Gross A, Graham N, et al. Massage for mechanical neck disorders. Cochrane Database Syst Rev 2012;(9):CD004871. http://dx.doi.org/10.1002/14651858.CD004871.pub4.
60. Kroeling P, Gross AR, Goldsmith CH. A Cochrane review of electrotherapy for mechanical neck disorders. Spine 2005;30(21):E641–8.
61. Graham N, Gross A, Goldsmith CH, et al. Mechanical traction for neck pain with or without radiculopathy. Cochrane Database Syst Rev 2008;(3):CD006408. http://dx.doi.org/10.1002/14651858.CD006408.pub2.
62. Graham N, Gross A, Goldsmith C. Mechanical traction for mechanical neck disorders: a systematic review. J Rehabil Med 2006;38(3):145–52.
63. van der Heijden GJ, Beurskens AJ, Koes BW, et al. The efficacy of traction for back and neck pain: a systematic, blinded review of randomized clinical trial methods. Phys Ther 1995;75(2):93–104.
64. Fouyas I, Statham P, Sandercock PA. Cochrane review of the role of surgery in cervical spondylotic radiculomyelopathy. Spine 2002;27(7):736–47.
65. Karjalainen KA, Malmivaara A, van Tulder MW, et al. Multidisciplinary biopsychosocial rehabilitation for neck and shoulder pain among working age adults. Cochrane Database Syst Rev 2003;(2):CD002194. http://dx.doi.org/10.1002/14651858CD002194.
66. Brison RJ, Hartling L, Dostaler S, et al. A randomized controlled trial of an educational intervention to prevent the chronic pain of whiplash associated disorders following rear-end motor vehicle collisions. Spine 2005;30(16):1799–807.
67. Sarig-Bahat H. Evidence for exercise therapy in mechanical neck disorders. Man Ther 2003;8(1):10–20.
68. Mior S. Exercise in the treatment of chronic pain. Clin J Pain 2001;17(4S): S77–85.
69. Mior S. Manipulation and mobilization in the treatment of chronic pain. Clin J Pain 2001;17(4S):S70–6.
70. Ellenberg MR, Honet JC, Treanor WJ. Cervical radiculopathy. Arch Phys Med Rehabil 1994;75:342–52.
71. Stav A, Ovadia L, Sternberg A, et al. Cervical epidural steroid injection for cervicobrachialgia. Acta Anaesthesiol Scand 1993;37(6):562–6.
72. Harland SP, Laing RJ. A survey of the perioperative management of patients undergoing anterior cervical decompression in the UK and Eire. Br J Neurosurg 1998;12(2):113–7.
73. Van der Velde G, Hogg-Johnson S, Bayoumi AM, et al. Identifying the best treatment among common nonsurgical neck pain treatments. Spine 2008;33(4S): S184–91.

Medically Unexplained Symptoms

Margaret L. Isaac, MD[a],*, Douglas S. Paauw, MD, MACP[b]

KEYWORDS

- Medically unexplained symptoms • Somatization • Somatoform • Depression • Pain

KEY POINTS

- Medically unexplained symptoms (MUS) are a significant cause of morbidity for patients and of resource use for the health care system.
- Multiple diagnostic categories exist for patients with MUS.
- Risk factors for MUS include female gender, low socioeconomic status, and a history of trauma (specifically childhood sexual abuse).
- A careful history and physical examination is required for all patients with MUS, with additional diagnostic testing dictated by the patient's symptom severity and chronicity.
- Treatments for MUS include cognitive behavior therapy, antidepressant treatment, and empathic, patient-centered care.

CASE 1: MS D

Ms D is a 71-year-old woman with a history of peptic ulcer disease, metabolic syndrome, major depressive disorder, and osteoarthritis who presents for clinical follow-up with pain all over her body. She states that she cannot remember a time when her entire body did not hurt. She is also concerned about chronic abdominal pain.

On examination, her vital signs are within normal limits. She is tender to light palpation in every major muscle group. She is diffusely tender to light palpation on abdominal examination, but without palpable masses, organomegaly, rebound, or guarding.

Her evaluation so far has included a basic metabolic panel, liver function tests, and a lipase, all of which were within normal limits, and a complete blood count that revealed a mild normocytic anemia (hematocrit, 34%), hand radiographs that showed advanced osteoarthritis at the first carpometacarpal joint bilaterally, lumbar spine radiographs that showed mild spondylosis, and an abdominal computed tomography (CT) scan significant for diverticulosis without evidence of diverticulitis. She has also undergone upper and lower endoscopy, which revealed no masses or ulcers, and mild diverticulosis as noted earlier.

The authors have no financial disclosures.

[a] Department of Medicine, Harborview Medical Center, University of Washington School of Medicine, 325 9th Avenue, Box 359892, Seattle, WA 98104, USA; [b] Division of General Internal Medicine, Department of Medicine, University of Washington School of Medicine, Seattle, WA 98195, USA
* Corresponding author.
E-mail address: misaac@uw.edu

Med Clin N Am 98 (2014) 663–672
http://dx.doi.org/10.1016/j.mcna.2014.01.013
0025-7125/14/$ – see front matter © 2014 Elsevier Inc. All rights reserved.

She is here to establish care with you after having seen multiple other physicians in your practice. She is concerned that she might have cancer in her abdomen or in her bones and expresses concern that her prior physicians have not taken her concerns seriously. What do you think is going on?

INTRODUCTION

Medically unexplained symptoms (MUS) are common in the outpatient and primary care settings. Although prevalence data vary, most studies suggest that more than 50% of patients presenting to primary care clinics with physical symptoms have no diagnosable organic disease.[1,2] Patients with a somatization disorder use twice as many outpatient and inpatient resources and have double the average health care costs per year, independent of psychiatric and medical comorbidity.[3] MUS are challenging to treat and can be frustrating for primary care physicians to address and manage. Risk factors for the development of multiple somatic symptoms include, but are not limited to, female gender,[4] low education,[5] abuse in childhood, and comorbid medical and psychiatric disease.[6] Having a specific and intentional diagnostic and therapeutic approach to patients with MUS can help providers build strong and effective therapeutic relationships with patients, manage limited health care resources wisely, and focus on improving long-term quality of life in the subset of MUS patients with chronic symptoms.

DEFINITIONS

The terms MUS and somatization refer to symptoms that have minimal or no apparent basis in physical disease. These terms can also apply to patients with underlying disease explaining the presence of physical symptoms, but with a symptom burden out of proportion to what is expected. Some investigators criticize the use of the term MUS because of the ambiguity inherent in declaring a symptom to be unexplained, or unexplainable, and the importance of including diseases that may have psychological underpinnings under the broad heading of medical illness.[7] Other disease classifications exist for patients with specific symptom constellations within MUS, including fibromyalgia, chronic fatigue syndrome, chronic pelvic pain, and irritable bowel syndrome. There may also be significant overlap with idiopathic environmental intolerance (IEI; also known as multiple chemical sensitivity), a poorly understood and subjective syndrome characterized by nonspecific, ambiguous, and recurrent symptoms attributed to low levels of chemical, biologic, or physical agents. Somatoform disorders are found in more than one-fourth of patients with IEI symptoms and some investigators think that IEI may be a variant of MUS/somatoform disorders.[8] Gulf War illness, which refers to a constellation of somatic symptoms in veterans of the Gulf War, is generally one of 2 types: chronic fatigue syndrome or multiple chemical sensitivity pattern,[9,10] and can be included additionally under the general heading of MUS.

The prior diagnostic criteria for somatization disorder in the Diagnostic and Statistical Manual of Mental Disorders, Fourth Edition (DSM-IV) were so specific and detailed as to exclude most patients with MUS. The Diagnostic and Statistical Manual of Mental Disorders, Fifth Edition (DSM-V), published in 2013, incorporates significant changes to these diagnostic criteria. Multiple prior diagnostic categories have now been subsumed into the classification somatic symptom and related disorders. The diagnostic criteria for somatic symptom disorder include:

A. One or more somatic symptoms that are distressing or result in significant disruption of daily life.

B. Excessive thoughts, feelings, or behaviors related to the somatic symptoms or associated health concerns as manifested by at least one of the following:
   1. Disproportionate and persistent thoughts about the seriousness of one's symptoms
   2. Persistently high level of anxiety about health or symptoms
   3. Excessive time and energy devoted to these symptoms or health concerns
C. Although any somatic symptom may not be continuously present, the state of being symptomatic is persistent (typically more than 6 months).

The diagnostic criteria require further specification if the patient has predominant pain and if the symptoms are persistent (>6 months), and also require specification of illness severity (mild, moderate, or severe).[11] The focus in this diagnosis is not the presence of somatic symptoms per se, but the psychological impact of symptoms on the patient. Other related disorders described in DSM-V include illness anxiety disorder, conversion disorder (functional neurologic symptom disorder), and psychological factors affecting other medical conditions.

PATHOPHYSIOLOGY

The pathophysiology of MUS is poorly understood. Controversy exists as to whether the syndrome is predominantly physical or psychiatric, or a combination of the two, and whether the various named syndromes within the broader category of MUS or functional somatic syndromes are physiologically distinct, valid, and meaningful.[12,13] In one small study, 1 in 3 physicians thought that the cause of MUS was likely spiritual.[14] Some evidence suggests a familial risk for somatization, although it remains unclear whether this link is genetic, epigenetic, or environmental.[15] MUS has also been linked to alexithymia, or an inability to verbally express emotions,[16,17] although causality has not been clearly established. Multiple studies suggest an association between MUS and a history of traumatic events, including abuse in childhood.[18-20] Other formative childhood experiences such as unexplained symptoms, parental illness (particularly poor paternal health), and increased parental illness behavior in response to children's symptoms are additional risk factors for development of MUS later in life.[21,22] A history of rape victimization is also strongly associated with the development of MUS.[20]

Somatization occurs across cultures, and no significant differences between cultural groups with regard to prevalence have been found.[23-25] However, there can be differences in specific symptoms between cultural groups.[26]

SYMPTOMS

The most common symptom attributed to MUS is pain,[1] including diffuse myalgias, arthralgias, low back pain, headache, and dysuria. Other possible symptoms include:

- Systemic symptoms: fatigue and insomnia
- Head and neck symptoms: tinnitus, pseudo–eustachian tube dysfunction, atypical facial pain, globus sensation[27]
- Cardiac symptoms: chest pain, palpitations, and dyspnea
- Gastrointestinal symptoms: bloating, nausea, abdominal discomfort, constipation, and diarrhea
- Genitourinary symptoms: chronic pelvic pain, dyspareunia, vulvodynia, and dysmenorrhea
- Neurologic symptoms: pseudoseizures, dizziness, weakness

The absolute number of physical symptoms is correlated with risk for depression and anxiety, and somatoform disorders additionally are strongly associated with mood disorders.[28]

CASE 2: MS L

Ms L is a 47-year-old woman with a history of hepatitis C and generalized anxiety disorder who presents with hemifacial pain and seizures. She states that she experiences episodes of throbbing pain that are migratory, occurring all over her scalp, lasting hours to days. It seems to occur more frequently when she has to leave the house to take her children to school or to come to medical appointments. No photophobia or phonophobia. No fevers, chills, or night sweats. No weight loss or nausea. Her seizurelike episodes usually consist of diffuse tremors followed by loss of consciousness, and she has had some mild trauma from falls related to this.

Her neurologic examination is normal. Routine laboratory tests were also within normal limits. A noncontrast head CT scan was performed and showed no masses or intracranial disorder. She has undergone multiple electroencephalograms, none of which show any epileptiform discharges.

Would you perform any further diagnostic evaluation?

DIAGNOSTIC TESTING/IMAGING STUDIES

A diagnosis of MUS can be made only after organic disease has been ruled out. It is therefore critical for clinicians to take a careful history and perform a thorough physical examination before making a diagnosis of MUS. History taking should be broad and comprehensive, with a specific focus on other symptoms that may suggest organic disease, and on patient attribution (to what does the patient attribute the symptoms?). The social history can be particularly useful in this setting as well, providing information on childhood factors that may predispose a patient to MUS, and on situational stressors that may be exacerbating mental and physical symptoms. However, in the absence of red flags in the history or abnormal physical examination findings, laboratory and radiographic testing should be used judiciously. Many physicians find themselves ordering tests they do not think are medically indicated in an effort to alleviate a patient's fears about underlying organic disease. However, extensive testing has not been shown to alleviate concerns about serious illness in patients with a low pretest probability of organic disease.[29] Some investigators recommend using MUS severity to dictate the intensity of further testing,[30] as follows:

- Normal to mild MUS: normal behavior, in which patients seek reassurance for infrequent and mild symptoms. Organic disease can be excluded through careful history taking, physical examination, and watchful waiting/observation over time.
- Moderate MUS: patients in this group may have either chronic or intermittent symptoms with significant physical and psychological distress and high health care use behaviors during symptomatic periods. Although these patients can be managed in a similar fashion to those with normal to mild MUS, increasing frequency of symptoms, ongoing chronic symptoms, and high use of health care resources may require clinicians to pursue further diagnostic evaluation.
- Severe MUS: patients with severe MUS have persistent symptoms, a high degree of physical and psychological distress, and high use of health care resources. In additional to a careful history and physical examination, these patients require additional diagnostic evaluation through consultation, laboratory

testing, or radiologic testing, if these tests have not already been performed at the time of evaluation.

Physicians frequently initiate further testing that is not medically indicated; failing to recognize clues offered by patients that the cause may not be organic. This failure can be detrimental to patient care, keeping the focus on making a diagnosis of an organic disorder that may not exist and overlooking the need to focus on treatment interventions that may lead to symptomatic and functional improvement.[31]

DIFFERENTIAL DIAGNOSIS

Somatization and major depressive disorder commonly coexist: 50% of patients with major depression present with MUS and between 45% and 95% of patients with major depression present with only somatic symptoms at the time of diagnosis.[32] Depressed patients who lack a consistent primary care relationship are more likely to present with exclusively somatic symptoms.[32] In addition, the severity of depression symptoms and decreased quality of life ratings are correlated with the presence of painful somatic symptoms.[33] The psychiatric differential diagnosis includes diseases such as malingering and factitious disorder. In factitious disorder, such as Munchausen syndrome, patients intentionally cause symptoms and disease (eg, injecting insulin to cause hypoglycemia). Malingering patients do not have organic disease, but intentionally feign or exaggerate somatic symptoms for secondary gain.

Panic disorder is another important consideration in the differential diagnosis of patients who present with multiple symptoms. Panic disorder is frequently undiagnosed: 70% of patients in one study with a diagnosis of panic disorder had seen an average of 10 physicians for symptoms before the diagnosis was made.[34] The most commonly seen symptoms in panic disorder involve cardiac, gastrointestinal, and neurologic systems, overlapping significantly with typical MUS presentations. Both patients with panic disorder and MUS present most frequently to primary care physicians and tend to be higher users of the medical system.

Many organic diseases can also present with multiple and vague symptoms. These organic diseases include, but are not limited to, multiple sclerosis, sarcoidosis, acute intermittent porphyria, hemochromatosis, Wilson disease, and connective tissue diseases such as systemic lupus erythematosus. Patients with these conditions may have symptoms involving multiple organ systems in the absence of specific abnormal findings on physical examination.

In addition, many patients with MUS also have significant organic disease. Their somatic symptoms may be unrelated to their chronic medical illnesses, or they may have symptoms out of proportion to or unexplained by their underlying disorder,[30] which can present a challenge in diagnosis.

CASE 3: MR C

Mr C is a 55-year-old man with a history of tobacco use, physical and sexual abuse in childhood, and Reinke edema. He presents to clinic for routine follow-up of postnasal drip, hoarseness, and a sensation that he needs to keep clearing his throat. He has had these symptoms for 2 years but only recently obtained health insurance, so presents to you for primary care follow-up. Five years before today's visit, he underwent direct laryngoscopy, which showed polypoid degeneration of the true vocal cords (Reinke edema), as discussed earlier, and a CT scan of his neck, which was unremarkable.

What would you do next to manage Mr C?

MANAGEMENT

Patients with MUS are highly variable with regard to their level of insight, focus of attention, and needs from medical providers[35] and may provide cues to their providers regarding their need for emotional support or explanation for their symptoms.[36] It can be particularly challenging for providers to discuss a diagnosis such as MUS, or one of its specific variants, with patients. The patient's experience is subjective, and the lack of objective evidence of organic disorder should not minimize providers' empathy for the patient's experience of discomfort or pain.

Multiple studies show the efficacy of cognitive behavior therapy for treating patients with MUS. There are some data to support the use of antidepressants for treating somatoform disorders[37] generally, and chronic fatigue syndrome[38] and fibromyalgia[39,40] specifically, with the bulk of evidence supporting their use for fibromyalgia. In addition, studies suggest that primary care providers can be trained by psychiatric colleagues to effectively treat MUS.[41] A multidimensional treatment program that included antidepressants, elimination of ineffective controlled substance medications, exercise, physical therapy, relaxation training, and medical management of comorbid conditions has shown promise in treating both mental and physical symptoms[42] in this setting.

In primary care practice, several principles can help guide providers in their treatment of patients with MUS (**Box 1** provides a summary)[43,44]:

1. Explain to the patient about the condition with care. Most patients have little understanding of terms such as somatization, and phrases such as MUS may or may not be useful, particularly in the setting of low health literacy. Specific labels for named MUS syndromes, such as fibromyalgia and chronic fatigue syndrome, can sometimes be useful to patients[45,46] as a mechanism to legitimize a patient's symptoms and to move on from diagnosis into the treatment phase of management. However, labeling a patient with a disease can also be detrimental, changing how patients view themselves, how they are viewed by family and close friends,[47] and even how they are treated by physicians.[48] Thus, the use of diagnostic labels is controversial[49] and clinicians are best advised to use their professional judgment and consider the needs of their individual patients before deciding on the type of language that will serve them best.

   Specific phrasing that may be useful includes "The good news is that with all the testing we've done so far, it does not seem that you have a life-threatening or dangerous diagnosis. Unfortunately, you do have an illness that is clearly affecting your life in a serious way. As doctors, we care for many patients with similar problems and unfortunately, at this point in time, we do not have a very good understanding of what causes these symptoms. I wish that I could provide you

---

Box 1
Therapeutic strategies for treating patients with MUS

1. Explain to the patient about their condition with care

2. Be explicit in expressing empathy for the patient's condition

3. Spend time each visit focusing not just on specific symptoms but on the impact that this illness has on the life of the patient

4. Include at least a brief physical examination as part of regularly scheduled follow-up visits

5. Establish frequent follow-up visits

6. Engage colleagues as a source of support

with a clearer explanation and understanding of what is causing your pain. Fortunately, there are things we can do as a team to start to work on getting you feeling better."

2. Be explicit in expressing empathy for the patient's suffering. Suffering, as a subjective experience, is always real even in the absence of an identifiable organic disorder.

3. Spend time each visit focusing not just on specific symptoms but also on the impact that this illness has on the life of the patient. In addition, time spent on the social history to better understand sources of stress can be helpful both in strengthening the therapeutic relationship and in better understanding external events and forces that may have an impact on the patient's symptoms.

4. Include at least a brief physical examination as part of regularly scheduled follow-up visits. In addition to being a useful diagnostic tool, the physical examination has profound significance as a therapeutic and healing ritual.[50] Examining a patient communicates sincere interest, concern, and care.

5. Establish frequent scheduled visits to provide stable, consistent care and to minimize the potential development of new symptoms (conscious or unconscious) to warrant frequent follow-up. Be confident in the diagnosis of MUS when it is present. Once an appropriate work-up has been done, testing or retesting of further symptoms should be approached cautiously.

6. Engage colleagues as a source of support. Treating patients with chronic disease is challenging, and it is common for providers to feel frustrated if a patient's symptoms do not seem to be improving. Negative patient affect is a strong predictor of symptom persistence in MUS,[51] and personality disorders are common in patients with moderate and severe MUS,[52,53] suggesting that many of the patients most affected by chronic symptoms may also be the most challenging for providers.[54] Physician frustration is correlated with the presence of somatization disorder in patients,[55] which again suggests the need for physician reflection, support, and self-care.

FUTURE CONSIDERATIONS/SUMMARY

In summary, caring for patients with MUS is challenging for health care providers. Even defining somatization syndromes is complex and controversial, reflecting the medical community's limited understanding of the pathophysiology for this group of disorders. Although risk factors for MUS have been described and are well understood, little is known about how MUS can be prevented. Uncertainty in medicine, as in any human enterprise, is a given, but the difficulties in identification and treatment of patients with MUS highlight the limitations in understanding the intersection between physical and mental health. Patients come to their physician looking for clarity, understanding, and relief of debilitating symptoms. The understanding of MUS will evolve, and perhaps an organic cause not yet understood or described may emerge to lend clarity and therapeutic opportunities to some patients with somatic disorders. In the meantime, the most powerful tools available are the ability to communicate the limits of current understanding, acknowledge the difficulties faced by patients with this disorder, and reinforce the willingness and desire of clinicians to partner with patients as the focus shifts from diagnosis to symptom management. Thus, the physician-patient relationship, still in its rightful place at the heart of the practice of medicine, lies at the center of effective treatment of patients with MUS.

REFERENCES

1. Katon W, Ries RK, Kleinman A. The prevalence of somatization in primary care. Compr Psychiatry 1984;25(2):208–15.

2. Kroenke K, Mangelsdorff AD. Common symptoms in ambulatory care: incidence, evaluation, therapy, and outcome. Am J Med 1989;86(3):262–6.
3. Barsky AJ, Orav EJ, Bates DW. Somatization increases medical utilization and costs independent of psychiatric and medical comorbidity. Arch Gen Psychiatry 2005;62(8):903–10.
4. Kroenke K, Spitzer RL. Gender differences in the reporting of physical and somatoform symptoms. Psychosom Med 1998;60(2):150–5.
5. deGruy F, Columbia L, Dickinson P. Somatization disorder in a family practice. J Fam Pract 1987;25(1):45–51.
6. Creed FH, Davies I, Jackson J, et al. The epidemiology of multiple somatic symptoms. J Psychosom Res 2012;72(4):311–7.
7. Henningsen P, Zipfel S, Herzog W. Management of functional somatic syndromes. Lancet 2007;369(9565):946–55.
8. Bailer J, Witthoft M, Paul C, et al. Evidence for overlap between idiopathic environmental intolerance and somatoform disorders. Psychosom Med 2005;67(6): 921–9.
9. Lange G, Tiersky LA, Scharer JB, et al. Cognitive functioning in Gulf War illness. J Clin Exp Neuropsychol 2001;23(2):240–9.
10. Smith BN, Wang JM, Vogt D, et al. Gulf war illness: symptomatology among veterans 10 years after deployment. J Occup Environ Med 2013;55(1):104–10.
11. American Psychiatric Association. Diagnostic and statistical manual of mental disorders. 5th edition. Arlington (VA): American Psychiatric Association; 2013.
12. Wessely S, White PD. There is only one functional somatic syndrome. Br J Psychiatry 2004;185:95–6.
13. Wessely S, Nimnuan C, Sharpe M. Functional somatic syndromes: one or many? Lancet 1999;354(9182):936–9.
14. Shin JH, Yoon JD, Rasinski KA, et al. A spiritual problem? Primary care physicians' and psychiatrists' interpretations of medically unexplained symptoms. J Gen Intern Med 2013;28(3):392–8.
15. Deary V, Chalder T, Sharpe M. The cognitive behavioural model of medically unexplained symptoms: a theoretical and empirical review. Clin Psychol Rev 2007; 27(7):781–97.
16. Gulec MY, Altintas M, Inanc L, et al. Effects of childhood trauma on somatization in major depressive disorder: the role of alexithymia. J Affect Disord 2013; 146(1):137–41.
17. Mattila AK, Kronholm E, Jula A, et al. Alexithymia and somatization in general population. Psychosom Med 2008;70(6):716–22.
18. Roelofs K, Spinhoven P. Trauma and medically unexplained symptoms towards an integration of cognitive and neuro-biological accounts. Clin Psychol Rev 2007;27(7):798–820.
19. Walker EA, Katon WJ, Hansom J, et al. Medical and psychiatric symptoms in women with childhood sexual abuse. Psychosom Med 1992;54(6):658–64.
20. Paras ML, Murad MH, Chen LP, et al. Sexual abuse and lifetime diagnosis of somatic disorders: a systematic review and meta-analysis. JAMA 2009;302(5): 550–61.
21. Hotopf M. Preventing somatization. Psychol Med 2004;34(2):195–8.
22. Hotopf M, Wilson-Jones C, Mayou R, et al. Childhood predictors of adult medically unexplained hospitalisations. Results from a national birth cohort study. Br J Psychiatry 2000;176:273–80.
23. Gureje O. What can we learn from a cross-national study of somatic distress? J Psychosom Res 2004;56(4):409–12.

24. Skapinakis P, Lewis G, Mavreas V. Cross-cultural differences in the epidemiology of unexplained fatigue syndromes in primary care. Br J Psychiatry 2003;182: 205–9.
25. Janca A, Isaac M, Ventouras J. Towards better understanding and management of somatoform disorders. Int Rev Psychiatry 2006;18(1):5–12.
26. Aragona M, Robetta E, Pucci D, et al. Somatization in a primary care service for immigrants. Ethn Health 2012;17(5):477–91.
27. Ullas G, McClelland L, Jones NS. Medically unexplained symptoms and somatisation in ENT. J Laryngol Otol 2013;127(5):452–7.
28. Kroenke K, Spitzer RL, Williams JC, et al. Physical symptoms in primary care. Predictors of psychiatric disorders and functional impairment. Arch Fam Med 1994;3(9):774–9.
29. Rolfe A, Burton C. Reassurance after diagnostic testing with a low pretest probability of serious disease: systematic review and meta-analysis. JAMA Intern Med 2013;173(6):407–16.
30. Smith RC, Dwamena FC. Classification and diagnosis of patients with medically unexplained symptoms. J Gen Intern Med 2007;22(5):685–91.
31. Page LA, Wessely S. Medically unexplained symptoms: exacerbating factors in the doctor-patient encounter. J R Soc Med 2003;96(5):223–7.
32. Simon GE, VonKorff M, Piccinelli M, et al. An international study of the relation between somatic symptoms and depression. N Engl J Med 1999;341(18): 1329–35.
33. Munoz RA, McBride ME, Brnabic AJ, et al. Major depressive disorder in Latin America: the relationship between depression severity, painful somatic symptoms, and quality of life. J Affect Disord 2005;86(1):93–8.
34. Sheehan DV. Current concepts in psychiatry. Panic attacks and phobias. N Engl J Med 1982;307:156.
35. Dwamena FC, Lyles JS, Frankel RM, et al. In their own words: qualitative study of high-utilising primary care patients with medically unexplained symptoms. BMC Fam Pract 2009;10:67.
36. Salmon P, Ring A, Humphris GM, et al. Primary care consultations about medically unexplained symptoms: how do patients indicate what they want? J Gen Intern Med 2009;24(4):450–6.
37. Muller JE, Wentel I, Koen L, et al. Escitalopram in the treatment of multisomatoform disorder: a double-blind, placebo-controlled trial. Int Clin Psychopharmacol 2008;23(1):43–8.
38. Pae CU, Marks DM, Patkar AA, et al. Pharmacological treatment of chronic fatigue syndrome: focusing on the role of antidepressants. Expert Opin Pharmacother 2009;10(10):1561–70.
39. Hauser W, Urrutia G, Tort S, et al. Serotonin and noradrenaline reuptake inhibitors (SNRIs) for fibromyalgia syndrome. Cochrane Database Syst Rev 2013;(1):CD010292.
40. Bellato E, Marini E, Castoldi F, et al. Fibromyalgia syndrome: etiology, pathogenesis, diagnosis, and treatment. Pain Res Treat 2012;2012:426130.
41. Kroenke K. Efficacy of treatment for somatoform disorders: a review of randomized controlled trials. Psychosom Med 2007;69(9):881–8.
42. Smith RC, Lyles JS, Gardiner JC, et al. Primary care clinicians treat patients with medically unexplained symptoms: a randomized controlled trial. J Gen Intern Med 2006;21(7):671–7.
43. Servan-Schreiber D, Tabas G, Kolb R. Somatizing patients: part II. Practical management. Am Fam Physician 2000;61(5):1423–8, 1431–2.

44. Epstein RM, Quill TE, McWhinney IR. Somatization reconsidered: incorporating the patient's experience of illness. Arch Intern Med 1999;159(3):215–22.
45. Woodward RV, Broom DH, Legge DG. Diagnosis in chronic illness: disabling or enabling–the case of chronic fatigue syndrome. J R Soc Med 1995;88(6):325–9.
46. Reid J, Ewan C, Lowy E. Pilgrimage of pain: the illness experiences of women with repetition strain injury and the search for credibility. Soc Sci Med 1991; 32(5):601–12.
47. Bergman AB, Stamm SJ. The morbidity of cardiac nondisease in schoolchildren. N Engl J Med 1967;276(18):1008–13.
48. Singh B, Nunn K, Martin J, et al. Abnormal treatment behaviour. Br J Med Psychol 1981;54(Pt 1):67–73.
49. Finestone AJ. A doctor's dilemma. Is a diagnosis disabling or enabling? Arch Intern Med 1997;157(5):491–2.
50. Verghese A, Horwitz RI. In praise of the physical examination. BMJ 2009;339: b5448.
51. De Gucht V, Fischler B, Heiser W. Personality and affect as determinants of medically unexplained symptoms in primary care; a follow-up study. J Psychosom Res 2004;56(3):279–85.
52. Rost KM, Akins RN, Brown FW, et al. The comorbidity of DSM-III-R personality disorders in somatization disorder. Gen Hosp Psychiatry 1992;14(5):322–6.
53. Stern J, Murphy M, Bass C. Personality disorders in patients with somatisation disorder. A controlled study. Br J Psychiatry 1993;163:785–9.
54. Hahn SR, Thompson KS, Wills TA, et al. The difficult doctor-patient relationship: somatization, personality and psychopathology. J Clin Epidemiol 1994;47(6): 647–57.
55. Walker EA, Katon WJ, Keegan D, et al. Predictors of physician frustration in the care of patients with rheumatological complaints. Gen Hosp Psychiatry 1997; 19(5):315–23.

Index

Note: Page numbers of article titles are in **boldface** type.

A

Abdominal migraine, 518, 525
Abduction test, for shoulder pain, 490–491
Abscesses, perirectal, 615–616
Acetaminophen
    for headaches, 519–520
    for low back pain, 424
Acetolamide, for headaches, 525
Achilles reflex, in low back pain, 416
Acid-suppression therapy, for dyspepsia, 557–558
Acne rosacea, 456, 460–462
Acne vulgaris, 455–459
Acotiamide, for dyspepsia, 558
Acromioclavicular joint, disorders of, 498
Actigraphy, for sleep disorders, 574
Acupuncture
    for dyspepsia, 559
    for headaches, 522
    for neck pain, 656
    for shoulder pain, 499–500
Adapalene
    for acne rosacea, 460
    for acne vulgaris, 458
    for periorifacial dermatitis, 463
Adhesive capsulitis (frozen shoulder), 489, 498, 500–501
Advanced phase sleep syndrome, 571
Albuterol, for cough-variant asthma, 398
Alcohol misuse, distal symmetric polyneuropathy in, 436–437
Allergic contact dermatitis, 474
Almotriptan, for headaches, 519
Alopecia, 446–455
    androgenetic, 449–452
    classification of, 447
    inflammatory, 447
    telogen effluvium type, 454–455
    treatment of, 450–452
Alopecia areata, 452–454
Amitriptyline
    for dyspepsia, 558
    for headaches, 519, 523
Amyotrophic lateral sclerosis, leg discomfort in, 437

Med Clin N Am 98 (2014) 673–695
http://dx.doi.org/10.1016/S0025-7125(14)00058-3
0025-7125/14/$ – see front matter © 2014 Elsevier Inc. All rights reserved.

medical.theclinics.com